SOCIAL BRAIN MATTERS

Stances on the Neurobiology of Social Cognition

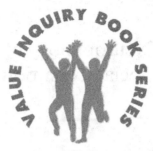

VIBS

Volume 190

Robert Ginsberg
Founding Editor

Peter A. Redpath
Executive Editor

Associate Editors

a volume in
Cognitive Science
CS
Francesc Forn i Argimon, Editor

SOCIAL BRAIN MATTERS

Stances on the Neurobiology of Social Cognition

Edited by

Oscar Vilarroya
and
Francesc Forn i Argimon

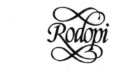

Amsterdam - New York, NY 2007

Cover Design: Studio Pollmann

The paper on which this book is printed meets the requirements
of "ISO 9706:1994, Information and documentation - Paper for
documents - Requirements for permanence".

ISBN-13: 978-90-420-2216-4
©Editions Rodopi B.V., Amsterdam - New York, NY 2007
Printed in the Netherlands

This study was financially supported by the Social Brain Chair at the Autonomous University of Barcelona, the Chair for the Dissemination of Science at the University of Valencia, the Barcelona City Council, and the Universal Forum of Cultures Foundation

CONTENTS

Foreword

Read the best books first, or you may not have a chance to read them at all.—Henry David Thoreau

The *Foundation Universal Forum of the Cultures* as a depositary for the intangible heritage of *Forum Barcelona 2004* is honored to co-sponsor publication of the discourses and documents comprising the dialogue *Social Brain Matters* and to help disseminate the knowledge generated and transmitted at this encounter.

This book is the result of the preparatory works and dialogic encounter *The Social Brain, Biology of Conflicts and Cooperation*, held within the *Universal Forum of Cultures* during 17–20 July 2004. The first *Universal Forum of Cultures*, held in Barcelona from May to September 2004, unveiled a new civic event on an international scale, an occasion which, without brandishing any particular flags, promoted common sense, creativity, and dialogue among cultures so that society could steer its globalizing processes towards the creation of a more prosperous, just, peaceful and freer world.

The Forum constituted a meeting among citizens. In Barcelona, each person expressed his or her attitude towards the challenges raised by globalization. Within a thirty-hectare enclosure, our common language was music, dance, theatre, cinema, workshops, games, exhibitions, ideas, and good practices. The city experienced a unique cultural blossoming that summer. Its people inaugurated a wholly new project for urban renewal. The territory itself formed part of an urban project on sustainability: a groundwater treatment plant, a waste incinerator, and a previously neglected area rebuilt to create a sustainable public space boasting new beaches and infrastructures favoring cultural convergence.

The main objectives of the *Universal Forum of Cultures* were fomenting cultural diversity, promoting sustainable development, and supporting conditions for peace. These objectives meet humanity's dire need to collaborate internationally in the face of new challenges in a continually more interdependent world where dialogue between peoples must be our priority. Humanity shares preoccupations on social, economic, and cultural themes that can only be confronted by gaining sufficient critical mass or by forming an alliance. Science must also contribute to this development.

The dialogue *The Social Brain, Biology of Conflicts and Cooperation* is a sample of the varied possibilities and enormous tasks ahead in constructing and understanding relations between society, biology, culture, and conflicts. Framed within the debate to contribute to constructing a culture of peace, the dialogue stemmed from four questions: Can we educate people to manifest solidarity? Is our brain ethical? Are we egoists or cooperators? Science: does it blaze trails towards coexistence?

These questions, accompanied by the documentary *Getting under the Skin of Conflict*—which, by relating common and intimate experiences, leads us to the roots of some of the great conflicts of our times—were the tools for the debate arising in the diverse spheres of cognitive science, psychology and philosophy. Among areas analyzed were the behavior of human beings, the capability they possess to adapt to changes and in what form the brain institutionalizes rules deriving from environment and social context. The dialogue brought together diverse professionals from contrasting work and study spheres—one of the main characteristics of the encounters carried out in the Universal Forum of Cultures.

Through a productive dialogue, scientists, politicians, thinkers, and civil society analyzed recent discoveries on the biological and cognitive mechanisms involved in human behavior of conflict and cooperation. They agreed upon bases for a modern social thinking focused on the knowledge, which science is unearthing regarding the biological roots of social behavior. The dialogue also revealed the importance of considering the interrelationship between biological, psychological, and social aspects, aiding understanding of human behavior, especially in questions relevant to current society.

The need to understand collective behaviors, increase the impact of educational or consciousness-raising campaigns, and improve the adaptability of societies to the uncertainty generated by globalization are some practical applications which this debate contributed to, argued by the most significant figures in the field.

The dialogue demonstrated the repercussions that research into the brain and behavior can have on individuals' quality of life and problem-solving. It also enabled the contributions we now present here, creating a permanent legacy in the constitution of the chair "The Social Brain" (Barcelona City Council-Autonomous University of Barcelona). Through this publication, we hope to provide a fertile continuity.

The *Universal Forum of Cultures Barcelona 2004* represented one step closer to constituting a new knowledge nucleus, allowing us to advance towards a better society for all people.

Mireia Belil, Director-General
Foundation Universal Forum of Cultures

Foreword

Throughout history, humankind has used science as a tool for the understanding of the laws of nature. Nowadays, at the beginning of the twenty-first century, it is not possible to understand our world without the help of science. The persistent search for the acquisition of knowledge has led to significant scientific, cultural, and social revolutions, which have provided us with a new approach to questions that, deep inside, we have been asking ourselves since we were born as a species.

Based on this conviction, the University of Valencia created the Chair for the Dissemination of Science. The initial intent was to provide a useful tool for the popularization of scientific knowledge and turn it into public knowledge of science. We firmly believe that the dissemination of science is a social need, which goes beyond making it possible for the public to value it properly. Our aim is for men and women to perceive an image of our world in a scientific, rational, and positive way.

The University of Valencia, through the Chair for the Dissemination of Science, found the most adequate way to actively participate in the *Forum Universal de les Cultures Barcelona 2004*. We produced the documentary *Getting under the Skin of Conflict*, which illustrated the dialogue titled *The Social Brain: Biology of Conflicts*. This wonderful documentary won the prize for Humanistic and Social Affairs at the 23rd International Biennial of Scientific Cinema in Ronda.

The celebration of that multi-disciplinary dialogue was so successful that only two years later, the Barcelona City Council, the University of Barcelona, and the Institute for Health Assistance made the creation of *The Social Brain Chair* possible. The University of Valencia is very pleased at this initiative, the intention of which is to gain and spread knowledge in the frame of social neuroscience. We firmly believe that society should welcome the studies and the activities carried out by this Chair; obviously, when we profoundly know how our brain works, it is possible to understand and reinterpret some social behaviors still incomprehensible.

The commitment of turning scientific outreach into one of our main lines of action led us to create the Chair for the Dissemination of Science. Similarly, we believe that The Social Brain Chair is a necessary tool to broaden our vision of the world with new, shared perspectives. Since the University of Valencia participated in the Forum Dialogues, we wish to be present in the first steps of this new Chair with the publication of this book, which reaps the benefits of that exciting initiative.

Francisco Tomás Vert
Rector, University of Valencia

Foreword

FROM DIALOGUE TO "THE SOCIAL BRAIN" CHAIR

Over several scorching days in July 2004, a group of scientists and thinkers came together in Barcelona. We had been invited by the Barcelona City Council to participate in an encounter carrying the peculiar name "The Social Brain: Biology of Conflicts and Cooperation," included within the events of the Universal Forum of Cultures Barcelona 2004. The organizers' concept was to bring together outstanding representatives from every discipline interested in the incipient knowledge field of "social neuroscience." This subject involves studying the neurobiological basis for social processes and includes different disciplines such as cognitive neuroscience, neuroeconomy, evolutionary anthropology, social psychology, artificial intelligence, and linguistics.

The disciplines to which the guest speakers belonged varied so greatly that many guests had never previously appeared together at the same event. The majority arrived with a lot of curiosity, not knowing exactly what was being asked of them, how they could contribute, or what they would take away from such an event. The best we can say about the meeting is that most speakers left feeling extremely glad to have come, as did the majority of the audience.

The success of this event and the development of social neuroscience in recent years have culminated in the creation of "The Social Brain" Chair, thanks to the sponsorship of the Barcelona City Council, and the welcome offered by the *Universitat Autònoma* [Autonomous University] of Barcelona and also the *Institut Municipal d'Assistència Sanitària* (Municipal Healthcare Institute). The interest of these institutions in a project of this nature came about, as Mayor Joan Clos explained, from the realization that many current social problems require an approach that incorporates knowledge of underlying neurobiological mechanisms.

Why is knowing how the brain works of interest to those involved in social research and social agency? This question's strong answer is that knowing how the brain works is essential to develop a social theory. The moderate defense is that such understanding may be useful. Both answers share the belief that to have an adequate theory regarding behavior and social events, we must understand social cognition in human beings. We define social cognition in the widest sense to include human beings' perceptive, motivational, and affective capabilities as social beings. For this to be possible, we must know the paths by which the brain conditions and produces these capabilities. To take seriously what we have learned from studying the brain forces us to deal with social subjects and everything social as limited by the way that we are motivated to empathize or compete with our fellows, how we think about them, and how we act according to those vectors. That implies that we must not only study the cognitive processes themselves on all possible levels, from genetics to psycho-social processes, but also that we must consider the brain's evolutionary past.

What type of contributions from social neuroscience could be useful in social science? Two examples can give you an idea. First, the concept of human reasoning, which cognitive neuroscience studies is delineating, corresponds to a complex system, an unconscious riddled with biases. The human brain is not a logical machine. We do not always reason from the given premises; our information is sometimes false or incomplete. Often, we have to fall back on highly contextual approximations, estimations, and heuristic rules that are dependent on our life experiences. Separation of reason and emotion does not appear to occur in the brain; we make decisions using neuronal networks that link the affective and cognitive dimensions of our intellects. So using traditional models to interpret and predict how human beings reason does not work. We need to understand reasoning on the basis of how we construct our world from our perceptions, how affective and cognitive dimensions are interlinked in thought, what the biases and heuristic rules we use, how we unconsciously evaluate the social situations in which we find ourselves—which influence our decisions—and how the state of our emotions affects our acts.

Social neuroscience has started to shed light on our moral brain. Application of evolutionary theory to social cognition implies that we must understand the brain as a system, which behaves in a moral sense exactly the way does because it is heir to a precise phylogenetic tradition. The brain our cranium protects is moral because its behavior used to comply with, and continues to comply with, highly specific adaptive functions. If we want to understand modern moral human beings, creating an idealized model of morality is insufficient. We must also understand evolutionary history and, through history, understand the moral functions our brain fulfilled within a particular environment. Biological anthropology has provided mechanisms such as selection of relatives, reciprocal altruism, and indirect and strong reciprocation that explain some of our moral behavior. Cognitive neuroscience has shown that moral cognition is emotional, socially directed, and dependent on context. It has identified its neurobiological mechanisms, such as identifying relatives using identity markers, detecting social emotions, operational memory to compare, judge, and foresee the results of social interactions, the capability of repressing immediate gratification, and many other factors, the development and dynamic of which condition moral cognition.

In sum, social neuroscience is enabling us to confirm that how we behave socially depends on how we are made and, above all, how our brain is made and works. This allows us to predict that scientific disciplines that study how the brain functions, how it evolved, and how it behaves biologically will help us to understand behavior and social actions.

"The Social Brain" Chair initiative is founded upon this belief. The success of the Dialogue in participation, proposals, and interactions, and the progress of social neuroscience as a scientific discipline have provided the stimulation for the creation of a research environment and periodic meetings in Barcelona to discuss many of the questions addressed. "The Social Brain" Chair constitutes, in this sense, a sphere for research and the transfer of knowledge in social neuroscience (NS).

The Chair aims to develop research within the realm of social neuroscience. It promotes contacts, interchanges, residences, and collaborations among researchers. It disseminates knowledge about social neuroscience to institutions and individuals who may benefit and to society in general, assessing any political, social, or cultural action that wishes to undergo analysis from a social neuroscience viewpoint. The challenge is to offer knowledge and tools in a manner that helps to refine political and social action in a world continually more at the mercy of scientific knowledge.

We would like to wish this initiative every success and extend an invitation to everyone interested in collaborating with the activities that the Chair will be instigating.

Oscar Vilarroya, Social Brain Chair Director; Antoni Bulbena, Joaquim Coll, and Adolf Tobeña, Social Brain Managing Commitee

ACKNOWLEDGMENTS

This book would not have been possible without the help of many people who have contributed to not only the writing, editing, and publication processes, but also to the conception, preparation, and carrying out of the "Social Brain" meeting that allowed the discussion and texts compiled in this volume. To be fair, then, we should list here so many names that it would probably take more space than the book itself. So we will just mention those who have been mostly directly concerned with the book.

First, we are tremendously indebted to the former Mayor of Barcelona, Joan Clos. He is the real artificer behind the whole project of the "Social Brain" meeting, Chair, and book. His vision, intellectual curiosity, and implication in the ideas and persons behind this project is a singularity which we have tried to deserve, if only in part, with the book we present here.

We would also like to mention the critical role professor Marina Subirats has played in bringing this project to fruition. Professors Jaume Bertranpetit and Ignacio Morgado also deserve credit. Nearly all the form and contents of the "Social Brain" projects stems from their previous work during many years in popularization activities and courses at the *Consorci Universitari Menendez y Pelayo* of Barcelona. They are first-rate researchers who have taken a lot of their time to transmit the scientific knowledge from the labs to the rest of the society. Professor Antoni Bulbena is also a decisive figure in this project. He has been a tireless supporter of all the "Social Brain" activities and active promoter of all the steps that have succeeded in creating the "Social Brain" Chair.

We are also thankful to Leonardo Valencia for his work at the "Social Brain" meeting and in editing the first draft of the book.

Bibiana Bonmati has blown wind in our sails, dealing efficiently with practical and organizational matters. In the field of practical concerns, Soledad Rubio deserves credit for making things easier with her accessibility and involvement.

Elizabeth Boepple's contribution to the book's readability and compliance with VIBS guidelines is hard to overemphasize. She has conceded us much more editing work and wisdom than we deserved.

We also would like to thank VIBS Executive Editor Peter Redpath and Managing editor Eric van Broekhuizen for their kind guidance and unwavering patience all the way through. In Robert Ginsberg's case, the debt is double, since he not only contributed to the Dialogue with a moving speech, and to the book with an excellent chapter, but also founded VIBS.

Finally, the authors of the chapters of this book have exerted an enormous influence on us, not only through their contributed chapters, but also as models of intellectual depth and integrity. We are infinitely thankful for their gracious contribution to this project, the most important of all, and for the opportunity that they have granted us to help spreading their valuable work.

Oscar Vilarroya and Francesc Forn i Argimon

INTRODUCTION

Francesc Forn i Argimon

This collected volume, the third in Rodopi's VIBS Special Series on Cognitive Science, may not be a standard work in academic philosophy. Most of its chapters are not strictly philosophical, and only some of the authors are trained philosophers. Others come from the fields of psychology, biology, neuroscience, linguistics, and anthropology. Yet all the contributions deal with philosophical issues concerning scientific practice. Despite the authors' widely diverse training and regular practice, this is a book of naturalist philosophy. A naturalist philosopher attempts to resolve philosophy's big questions, taking into account the results of scientific activity. Naturalism is firmly rooted in the origins of philosophy in ancient Greece, and it gained substantial momentum during the so-called Scientific Revolution of the sixteenth and seventeenth centuries.

Contemporary philosophy cannot ignore scientific progress or its impact on society and culture. Neither should it be science's mere reflexive appendix. One of the forms under which this belittling of philosophy occurs is through casual references to philosophical theories in scientific essays, on the assumption that nowadays philosophy is an anachronism from which we must free ourselves. Some such references are so common that they have become received wisdom. In cognitive science, critics often level charges of this ilk against René Descartes' philosophy. In texts of contemporary social science or ethics, Immanuel Kant is usually the target. Some thinkers criticize these authors and the whole philosophy of subjectivity as the source of many philosophical obstacles to a scientific approach to cognition and morality. The Cartesian divide between the physical world of everyday objects and bodies, and the mental sphere, equally immediate to us but apparently unattainable from an objective, third-person perspective, would be one of these obstacles. According to these critics, we can only deal appropriately with the mind-body relationship after rebutting the dualism held by Descartes and his contemporary heirs. Cartesian dualism is the claim that mind and body are made of different stuff, and that we know of them by different means.[1] Some authors argue a similar case against the Kantian categorical imperative, which they construe as the requirement to obey the moral law in disregard of any objective circumstances. They consistently present it as an example of aprioristic reasoning in ethics.[2]

In this introductory chapter, we follow the customary practice of making a brief reference to these two early modern philosophers, but our motivation is the opposite of the usual critiques. Our aim is to reclaim Descartes and Kant into the naturalist philosophical tradition of cognitive science, while noting that the above criticisms are, in some senses, deeply unfair. One of these senses is exemplified in the depiction of these authors as symbols of an intrinsically obscurantist, anti-scientific worldview.

The Descartes and Kant so described are not in accordance with their historical figures or with the logic of their thought. Descartes, the creator of analytical geometry, was convinced that philosophy would benefit from the use of scientific concepts and reasoning, such as to proceed inductively from empirical data, or deductively from unambiguous evidence.[3] Although he viewed mental content as irreducible to physical terms, he also believed that some of mind's essential aspects, such as our mental health, depended on our bodily organs.[4] He did not hesitate to dissect corpses in search of the physiological basis for the two-way communication between mind and body. We can consider him one of the first experimentalists in a modern sense, since he explicitly collected empirical data to test hypotheses, such as whether we can liken bodies to mechanisms.[5]

In his turn, Kant took modern physics as a model of true knowledge, on which he based his attempt to lay the foundations of wisdom.[6] He declared that the structure of our cognitive apparatus imposes some constraints on our representation of reality, constraints that are apparent in the results of Newtonian physics. He also argued for a dichotomy between the realms of nature and morality, claiming that different laws govern each sphere.[7] This claim, which is in the basis of the concept of the categorical imperative, appears to be uncontroversial to many contemporary scientists and moral philosophers, including some of the contributors to this book.

Neither Descartes nor Kant thought that scientific knowledge was irrelevant to ethics. In the famous metaphor of the tree of knowledge in his *Principles of Philosophy*, Descartes described moral doctrine as one of the main branches arising from the tree's trunk, physics, while its roots were metaphysics.[8] Kant wrote the *Critique of Practical Reason*, his major work on ethics, according to the canon of treatises on geometry of the epoch, demonstrating propositions from axioms or postulates and deriving corollaries and theorems from these propositions.[9] This form could have served communicative purposes but might have also been a satire from Kant, who was a fierce opponent of the deductive method in philosophy.[10] He would have used the deductive form to demonstrate human autonomy and freedom, which Benedict (Baruch) Spinoza had denied using the same method.[11] In any case, the logical structure of the *Critique of Practical Reason* is an example of the degree to which Kant intertwines science, philosophy, and ethics in his discourse.

Descartes and Kant were naturalist philosophers, even though their claims may often appear misguided to us. Yet in some of their contentions, they pointed in the right direction. Despite their differences, both were convinced that studying the mind—what it can know and which methods were the best to get at this knowledge—was an essential part of research on the real world and the stuff of which the world is made.[12] Descartes spoke of innate mental mechanisms—not only of innate contents, as many scholars commonly misunderstand—related to symbolic language, arithmetic, and geometric intuitions. Even though this thesis is still the object of acrimonious debate, many outstanding cognitive scientists hold that higher cognitive functions are contingent on innate modules in our minds. Science has also verified Kant's insight that perception is the product of an active process of construction of the sense data, which requires the use of concepts.

Still, much of what Descartes and Kant proposed on these and other subjects has proved to be wrong. To separate current-day wheat from obsolete chaff, we must consider the huge scientific progress made since their time. Some impressive technological advances have uncovered previously unobservable and un-measurable data: cerebral processes accompanying cognition, the brain's biology, and the location and functioning of activity-specific neuronal circuits. These technologies, and the empirical findings they have made possible, motivated a substantial change in our approach to the problem of knowledge and moral questions. We know, for instance, that neuronal circuits are involved in the active construction of knowledge that Kant postulated. The plasticity of the human brain, and the evidence that mental capabilities depend on diverse mechanisms located in different cerebral zones, confirms the functional approach embedded in the Kantian language of the faculties of the mind.[13] Yet several studies, carried out using the aforementioned technologies, have identified particular cerebral structures required to accomplish these functions.

Another scientific breakthrough that has radically modified our conceptual perspective on these problems is Darwinism, one of the most significant modern theories of naturalist philosophy. It provides a scientific answer to the all-time big philosophical question: Why do we exist? It is also one of the soundest and more comprehensive theoretical models from which to account for the results of contemporary science. The latest version of Darwinism, the Synthetic Theory of Evolution, is the result of the combination or synthesis of Darwin's ideas and recent developments in genetics and molecular biology. Due to this theory, we know that the innate modules, which allow us to develop higher cognitive functions, including moral knowledge, are the product of our evolutionary history. Darwinism is the best reason for claiming, against Descartes and some current religion-based theories, that higher cognitive capabilities are not divine seeds implanted in us by an intelligent, omnipotent, and provident Designer.[14]

The scientific and philosophic implications of Darwinism are still wanting for a more comprehensive development. This book examines those implications most relevant to the study of our social behavior, while maintaining the Cartesian and Kantian emphasis in the need of a thorough examination of the mental capabilities involved. The first part focuses on how we learn social and ethical values. In the opening chapter, and after a lively introduction, Núria Sebastián Gallés discusses how neuroscience has considerably extended our knowledge of learning processes. The key role of emotion and the determination of sensitive periods when learning becomes more efficient, rely on the incredible plasticity of the brain structures involved, and the multiple connections between them. Within the framework of a neural Darwinism, Sebastián Gallés defines learning as the product of the selection, especially active during the first years of life, of the most active circuits of neurons and synaptic connections involved in those tasks required most frequently. Such tasks, and the environments and situations that activate emotional paths in the brain, determine what behaviors we learn most permanently and deeply.

Daniel C. Dennett explores the prospects of Darwin's brilliant intuition, as it applies not to intra-individual processes at a molecular level, but to cultural phenomena. He explores the consequences of such application in learning altruism. Cultural transmission, which allows innovation at a much faster rate than genetic inheritance, is also present in other animals. But only in *Homo sapiens* can the products of this cultural evolution modify their biological conditioners. The bad news is that memes, the units of cultural transmission, parasitize the human brain to the benefit of their reproductive fitness, oblivious to our wellbeing. The concept of a person and religious or political fundamentalism are significant illustrations of this process. On the other hand, and this is the good news, these spiritual parasites enable us to aim at goals and values, such as altruism, other than mere survival and reproduction of the species. Ethical learning is the product of an unconscious, involuntary selection process. Human freedom would consist in our being slaves to the appropriate ideas. The following chapters in this first part take up and develop, from different perspectives, the critical issues of how to define those ideas and the procedures for instructing people to comply with them. In doing so, these authors each discuss the explanatory levels, content, and methods involved in learning ethics and social values.

Supporting her claim with thinkers such as Ludwig Wittgenstein and Lev Semenovich Vigotsky, Katherine Nelson proposes to combine the focus on brain mechanisms with a socio-cultural perspective. Learning results from the interaction of cerebral, somatic, and symbolic processes, and occurs in the confluence of the individual's physical, relational, and cultural environments. The child learns contents not as isolated mental representations, but in the context of concrete activities and narratives, inserted in forms of life and ways of doing things distinctive of social and culture groups. What the child can learn depends on its degree of physical and mental development and previous experiences. In this context, the scaffolding metaphor suggests that the best teacher is not an external guide to the process, but a participant in the activity of learning. The teacher assists and controls the child's advances, introducing new capabilities appropriate to the child's developmental level.[15] When learning to speak and to perform higher cognitive capabilities, the child incorporates the values of the family and other social and cultural environments where learning occurs. But the occurrence of learning, ethical or other, will rely ultimately on factors Nelson terms as *historic*, namely the development and previous experience of the learner.

From a similar focus on concrete situations and the individuals' interaction with their environment, Eric Bredo's "*When* is Ethical Learning?" submits the approach underlying the search for the biological basis of ethical learning to philosophical examination. According to him, the purportedly inherent conflict between human nature and morality derives from the delimitation of entities (genes, neurons, organisms, groups) and levels of analysis (molecular, genetic, individual, social) in the description of this nature. Taken in isolation, the needs and objectives of the selected units always appear to collide with those of other units, belonging to the same or another level. Most authors argue for the explanatory superiority of their level of analysis with respect to others. Adhering to this sort of position hinders and obscures cooperative efforts and mutual consideration of all the interests at stake that define the ethical perspective. In contrast with this competition of views, Bredo stresses the theoretical and practical advantages of the swift of emphasis the chapter's title suggests. Instead of attempting to determine *where* ethical learning takes place, through a cross-situational study of the relevant units and levels of analysis, he urges us to stress *when* such learning takes place. We should define the (ideal) situations in which learning is likely to occur and favor the cooperation of the agents involved and other conditions that facilitate it in a (real) given situation.

Lawrence Barsalou and Emily Parker's contribution, grounded in social and cognitive psychology, introduces a double distinction between types of certainty and proper domains where we should apply each type. Our judgments about beings, things, and events of the everyday world, and the beliefs upon which we base those judgments, rely on low-level perceptions that require nearly no conceptual processing. From this fundamental perceptual domain, Barsalou and Parker distinguish the social and cultural sphere, where beliefs depend on perceptions that are much more dependent on concepts and stem from the interaction of different cognitive modalities. In the cultural domain, the social and cultural context is much more influential, and certainty is inseparable from a given perspective. The authors view the attribution of the wrong kind of certainty to each perceptual sphere, of perspectiveless certainty to ethical judgments, and perspectival certainty in the basic perceptual domain, as a source of conflicts. They conclude by turning from the theoretical to a more applied point of view. They propose interventions aimed at favoring the covariance of certainties and domains, the reasoned attribution of each type of certainty to its corresponding domain.

Stevan Harnad intertwines the issues of implicit learning of values, introduced by Sebastián Gallés and Nelson, and the impact on our beliefs of the conceptual processing of sensory data, which Barsalou and Parker discuss. The difficulties of altruism towards all human beings derive, according to Harnad, from the behavioral effects of the implicit learning of the fundamental "We/They" category. A concept unifies the set of things that underlies it, but in doing so, it establishes a dichotomy with respect to its complement, the set of all things not included under the rubric of the concept. For a concept to be functional, competent use requires us to be able to distinguish between examples and non-examples of things that are included in it. Harnad holds that the acquisition of the "We" concept is related to the phenomenon of imprinting, by which infants identify and bond with the first protective figure they perceive. Accordingly, we tend to categorize any individuals physically or otherwise different from those who formed the original "We"—normally our parents and siblings— as members of the "They" category, and so unworthy of social or moral consideration. Inspired by Jonathan Swift's irony, and in the spirit of more recent social experiments, Harnad ends with a proposal, which appears unrealizable but still worthy of consideration insofar as it enables us to discern the intricate complexities of the problem.

The second part of the book focuses on the neurobiological basis of moral behavior, paying special attention to two anomalies in such behavior: suicide terrorism and moral indifference. Through a careful reading of these chapters, we can also find the traces of the debate opened in the first part on the relative significance of explanations of altruism from evolutionary and cognitive psychology, neurobiology, and social and symbolic interactionism. The section opens with several analyses of the deadly martyrs phenomenon from neuroscientific, anthropological, and cognitive perspectives.

Adolf Tobeña takes as starting-point Darwin's observation that human morality is a product of *Homo sapiens*'s sociability conditions and affective and cognitive mechanisms. Consistently, morality is often limited to the members of the in-group, the group to which the individual senses belonging, thereby exerting a normative influence over the individual. Suicide terrorism is the result of a radicalization of this in-group bias, consisting of extreme altruism towards the terrorist's in-group and complete amorality with respect to competing groups. To discuss it, Tobeña resorts to an experimental ethics combining explanatory levels (individual organisms and groups) in the framework of multidisciplinary cooperation (evolutionary biology, neuroscience, social psychology, and differential psychology). The challenge for an evolutionary explanation is to account for the adaptive value of such extreme altruism. In addition, evidence from neural imaging shows a significant correlation between the cerebral areas involved in moral decisions and those related to emotional control. Whereas dysfunctions observed in these areas may explain the behavior of psychopaths, such dysfunctions are of no use in the case of deadly martyrs, who exhibit a striking mix of lack of moral feelings toward out-groups and intense empathy with respect to the in-group. Social neuroscience has made considerable advances in the study of the affective and cognitive biases underlying this moral asymmetry. To satisfactorily explain suicide terrorism, we need to collect precise data about its neuro-physiological basis and to discern general tendencies and individual differences.

According to Scott Atran, we must understand deadly martyrdom within the context of religious phenomena. Religions are belief systems that appeared in the latest stages of human beings' evolution as social animals. What is crucial in this cultural evolution are not the memes but the structure of the human cognitive apparatus, which, as Barsalou and Parker remarked, grants an almost universal validity to our typical expectations regarding the behavior of things and people in everyday settings. Religions are characterized by contradicting any of these expectations; they attribute intentions to objects or postulate the existence of insubstantial agents. In this way, they give a supernatural foundation of values hard to justify on rational grounds, like what we must consider good or bad, or why birth must determine social hierarchy. They help us to confront frustration, suffering, and existential anxiety, reinforcing the bonds with our group and the disregard of alien groups. Deadly martyrs are not the children of misery, illiterate, or morally derailed, but educated, young altruists, living unfulfilled lives in corrupt or threatened societies. These conditions result in them being easily manipulated by organizations with a hidden agenda, which use religion in the combat against the Western societies who support their dictators and/or aggressors. Conversely, the best recipe for preventing suicide terrorism is respect for cultural and religious diversity, along with the encouragement of political participation and economic opportunities around the world.

The psychological mechanism underlying the moral insensibility of suicide terrorists toward their objectives is at the core of Shaun Nichols's analysis. He distinguishes three types of indifference when faced with alien suffering, of which only one, the indifference characteristic of psychopaths, derives from deficient psychological functioning. The other two types derive from habituation to the situations that usually trigger the emotional display, and from strategies to cope with that display. Nichols offers representative cases of a dentist, accustomed to patients' suffering during particular operations, and the process by which the repetition of a word inhibits its semantic processing. These cases of inhibition by habituation and that of psychopaths' abnormal cognitive and emotional functioning share the common feature that inhibiting effects occur in the intermediate processing stages, what he terms *midstream effects*. In still another case, *upstream effects*, such as previous subjection to social or cultural norms, impose the use of strategies for inhibiting emotion. For example, a father controls his nausea as he cleans up his sick child's vomit; the soldier avoids thinking about the damage he inflicts on the enemy. Deadly martyrs fit the same description as that of the soldier's avoidance, and therefore, as Atran and Tobeña observed following Darwin, they are not amoral psychopaths, but agents of an all too human morality.

Moral indifference of another sort, less sanguinary but much more widespread than that of suicide terrorists, is the insensitiveness of affluent First World citizens with respect to the poverty and deprivation of the rest of humanity. William S. Rottschaefer examines this indifference from the perspective of a naturalist moral philosopher. He starts from Peter Singer's ideal of extending the moral community to the whole of humanity, and he resorts to the results of cognitive science to evaluate the chances that we could achieve this ideal, accept it as normative, and implement it.

Singer claims that reason predisposes us to endorse a minimum moral rule, which dictates that we give a small share of our income to the poorest. Yet cognitive science teaches us that reason cannot motivate people to translate the moral rule into action, and moral emotions,—which do have the motivational power required—are restricted to family, affinity, and reciprocal interaction relationships. A promising approach for us to bridge the gap between reason and emotion is Albert Bandura's cognitive social theory. According to Bandura, we acquire the concept of the self as a moral agent, capable to push rational impartiality beyond the restricted reach of emotional motivation, through practice, observation of role models, and symbolic learning. Moral action is highly sensitive to situational factors, to the social and institutional practices and contexts that can favor or hinder the individuals' acquisition of the concept of a universal moral community.

Tobeña, Atran, Nichols, and Rottschaefer's contributions are nice instances of the naturalistic turn in social and ethical studies. Félix Ovejero explores the scope of this turn, namely the prospects for social neuroscience to resolve problems such as terrorism, apparently unsolvable within classical models. On the positive side, the results of neurobiology and evolutionary biology have enabled us to discard theories based on inadequate concepts of human dispositions as purely unselfish or calculating. Evolutionary theories on the origin of moral behavior in emotions have revealed sociological and economic fallacies, such as invoking social or individual benefits as causes of morality. A new, more accurate description of human dispositions allows us to surpass restrictions and problems in implementing the principles of ethics and social justice. But social neuroscience does not contribute nothing to the definition and justification of these principles. In the case of terrorism, for a naturalist approach to be productive, we need a concept that, according to Ovejero, we are still a long way from defining. An operational concept should provide necessary conditions (without which terrorism would not exist), and sufficient conditions (those that, when present, produce terrorism). Ovejero's conclusion is that we need more science, in the sense of experimental research and conceptual analysis.

Other shortcomings of current neuroscientific ethics stem from its theoretical inheritance. The experimental designs based on purported moral dilemmas (the trolley and footbridge dilemmas and the ultimatum game) exhibit excessive dependency on game theory, and its bearing on an utilitarianist conception of moral decision as a reckoning of costs and benefits. Antoni Gomila proposes a revision of these designs, and of the theoretical model on which they are grounded. He focuses on the complexities of the relationship between anomalous moral behavior and psychopathology. Customary identification of both arises from a conceptual confusion: the failure to distinguish different levels in morality. The basic level corresponds to personal inclinations and primary moral emotions, such as empathy, while the higher level is related to rule awareness and reflection, and more sophisticated moral feelings such as remorse. Without this distinction in mind, we do not fully understand that our considerations of the moral significance of an action and our motivations to perform that action do not always coincide.

In concluding, Gomila exhorts us to support empirical research in a more adequate understanding of the self as moral agent. The pilot who suffered guilt for his part in flying reconnaissance flights over Hiroshima before the atom bomb was dropped, and the young British poet who refused to return to the trenches after being decorated for his heroism, are examples of how the strength of moral values cause mental and social conflicts. These conflicts do not indicate moral pathology; on the contrary, they evince the sufferer's determination to maintain his or her ethical standards.

Based on empirical evidence, David J. Premack claims that the basics of morality in Gomila's sense are present in infants, in the form of the three principles: do not harm the others, help others when they are in distress, and be fair to others. The most satisfactory explanation of this early moral knowledge is that it is a product of the evolution of the species. The long time our ancestors spent in small groups of hunter-gatherers accounts for these basic moral principles, as it does for the cognitive equipment that capacitates us to use language, calculate, or attribute mental states to others.

Yet in any of these capabilities, we consciously violate our competence as we do in morality. According to Premack, the reason for this gap between moral competence and moral performance originates in the hunter-gatherer lifestyle, which would have favored an inclination toward social control and group bias, but not self-control. The higher level of morality, requiring self-control and the induction of moral rules, comes from the mother, who employs her tight bond with the child to teach him or her to suppress natural impulses. Women appear to have a natural disposition toward altruist exchange, acquired in the context of their collecting and sharing plants and fruit. In their role as mothers and with their intrinsic disposition to give, women are the privileged repositories of a uniquely human morality. Classical evolutionary models that only explain kin, reciprocal, and group altruisms largely ignore this level of morality.

The third, final section of the book includes different perspectives on the evolutionary origin of social and moral behavior, and some practical teachings derived from the scientific and philosophical study of this origin. Arcadi Navarro introduces a comprehensive perspective on all the evolutionary models cited by Tobeña, Ovejero and Premack, namely kin and group selection, reciprocal altruism direct and indirect, and altruist punishment. After emphasizing the shortsightedness of strictly competitive views of evolution, Navarro depicts a hierarchical schema, in which interaction of different biological entities at lower levels results in the emergence of more complex levels. Collaboration and specialization of different cells gives rise to the existence of organisms, some of which organize themselves as social entities competing or allying with each other. This mix of conflict and cooperation on multiple levels explains natural evolution and the evolution of contemporary societies and cultures.

Similarly, in the heat of conceptual debate, the flaws of genetic and individualist models have prompted theorists to integrate the normative and group effects of the social level into their explanations. This level is, in its turn, unintelligible without recourse to the lower levels, so the whole picture constitutes a comprehensive model of great explanatory power. Navarro extracts valuable practical lessons from this model and signals the ethical import of aspects still unknown to us, such as the details of the intricate system of identity markers behind group selection.

Group-identity markers are crucial because the biological dispositions in the last hierarchic level lead us to cooperate only with those we perceive to be members of our in-group. As Harnad indicated, to expand morality beyond in-group limits, we need to favor a universal human identity. But before we do, we should understand the relationship between cultural factors like this identity on the one hand and individual minds on the other. Sandro Nannini compares this relationship with the one between mental states and brain states: as no mental states occur in the absence of cerebral activity, cultural traits or memes only exist as a function of human individual minds. Both relationships are distinguished by the place they occupy in the biological hierarchy: social and cultural factors have a kind of second order existence. They depend on individual mental states, which, in their turn, depend on cerebral states.

Yet we always have ways of speaking about mental states, and about memes, which do not presuppose this ontological dependence with respect to their respective cerebral and mental correlates, rationalizations of mere epistemological value. Folk psychology postulates mental states, such as beliefs and desires, as causes of behavior, without implying they have neurophysiological correlates in the brain. Analogously, the concept of a rational agent is useful for economic theory, but it need not correspond with factual people. Nannini concludes that the meme for universal human identity may have causal efficacy in behavior, but if not based on biological markers in existent individuals, this efficacy will be limited and fragile.

Nannini is suggesting a revision or elucidation of the ontological framework of the model Navarro proposes. In the next chapter, F. John Odling-Smee argues for an epistemological, as opposed to ontological revision of Standard Evolutionary Theory, and its full development in an Extended Evolutionary Theory (EET). Though preserving Darwinian orthodoxy with respect to transmission of inherited characteristics, EET introduces the consideration of a driving force of evolution mainly disregarded by Standard Theory. This force is the effect of the behavior of organisms on the environment, and so their contribution to the selective pressures over the genetic make-ups that will pass to new generations. Odling-Smee calls niche construction the process by which many species, through their physical interaction with the environment, modify the conditions to which they are later to adapt themselves genetically. For example, earthworms compensate the inadequacy of their kidneys by actively changing the soil's composition. In *Homo sapiens*, niche construction is immensely empowered by culture. This empowerment is one of the rationales behind the extension of Standard Theory, which fails to account for the two-way causality between organisms and environment. EET also describes how niche construction can become niche destruction by not being adaptive; in cases like climate change, it may trigger a future genetic mutation in response to its adverse effects in the ecological niche.

The interaction of biology and culture is so complex that it overcomes our ability to make precise predictions of future ramifications. For example, a current effective cultural response to global warming caused by human activity may prevent natural biological adaptation to global warming in the future. Large, complex brains have enabled human beings to develop cultural technologies, like meal cooking, to compensate for the limitations of their digestive apparatus. In doing so, they could have liberated energetic resources, which favored the evolution of still larger and more complex brains, more efficient in cultural and social cognition. Camilo José Cela Conde, Miguel Ángel Capó, Marcos Nadal and Carlos Ramos delve into the essential findings and different perspectives in the scientific research on this sophisticated social brain. Phylogenetic studies, sociobiology, evolutionary psychology, and moral neurobiology agree in focusing on the brain as the key of human sociability and morality. Yet each of these approaches places the main source of social cognition in different structures or systems. In their review of the diversity of viewpoints and experimental models, Cela Conde and his collaborators provide a comprehensive survey of the current state of affairs in the social and moral province of cognitive science. Concerning the phylogenesis of the human social brain, its functional superiority with respect to those of other species, is said to depend mostly on the increment of the relative size and degree of gyrification of the brain, which occurred during the evolution of our lineage. Scientists have not yet related cognitive and affective capabilities to fixed neural areas and circuits, but to different combinations of structures and mechanisms.

Similarly, in spite of their ignorance of the details of the interaction of genes and environment in the social brain development, researchers firmly believe that neither genetic dispositions nor environmental conditions are determining factors in isolation each from the other. Cela Conde and his collaborators distinguish several methodological trends in the research on the origin and genesis of the human mind: field study of animal behavior in natural settings, analysis of fossil evidence, laboratory experimentation, and the use of neural imagery devices. Those methodologies have allowed us to study imitation and representation abilities in the context of ecological and cultural niches, and the plasticity of the cerebral structures involved.

Merlin Donald proposes a compelling conceptual framework to understand and integrate the findings of those sometimes-independent lines of research. According to him, three critical evolutionary transitions that occurred in succession during the last two million years separate us from other animals, including the other higher primates. The first transition was our acquisition of mimesis, which includes the cognitive, sensory, and motor capabilities activated in practices such as dance, pantomime, and nonverbal expression. The second evolutionary breakthrough occurred when brains evolved anatomical structures that enabled human beings to narrate stories in articulated language, and the third refers to the invention of symbolic notational systems to record and convey those stories. Donald draws an analogy between the relationship of individual minds and their social and cultural interactions that emerged with those transitions, with the relationship between individual computers inter-connected in a network and, through this network, to the World Wide Web.

Oral cultures, like other products of the appearance of language in the second transition, amplify the cognitive abilities of individual minds, while imposing organization and worldviews on them. Finally, writing and literacy advanced even further the overcoming of cognitive and biological boundaries of human beings as individuals, making more powerful and oppressive the link that unifies them in communities of minds.

Not surprisingly, Donald concedes a significant role in the evolution of our social behavior—of our sharing of minds—to symbolic language. The understanding of language, a decisive test for every philosophical or scientific theory worth its name, is a crucial component of the new perspective underlying Social Neuroscience. Recent empirical and conceptual findings regarding the Social Brain, which appear to challenge most of the assumptions of mainstream linguistics, serve to further amplify its significance.

Luc Steels proposes a framework that accounts for theoretical difficulties of an evolutionary explanation of our language-apt brain and some practical difficulties arising in the development of communication systems in Artificial Intelligence devices. In the précis of his Complex Systems' Approach, he postulates a set of hypotheses, which explains quite elegantly all the complexities involved. In sum, Steels depicts the language faculty and its elements as tools, which our ancestors invented and which we are still adapting and reinventing to fit the unstable requirements of successful communication in diverse social contexts and changing physical environments. Accordingly, Steels hypothesizes that our social brain evolved the neural subsystems accountable for those linguistic details, not as an innate and genetically predetermined language organ, but as a flexible bunch of diverse, non-specific cerebral mechanisms selected and disposed to maximize communication while minimizing energetic resources.

The ultimate condition for the emergence of this sophisticated toolbox would be deep sociability, which freed humanity from the Darwinian world of the survival of the fittest while exposing most of us to the deception and manipulation of the greedy for power and the morally indifferent. Our social nature has then this double significance of deliverance and bondage, of enhancement and restraint, which is apparent to us in the study of more ancient cultures in history and anthropology.

In contrast to Donald's epochal transitions, Derek Bickerton emphasizes the recent evolution of the concept of time and how our understanding of this concept changed our worldview. Some contemporary trends in philosophy, anthropology, and cultural psychology have labeled as specious the notion of progress applied to worldviews. But our discovery of the depth of time, of the enormous time that had passed since life appeared on Earth, and of the profound changes occurred in that time, has allowed us to see things in a way we previously could not.

One such conceptual advance made possible by the acquisition of the time concept has been Darwin's idea of the evolution of species and its extension to, and interaction with, cultural development. Like Daniel C. Dennett in the first section, David Premack in the second, and F. John Odling-Smee earlier in the third part of the book, Bickerton more deeply analyzes the implications of Darwinism for our self-understanding. According to him, while the effects of agriculture on niche construction and population numbers have turned contemporary human societies into something close to anthills, the nature of human individuals within those societies still resembles the nature of apes. This clash between ant-like forms of social organization and individual dispositions characteristic of primates is the source of many inter-group conflicts and much personal dissatisfaction. When facing these problems from this developed neo-Darwinian perspective, we encounter a formidable dilemma, which Bickerton expresses in its most straightforward, uncomfortable terms.

In some respects, the final chapter is *sui generis*. It does not deal with the evolutionary origins of the social brain or the philosophical implications of those origins, as the rest of the chapters in this third section did. Neither does it try to make sense of discursive language and self-concept, morality, religion, art, and other uniquely human phenomena in scientific, objective terms, as contributors to the first two sections of this book—Sebastián Gallés, Dennett, Scott Atran, Tobeña, or Premack—did. Instead, Robert Ginsberg goes just the other way around, and proves that his direction is as significant as the others' are. He holds that while we, as philosophers and scientists, need to get an objective grip on the social and ethical issues here at stake, our sensitive nature as human beings requires us to attribute a personal, subjective meaning to the resulting knowledge.

In other senses, Ginsberg's chapter is completely in tune with the rest of the book. Nelson, Bredo, and Harnad signaled the extent to which cognitive and ethical learning are intertwined, while Parker and Barsalou, along with Nichols, emphasized the links of cognition and emotion in the highest levels of their processing. In doing so, they all resume the Cartesian endeavor of grounding ethics on a philosophical and scientific inquiry into the mind-body communication and mutual influences. On the other hand, Atran, Ovejero, and Gomila assume the Kantian dichotomy by which objective knowledge cannot rule over ethical considerations in the justification of moral laws. Ginsberg also builds upon Descartes and Kant, among others, to focus on Harnad and Rottschaefer's concern for the extension of the moral community to the whole of humanity. Ginsberg resorts to some of the best classical and contemporary philosophy to make a strong argument for this extension, invoking both levels of morality, which Rottschaefer, Gomila, and Premack singled out: the rational, more sophisticated, higher level, and the basic, motivating one. Finally, he proposes three ways for attaining that human moral community, a methodological triad to learn by and through the heart.

In addition to its content making an undeniable contribution to naturalist science and philosophy, the Social Brain Dialogue also unearthed less obvious results. We can view it retrospectively as a large experimental laboratory, where the subjects were some of the best philosophers and scientists involved in the multidisciplinary endeavor to which the prologue termed Social Neuro-science. The organizers and the audience attending the debates enjoyed these experts making the results of their thought and research activity explicit while watching how they interacted with each other and with their listeners, how they translate their vast knowledge into words, looks, facial expression, and gesticulation. We cannot easily convey this unique experience of direct com-munication of the work of years, sometimes a lifetime, of research and delib-eration, through written word. That is why we refer every interested reader to the documentary, which opened the Dialogue (available free of charge on DVD for only the cost of shipping: contact *Càtedra per la Divulgació Científica* (Chair for the Vulgarization of Science), Valencia University, cdciencia@uv.es), to serve as an introduction to the book's readings, and to give a hint of that special atmosphere.[16] This introductory chapter and its at-tempt to recreate some of the debates within the philosophical and scientific elite who met in Barcelona that summer points in the same direction. One of our aims was then, as it remains, to demonstrate the benefits of cooperative discourse. We are convinced that efforts to resolve conflicts through the dis-cussion of views, regardless whether we achieve immediate resolution or agreement, is always of mutual advantage for all the stakeholders. Influence and conversion, the social phenomena by which even a minority can induce change in the beliefs and identities of the majority, sometimes affects such an advantageous approach. We editors hope to contribute to a change for the better, small though it may be, in the individual minds of the readers of this book, which is the result of thorough revision and updating of the authors' original papers. Massive social and cultural changes, of the kind we need to-day, could require something more, but in any case nothing less, than many individual changes.

Notes

1. Gilbert Ryle, *The Concept of Mind* (London: Hutchinson, 1949), pp.11–24; David Rosenthal, ed., *The Nature of Mind* (New York: Oxford University Press, 1991), pp. 51–81.

2. Thomas E. Hill, Jr., "Kantianism," *The Blackwell Guide to Ethical Theory*, ed. Hugh Lafollete (Oxford: Blackwell, 2000), pp. 227–246.

3. Lewis J. Beck, *The Method of Descartes: A Study of the Regulae* (Oxford: Clarendon Press, 1952), pp. 83, 215; and Michio Kobayashi, *La Philosophie Naturelle de Descartes* (*Descartes' Natural Philosophy*) (Paris: Jean Vrin, 1993), p. 13.

4. René Descartes, *Œuvres De Descartes* (*Descartes' Works*), vol. 11, eds. Charles Adam and Paul Tannery (Paris: Librairie Philosophique Jean Vrin, 1983), p. 327; and *The Philosophical Writings of Descartes*, vol. 1, trans. John Cottingham, Robert Stoothoff, and Dugald Murdoch (Cambridge, UK: Cambridge University Press, 1988), pp. 338–339.

5. Alfred Rupert Hall, *The Revolution in Science 1500–1750* (London: Longman, 1983); and Salvi Turró, *Descartes: Del Hermetismo a la Nueva Ciencia* (*Descartes: From Hermetism to New Science*) (Barcelona: Anthropos, 1984), p. 295.

6. Immanuel Kant, *Kants Gesammelte Schriften* (*Kant's Collected Writings*), vol. 3, *Kritik der reinen Vernunft* (*Criticism of Pure Reason*), 2nd ed. (Berlin: G. Reimer, 1902), Preface, pp. xii–xv; and *Critique of Pure Reason*, trans. Norman Kemp Smith (London: MacMillan, 1929, rev. 1933).

7. Kant, *Kants Gesammelte Schriften*, vol. 5, *Kritik der praktischen Vernunft*, (*Criticism of Practical Reason*), pp.1–163; *Critique of Practical Reason and Other Writings in Moral Philosophy*, trans. Lewis White Beck (New York: Garland, 1976); Felipe Martínez Marzoa, *Releer a Kant*, (*Rereading Kant*) (Barcelona: Anthropos, 1989), pp. 95–105.

8. Descartes, *Œuvres De Descartes*, vol. 9B, p.14; *The Philosophical Writings of Descartes*, vol. 1, p. 186.

9. Kant, *Kants Gesammelte Schriften*, vol. 5; *Critique of Pure Reason*.

10. Dieter Henrich, *Between Kant and Hegel: Lectures on German Idealism*, ed. David S. Pacini (Cambridge, Mass.: Harvard University Press, 2003), p. 61.

11. Salvi Turró, personal communication, circa 2000.

12. Geneviève Rodis-Lewis, "Preface" René Descartes, *Discours de la Méthode* (*Discourse on the Method*), ed. G. Rodis-Lewis (Paris: Flammarion, 1992); Wayne Waxman, *Kant's Model of the Mind* (New York: Oxford University Press, 1991), p. 272.

13. Andrew Brook, *Kant and the Mind* (Cambridge, UK: Cambridge University Press), 1994), chap. 1.

14. Descartes, *Œuvres De Descartes*, vol. 6, pp. 63–64.

15. David J. Wood, Jerome Bruner, and Gail Ross, "The Role of Tutoring in Problem Solving," *Journal of Child Psychology and Psychiatry*, 17 (1976), pp. 89–100.

16. *Bajo la Piel del Conflicto* (*Getting under Conflict's Skin*), DVD, Artistic Director and Co-author, H. Carmona, Scientific Director and Co-author, O. Vilarroya (Valencia, Spain: Universitat de Valencia, 2004).

Part One

LEARNING PROCESSES
OF SOCIAL VALUES

One

LEARNING: A BRIEF INTRODUCTION FROM THE NEUROSCIENCES

Núria Sebastián Gallés

SCENE I. A desert place.
Thunder and lightning. Enter three Witches.
First Witch:
When shall we three meet again
In thunder, lightning, or in rain?
Second Witch
When the hurlyburly's done,
When the battle's lost and won.
Third Witch
That will be ere the set of sun.[1]

William Shakespeare chose the following words to start Macbeth: "A desert place. Thunder and lightning. Enter three Witches." With just these nine words, he is able to describe a fearful scene. Human beings do not like to be in desert places, much less during a storm. Not at all if three witches enter the scene.

Why do people consider some situations scary? Many children (and adults) panic in the dark. Others freeze in front of a snake. Fear is not a good companion of reason and happiness. But in many circumstances, it helps to make permanent memories: a traumatic situation is almost impossible to forget.

The Gileadites captured the fords of the Jordan River opposite Ephraim. Whenever an Ephraimite fugitive said, "Let me cross over," the men of Gilead asked him, "Are you an Ephraimite?" If he said, "No," then they said to him, "Say 'Shibboleth.'" If he said, "Sibboleth," and could not pronounce the word correctly, they grabbed him and executed him right there at the fords of the Jordan. On that day forty-two thousand Ephraimites fell dead."[2]

Judges tells us that forty-two thousand Ephraimites were killed because they could not pronounce the word "Shibboleth." Put yourself in the shoes of an Ephraimite for a moment. You see that all your fellows are killed because of their failure to say "sh," and you hear the Gileadites saying "Say 'Shibboleth.'" Despite facing the possibility of losing your life and the examples provided by your enemy, you cannot learn to pronounce "sh."

These two examples show two of the most extreme situations in learning. The first refers to circumstances that, even though experienced only once in your life, leave permanent memories. For traumatic experiences to create these types of memories is not unusual. The second refers to a situation where, in spite of multiple instances and a high motivation to learn, to modify our behavior is impossible. Learning a second language is just one case of this category.

What is learning? How do we learn?

1. Multiple Definitions of Learning

As the reader might have guessed from the above quotation, to define learning is a difficult task. From a biochemical perspective, we could say learning is what happens when some molecules are modified. At a more global level, learning can be described as the increase in association between two events. The term "association" has been traditionally linked to the concept of "learning." In 1949, one of the fathers of computational neurobiology, Donald Hebb, postulated a computational rule, known as the "Hebbian Rule," which makes explicit this assumption. This rule postulates that learning implies coincident pre- and post-synaptic activity. Although many of Hebb's ideas were not right, recent research on neurobiology has shown that this coincidence of activities causes synapses to change, and therefore, they constitute the basic mechanism of learning. But, can learning be defined just by making reference to biochemical changes?

One of the main problems in defining learning has to do with the more general issue of relating "mind" and "brain." A long tradition in Western culture separates these two levels. We can travel back to Greek philosophers, René Descartes, and even contemporary philosophers. One attempt to relate brain and behavior was phrenology. During the late nineteenth century, that movement tried to locate each cognitive function and personality trait at precise brain locations (see Figure 1).

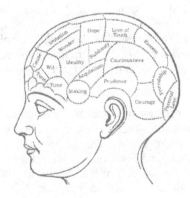

Figure 1. Brain map proposed by Phrenologists.

This approach was wrong, but it helped society to accept the notion that cognitive functions could be related to particular brain structures. Modern neuroscience has provided an appropriate background to address these issues. We now know that our cognitive functioning is quite complex. To present any comprehensive account of it that only considers one level of description would be impossible. We must give problems the right level of explanation, but what is the proper level to explain "learning"?

2. Learning at a Molecular Level

What is the relationship between synaptic changes and behavioral changes? We are far from being able to answer to this question, but, as in other fields of neuroscience, we are getting increasingly closer to it. In 1973, Timothy Bliss and Terje Lomo described, for the first time in the mammalian brain, the existence of Long-Term Potentiation (LTP).[3] Science considered this a great finding. Why was this discovery so significant?

The basic unit (cell) of our nervous system is the neuron. Neurons can have many different shapes, some of them quite spectacular (see the cerebellar Purkinje cell in Figure 2).

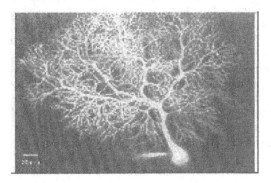

Figure 2. Cerebellar Purkinje cell.

Although we can think of our nervous system as a road network, where electric impulses (or information) travels, one particular property makes it radically different from most networks of which we are used to thinking. Ramón y Cajal was the first to describe our nervous system as a *discontinuous* network of neurons: neurons do not "touch" each other. Instead, they stand next to each other, with gaps between them. For the nervous signal to travel across the system, it needs to "jump" over those gaps. This is done through synapses (see Figure 3). When the nervous signal reaches one end of a neuron (the end of an axon), it causes some substances (neurotransmitters) to be released into the gap. These neurotransmitters induce some chemical reaction on the end of the adjacent neuron (a dendrite). This chemical reaction triggers the transmission of the nervous signal in the second neuron, so the signal continues to travel through our brain. Our brain being not a "solid," continuous network, but instead needing biochemical changes at crucial points to have the signal traveling across it, is the foundation of learning.

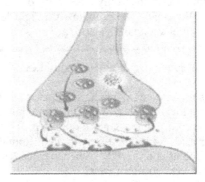

Figure 3. Neuron synapse.

Different factors (like drug or alcohol consumption) can modify these biochemical reactions, but the repetition of the transmission also modifies their properties. In a sense, we can think of synapses as "living" connections; they will evolve and adapt themselves as a function of their past experiences. Our brain is a "plastic" structure. In this context, plastic refers to its ability to change its functioning as a consequence of past experiences. Our brain is "plastic" because the activity at the synapses changes. Now we have a hint about why the discovery of LTP in the mammalian brain was so significant.

One current view of learning at a molecular level is that it involves molecular changes that occur at the synapses. One of the best candidates for this molecular change is LTP, operationally defined as a long-lasting increase in synaptic efficacy which follows high-frequency stimulation of afferent fibers. This form of synaptic plasticity may participate in information storage in several brain regions.

We are far from understanding all the complex mechanisms involved in these processes. We understand, even from personal experiences, that our brain operates better when our basic needs are satisfied (sleep, food, water). Fear has strong consequences (at a molecular level) in the way learning occurs. It has the consequence of modifying the biochemical properties of the neurotransmitters, making some experiences especially salient (the basis of traumatic experiences, which individuals are unable to forget throughout their entire lives).

Until now, we have been talking about learning as if just one type exists. But this is not the case. To assume that our brain is a homogeneous structure and that all of its parts have equivalent roles in learning is inaccurate. True, learning happens throughout our brain, but to disregard differences in learning how to play tennis, how to get around in a new building, or how to speak a new language is erroneous. Our mature brain is a highly specialized "device," different parts of which carry out different types of knowledge and "activities." To better understand how learning takes place, we must consider not only "what" biochemical changes are taking place, but also "where" these changes happen.

3. Is Learning More than Changes in Synaptic Strength? Learning and Brain Systems

If we broadly define learning as gathering knowledge, it bears a strong relationship with memory, as it refers to our capability to store knowledge. Research in cognitive psychology showed that different types of "knowledge" exist. Neuroscience has confirmed and extended these findings by providing evidence of how different brain systems support different memory types. We can gain an initial understanding of the diversity of memory types and learning and storing mechanisms by considering the case of amnesiac patients. We all know that under some circumstances, individuals can forget their past life. Writers and moviemakers have used this topic. They write about people who, after suffering some traumatic experience, have forgotten "everything." But have these characters completely forgotten all of their memories? Amnesiac patients usually have trouble remembering their names, where they live, work, or facts such as where they went on vacation last summer. Usually they forget information about their personal life. They may suffer a highly selective memory deficit by forgetting what happened during a particular traumatic experience, but without any "learning" problem.

Neuroscientists have proposed a fundamental division between two memory types: "declarative memory" and "procedural memory." Broadly, declarative memory corresponds to what cognitive psychologists call "explicit learning." Explicit learning is usually related to our ability to put into words something that we are learning—for instance, when describing the set of instructions that have been followed to acquire new data (for example, how to cook a new dish). Therapists can teach many amnesiac patients some skills, but they fail to explicitly state the sequence by which they manage to do so. At an anatomical level, declarative (explicit) memory involves the hippocampus, several surrounding cortical areas, and other cortical areas.

If declarative memory corresponds to explicit learning, procedural memory corresponds to "implicit learning." Implicit knowledge is involved in many different aspects of our lives. We have an implicit knowledge of the grammar of our language that makes us to reject a sentence like "the boy open the window" because "it is not correct." Different studies have shown that implicit learning is involved even in classification tasks, which we may at first consider as an example of declarative knowledge: participants can sort items (exemplars) into two categories, without being able to tell what criteria they used. Implicit learning is also involved in slight changes in motor skills that accompany, for instance, our improvements when learning a new sport. From the point of view of brain structures being involved in this type of learning, two subsystems operate: the neostriatal subsystem (belonging to the basal ganglia) and the cerebellar subsystem. Although both subsystems subserve different functions, they share the property of being essential in the processes of learning without conscious recollection. Figure 4 illustrates the relationship between brain areas and memory systems. In this diagram, a third memory system has been added: emotional memory.

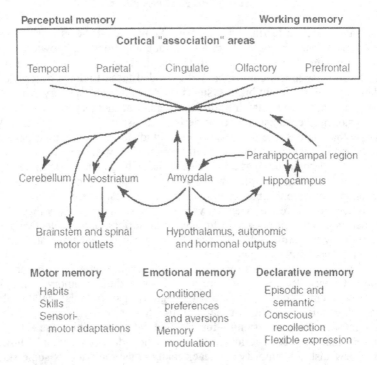

Figure 4. Relationship between Brain Areas and Memory and Emotion Systems.
Copyright 2002, Elsevier Science (USA). All rights reserved.[4]

Emotional memory is the learning and recollection of knowledge about our emotional state in a designated circumstance. The scene described by Shakespeare in the first words of Macbeth causes us to contact different fearful experiences that left strong memories in our brain. Investigators have well documented the consequences of emotional states in learning in recent years. One central structure in emotions is the amygdala, a small structure located in the inner part of the brain, which resembles an almond (this is where the name comes from). The amygdala, as can be seen in the Figure 4, receives inputs from many sensory and secondary centers and is responsible for increasing our heart rate, blood pressure and, together with the hypothalamus, controls a wide variety of hormones. We can view the amygdala-hypothalamus complex as a powerful "drug-triggering" center in our brain. Changes in the neurotransmitters may have key consequences in the learning processes. These effects can involve increasing the efficiency of storage, as in the case of the increase of arousal induced by emotional changes.[5] Generally, the strength of a memory (learning) should correlate with its importance to the organism. We can view the consequences of emotions as a successful evolutionary mechanism for learning and remembering the more important things of our lives.[6]

Research in cognitive neuroscience has shown that individuals suffering Post Traumatic Stress Disorder (a highly disabling condition, associated with intrusive recollections of a traumatic event, avoidance of situations associated with the trauma and psychological numbing) show abnormal functioning of the amygdala, hypothalamus, and the medial frontal cortex. These studies have shown that the amygdala overreacts to stimuli associated with the traumatic experience, and the hypothalamus and medial frontal cortex appear to be unable to compensate for this.

Although all human beings may suffer a traumatic experience they may not forget throughout their entire lives, also undeniable is that infancy and childhood are especially sensitive periods for learning.

4. Learning at Different Moments in Life

Up to this point, we have been presenting evidence about learning at a time when the brain is a relatively mature, stable structure. In this context, the changes occurring at the molecular level would not represent major transformations in its structure and overall functioning. As living entities in general, and as humans in particular, we experience a long period of growth. That we cannot learn all types of knowledge in the same way at different moments in life is indisputable. One of the most frustrating experiences as an adult learner is that of trying to acquire a new language—even more so if we compare ourselves with infants and young children, who are able to acquire a new language without apparent effort. Remember the example of the Ephraimites and their inability to pronounce the sound "sh." But not all learning is more difficult for adults than for children. Both experience and our mature brain help us in most of situations. To learn to play chess at age twenty is plainly easier than to learn the game at age three. Why is it that for some types of knowledge (like learning a new language) having a "young brain" appears to be an advantage, while not for others? Many researchers have related the answer to this question to the existence of "critical periods" in brain development. Because this is a quite controversial issue, I will briefly address it here.

One general property of the developing brain is that just before and after birth, an exuberant growth of neurons and synapses occurs (although the precise timing depends on the particular area of the brain in question). The number of neurons and synapses is much larger during this period than in the adult, highly functioning brain. During this phase, a "crude" competition for both neurons and synapses to "survive" happens and only a subset of them (those better suited for the intended processing) will manage to succeed. We find an example of this neuronal struggle for survival in the development of the neocortex of a transgenic mouse over the first days of life. At the beginning of the sixth day in postnatal development, the axon cone pictured in C in Figure 5 includes two axons; nineteen hours later (C'), only one axon is left. We could say that the leftmost axon "won the battle."[7]

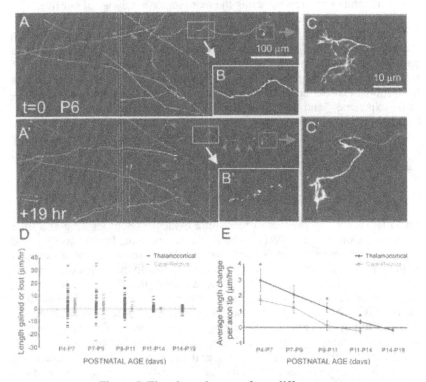

Figure 5. Time-lapse images of two different axons.

The great advantage of this cell death and axon "pruning" is that our brain increases its efficiency. To believe that "more neurons" or "more synapses" is better than having less is incorrect. The purpose of synaptic overproduction may be to capture and incorporate experience into the developing synaptic architecture of the brain. Figure 6 shows the evolution of the mammalian visual system, with the improvement in functioning produced by axon pruning (and the consequent reorganization of neuronal projections).

In the immature brain, retinal projections are unspecified, while in the adult brain, we see a highly ordered and structured organization. Often, this specialization is the outcome of both internally driven information ("innate" specifications) and externally driven activity (the influence of experience). We can say that during this neuronal reorganization, our brain is highly plastic, in the sense that relatively small amounts of experience have a great impact.

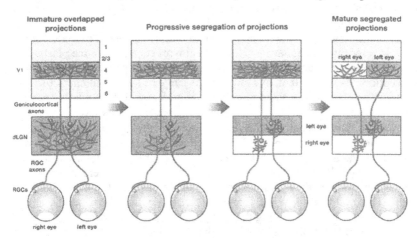

Figure 6. Evolution of the mammalian visual system, with the improvement in functioning produced by axon pruning.

At the same time, to believe that the entire brain develops in a homogeneous fashion would be wrong. These periods of cell death and synapse pruning vary significantly from one area of the brain to another. For example, at around age five or six, the number of synapses in the visual and auditory areas of the brain resembles those of the adult. Not until mid to late adolescence does the number of synapses in the areas of the brain that subserve higher cognitive functions and emotions (prefrontal cortex) approach adult patterns.

"Critical period" means that, because of biological constraints—related to cell death and synapse pruning among other things—our brain would be especially fit to learn some things during a relatively short period as compared with any other time in development. Experience before, or more importantly, after this period would be less efficient, or completely inefficient. Although nobody denies the existence of critical periods in development, the way commentators usually present the concept is wrong.

Our brain is a highly specialized machine. The hippocampus is involved in learning processes that make use of declarative memory. The amygdala is involved in emotional processing. In the same way, the different cognitive processes involve different brain systems. For instance, complex reasoning and planning chiefly involve frontal structures. These structures do not reach adult levels until almost adulthood. To think of the existence of a "critical period" for learning cognitive abilities that rely heavily on these structures would be difficult. Yet, a few "sensitive periods" exist (to use a more modern term) in human development, most of which are related to basic functioning (like the reorganization of the visual cortex presented above). Significantly, proper functioning does not depend on having "more" experience. In the past years, this notion has received a lot of attention, For example, music "to stimulate your baby's brain" have become commonplace. But we have no scientific evidence that over-stimulating a normal, healthy infant has any beneficial effect. On the contrary, evidence suggests that it may be a waste of time.

In a recent article, Patricia Kuhl and coworkers explored the plasticity of human infants to acquire foreign sounds.[8] Research studying infant speech perception has shown that, at birth, infants can distinguish all speech sounds, even if they do not hear them in their environment and if, as adults, they will be unable to reproduce them. For instance, Spanish adults have trouble perceiving the Catalan contrast /e-ɛ/, but at four months, Spanish babies can easily discriminate the two sounds.[9] Parallel results have been reported comparing infant and adult data with a wide variety of foreign contrasts, such as the /r-l/ contrast, which Japanese adults have great difficulty perceiving. During the first months of their lives, Japanese infants have no trouble telling them apart. This ability to perceive foreign contrasts declines between the ages of six and twelve months. During the first year of their lives, infants modify their brains to start to become highly competent listeners and speakers of their maternal language. So, the acquisition of the speech sound repertoire of the maternal language is characterized not by adding new sounds, but by "forgetting" those sounds not used (The parallels between this process, cell death, and axon pruning are obvious).

We might ask to what extent this "forgetting" is reversible. Popular wisdom assumes that acquiring a second language before puberty usually leads to a native-level performance. Scientific research has proven that this is not the case. When sensitive measures are used, we can find significant differences in some linguistic domains between natives and bilinguals who acquired their second language during the first three years of their lives. Kuhl and co-workers have analyzed the effect of exposing nine-month-old American infants to Mandarin Chinese. They tested them with a Mandarin Chinese contrast that adult American listeners have trouble perceiving. Investigators exposed infants to twelve twenty-five minute sessions (the total exposure period lasted about four weeks). The results showed that at this early age, reversing the decline is possible. Compared with a control group not exposed to Mandarin Chinese, the infants exposed to Chinese better discriminated the Chinese contrast.

In this experiment, investigators exposed infants to "life" materials: native speakers of Mandarin talking and playing with the infants. In an additional experiment, researchers exposed two new groups of American infants to recorded materials, equivalent to the "life" ones, either with audiovisual exposure or with just audio exposure. The results showed that these two groups did not benefit from being exposed to Mandarin Chinese: they found no significant difference in their discrimination of the Chinese sounds by infants who heard recordings and American infants not exposed to Chinese.

What does a live person provide that a recording does not? Although science cannot yet provide a definitive answer, we can advance some proposals. We have seen that brain systems responsible for emotions play a significant role in learning. During the first few months of life, crucial "rewiring" and "reconfiguration" processes occur that affect the way these structures connect with other brain areas (especially with the control of attention). Accordingly, concluding that emotions may play a more significant role in learning in infancy and early childhood than in adulthood would be a reasonable assumption. Plainly, interacting with a human being is more likely than a Digital Video Disc (DVD) to create emotions in a nine-month old.

5. Researchers, the Ivory Tower, and Real Life

We have made significant advances in our comprehension of learning processes and quite likely, these advances will increase even more in coming years. We have allocated significant amounts of money to continue these studies, but will it be enough for the actual improvement of how we learn?

In addition to advancing our knowledge in the basic mechanisms of learning, advancing our knowledge of how society can use our understanding is crucial. Neuroscience is in its infancy, and building bridges from theory to practice is not easy. Usually, educators and practitioners receive "brain-based" applications with skepticism. True, we have not validated many of the commercially available programs that claim a "scientific" basis, for instance, the putative benefits of early stimulation. "Neuromyths" abound and have a tremendous negative impact on how society perceives science.

To solve both the problem of building bridges between science and society and to guide the non-specialist, different administrations need to become involved. Fortunately, we appear to have taken some steps in that direction. On one hand, the United States National Science Foundation has launched the program "Science of Learning Centers." Realizing the need for interdisciplinary approaches, these centers are designed to put together all disciplines that relate to this topic, ranging from psychologists and biologists to mathematicians, anthropologists, and educators. A second initiative that deserves mention is the Organisation for Economic Co-operation and Development (OECD) "Brain and Learning" project. According to their Internet website:

> Over the past few years, science has made substantial advances in understanding the brain. Consequently, the challenge facing us today, is to explore the relevant research in order to develop a pathway towards a neuroscientific approach to the question 'how do we learn?' Our objective is to formulate a sounder basis for the understanding (and, over time, an improvement) of learning and teaching processes and practices, notably in the areas of reading, mathematics and lifelong learning.[10]

These are ambitious initiatives, but understanding what learning is and how it is affected at all levels is a huge challenge. Undoubtedly, we need large-scale teams and programs to address the question.

Notes

1. William Shakespeare, *Macbeth*, Act 1, scene 1.

2. Judges, 12.

3. Timothy Bliss and Terje Lomo, "Long-Lasting Potentiation of Synaptic Transmission in the Dentate Area of the Anaesthetized Rabbit following Stimulation of the Perforant Path," *Journal of Physiology*, 232:2 (1973), pp. 331–356.

4. Larry R. Squire, *Fundamental Neuroscience* (New York: Academic Press, 2003), p. 1303.

5. James L. McGaugh, "Memory: A Century of Consolidation," *Science*, 287, (2000), pp. 248-251.

6. L. Helmuth, "Fear and Trembling in the Amygdala," *Science*, 300 (2003), pp. 568–569.

7. Carlos Portera-Cailliau, Robby M. Weimer, Vincenzo De Paola, Pico Caroni, and Karel Svoboda, "Diverse Modes of Axon Elaboration in the Developing Neocortex," *Plos Biology*, 3:8:e272 (2005), pp. 1–15, http://www.doaj.org/doaj?func= abstract&id=121845&recNo=11&toc=1 (accessed 29 December 2006).

8. P. Kuhl, F. M. Tsao, and H. M. Liu, "Foreign-Language Experience in Infancy: Effects of Short-Term Exposure and Social Interaction on Phonetic Learning," *Proceedings of the National Academy of Sciences*, 100 (2003), pp. 9096–9101.

9. L. Bosch and Núria Sebastián Gallés, "Simultaneous Bilingualism and the Perception of a Language Specific Vowel Contrast in the First Year of Life," *Language and Speech*, 46 (2003), pp. 217–244.

10. Organisation for Economic Co-operation and Development "Brain and Learning" http://www.oecd.org/department/0,2688,en_2649_14935397_1_1_1_1_1,00.html (accessed 15 October 2006).

Two

CAN UNSELFISHNESS BE TAUGHT?

Daniel C. Dennett

Can unselfishness be taught? Well, why not? We can definitely teach calculus, can we not? Not everyone can learn everything, but we can teach many things. As Núria Sebastián Gallés points out, we have evolved highly efficient organs of learning, our brains, with the capability to process huge amounts of information at an impressive speed.

Some human abilities appear to be difficult or even impossible to teach, like style or wit. We consider musical talent generally to be a natural gift, something innate. So we can put the question in this form: is unselfishness learned like calculus or innate like wit?

Let us take another example: can Catalan be taught? Catalan native speakers do not merely learn the language in instructional contexts, they acquired it by listening and hearing it spoken to them at an early age. For me to learn it would be much more difficult and, according to Sebastián Gallés, I will never speak it fluently regardless of the degree of my effort or practice. For the rest of my life, I will remain unable to discriminate phonemes which sound quite distinguishable to native speakers.

Can we be fluently unselfish or must we learn unselfishness as we learn a second language? Intriguing as this question may be, I am not going to pursue it here. What concerns us here is what we can do to teach unselfishness in whatever way we can demonstrate to be effective. Do we need to teach it at all? Maybe we are born with an innate sense of unselfishness, as some are born with a natural talent or wit. Such a belief, if true, would be wonderful, but believing something does not necessarily make it true.

We know from evolutionary biology that a variety of unselfish behaviors is apparently innate, commonly occurring in the animal world, for example, affectionate behaviors exhibited by parents for their offspring. Scientists try hard to provide an evolutionary explanation of the many evidences of parental sacrifice towards their breed. But upon closer examination, we will find something with quite shocking implications for the caring mothers and fathers who may be reading these words. Not only do we observe unselfishness out of love, we also observe conflicts that arise between parents and their young, conflicts so intense that they lead to behavior akin to an arms race between them.

A much-discussed example is how nestling birds blackmail their parents by desperately crying for food. Apparently aware of the high risk that noise will attract potential predators, the parents are compelled to feed their young as quickly and repeatedly as possible to minimize their cries, thereby preventing them from being eaten.

Parents may not be as unselfish as they may appear. Consider the interaction between the human mother and her unborn child during pregnancy. In a key sense, its development progresses as a conflict, starting with the fetus sending out invasive hormones into the mother's bloodstream to obtain the maximum share of nutrients. The mother counteracts, by unwittingly introducing in her circulatory system hormone antagonists, which in turn, can affect the fetus. This alternating escalation of offensive and defensive actions occurring in the prenatal environment has been exquisitely studied by the Harvard evolutionary biologist David Haig, who argues that we must be especially cautious in construing the interaction between mother and baby as a straight case of biologic unselfishness.

A significant distinction exists between learning and being taught. Learning, not teaching, can occur without information being culturally transmitted. As Sebastián recalls, most of what we learn is not by formal instruction but by imitation, by copying role models. What can we learn in this way? A non-exhaustive list includes learning facts and learning habits. The documentary, *Bajo la Piel del Conflicto (Getting under the Skin of Conflict)* explores some interesting insights derived from the double sense of the term "habit" in English, and I guess in Catalan and Spanish too: habit can connote either a costume such as the garb worn by some monks, or routine behavior done in much the same way upon each occurrence and at regular intervals, such as brushing teeth upon arising in the morning. We learn the habits in the second sense by mere repetition, which facilitates and strengthen the behavior until we execute it fluently; then it becomes part of us as the garb monks wear becomes part of their identity. And just as we can learn habits, we can learn methods of thought as well.[1]

All kinds of methods are culturally transmitted, not only in *Homo sapiens*, but also in birds and other mammals. A major component of instinctive know-how passed on to new generations is transmitted by social learning. For instance, diet preferences or mating strategies do not spread through genes or direct instruction, but by something closer to imitation. Traditions exists even in the non-human world: we find arguments and wonderful examples in a book titled *Animal Traditions* that thoroughly surveys the scientific knowledge in the field.[2] It concludes that we are not the only species able to transmit information non-genetically, through environmental and social interaction with our young and other members of our species.

While non-human animals transmit behavioral traditions from one generation to the next, we human beings are unique in the learning of thought habits. Behavior and thought habits are crucially different in kind; I will concentrate now on the second. Methods of thought are special in that they are always designed, intended to serve designated functions. They are optimized to accomplish the tasks for which they are designed, but not necessarily by a single human agent, composer, or author.

Charles Darwin described such patterns of transmission in *Origin of Species*.[3] He illustrates the then-astonishing new concept of natural selection by an exemplar with which he expects his audience to be familiar, the concept of *methodical selection*, the foresighted, purposeful, and deliberate design of varieties of pigeons and dogs by animal breeders, or of plants by farmers and plant breeders.

Against methodical selection, Darwin opposes *unconscious selection*. Long before our ancestors discovered that they could obtain stronger or meatier animals through methodical selection, they unconsciously selected the best individuals for breeding. The origin of our domesticated species evinced not a brilliant technology or human capacity for foresight, but the mindless favoring of the best or the prettiest individual of the litter for breeding, while the others they ate. Their process was a gradualistic and unpurposeful creation of new varieties and eventually new species due to the cumulative effect of undeliberate breeding preferences.

A superb example quoted by Darwin is the King Charles spaniel, who became a much larger dog in only a few generations due to unconscious selection. Nobody deliberately and permanently attempted to alter the breed to obtain a bigger species; the changes were instead the outcome of several random choices. Darwin cited this unconscious selection, in which a human agent is unwittingly producing the modifications, as the link between foresightless and foresighted breeding. The element of intelligence is thereby introduced, but to a lesser extent than in methodical selection.

What is produced in an unpurposeful manner, due to the unconscious intervention of human agents, Darwin notes, can be done by nature's mindless mechanisms. And so he teaches us about natural selection.

What I am suggesting is that the same trio of kinds of natural selection, strictly natural, unconscious, and methodical applies to the evolution of human culture. In human culture, we have many things excellently designed but which no one has intentionally designed. Some are no doubt the foreseen, intended products of human intelligence, but many others lack any foresight or intention. We cannot identify an author, composer, or finder who designed the invention; instead, the improvement occurred by no deliberate intention through centuries.

So evolution can redesign and add idiosyncratic features to culture without any deliberate authorship. Consider the case of language, which we have also discussed in the Universal Forum of Cultures, Barcelona, 2004. Romance languages share a common ancestor, Latin, from which they diverge into separate tongues. We know a lot about the moment of their differentiation, but in no case was the diversion foresighted or intended by any human group. Sometimes a pronunciation characteristic of a linguistic subgroup, their language, became fashioned and integrated in the language of the entire population. Sometimes, as Yiddish linguist Max Weinreich instructs, a language is a dialect with an army. But more often the boundary between one language and another is crossed by nothing more or less than a series of cumulative variations. No ingenious designer exists: that's the import of the Darwinian idea of evolution by natural selection.

We find a nice illustration in folk music. We know of many authorless melodies which have evolved from ancient times, without any identifiable composer. If we could build a time machine to trace back the origin of one of those songs, we would discover many gradual changes until we could not recognize the song as we know it today. They have undergone so much modification, their authorship spread through so many eras and generations, that no single composer deserves the title of author of these songs. Ironically, to make these changes does not require the cleverest of musicians, but only mediocre ones, with poor memory or those unable to sing the song properly as originally composed. They transmitted the song not as it was passed to them but as they knew it or remembered it, possibly making unconscious errors in the replication process that come down to us as the version with which we are familiar.

We can apply all of this to ethical behavior, to this concept of unselfishness. In ethics, we have the Golden Rule: do unto others as you would have them do unto you. Compare the Golden Rule with an imaginary Rule that I will call the Tin Rule: Do what you would have members of the community of rational agents do when their actions have positive or negative effects on the self-concept, physical integrity, possessions, and quality of life of other members of the community such as yourself. The Tin Rule means exactly the same that the Golden Rule. Some philosophers would probably prefer the Tin Rule because they are familiar with this sort of language in their lives, frequently uttering this kind of statement. My point is that, both having the same meaning, the Golden Rule is far better designed than the Tin Rule, much more succinct, easier to remember, and by all means, a better candidate for replication.

Each statement, in its own way, conveys the same message; their propositional contents are identical. The endorsement of one implies that of the other. If the Golden Rule enhances, say, your biological fitness, so does the Tin Rule, to the same degree. The lack of applicability of the Tin Rule does not depend on its content, since is the content is exactly the same that of the Golden Rule, but on its poor replicability. The Golden Rule's better fitness, our likelihood to replicate it more than the Tin Rule, is the key to its success. This is true for reasons which have nothing to do with the ability or strength of those who adopt the rule. What then is the cause of this cultural fitness of the Golden Rule?

One possibility is that it was consciously designed by an expert, a kind of creative publicist. Advertisers owe their livelihood to devising successful slogans, phrases that may trigger emotional pathways as the ones cited by Sebastián, compelling us to hum them repeatedly. Some of those slogans do their job quite well, but most do not. Coming up with a successful slogan is quite difficult. Professional publicists produce many slogans of which only a few will capture our attention through a gradual process of undeliberated selection.

Most probably the Golden Rule is authorless, in much the same way some folk songs are. It evolved from something else, replicated, and gradually acquired the form it now has. It has no single human designer, no need of improvement or redesign. "Mother Nature is cleverer than you are," to use the words of Leslie Orgel, epitomized by Francis Crick as Orgel's Second Rule.[4]

What I have sketched so far is a Dawkinsian theory of cultural change, the theory of cultural entities as memes suggested by Richard Dawkins in *The Selfish Gene*.[5] We can use this conceptualization to argue that cultural evolution is as mindless as biological evolution. Fascinatingly, the "meme" story has provoked a harsh reaction in many people, perhaps because of its being a bad theoretical idea, but I do not think so. I believe instead that people reject the theory because it diminishes the role of human authorship, the contribution of individual geniuses to the masterpieces of our cultural heritage.

To present a sound defense of the meme theory here would be beyond the scope of this chapter, but I will point out one of its major advantages: it excuses us from any explanation of unselfishness in terms of human fitness alone. Some would like to argue for a natural cultural selection, in which cultural entities are selected in view of their contribution to the biological fitness of the organisms that adopt them. From this perspective, a better fishhook is selected because it enables its user to catch more fish, like a stronger arm enables its owner to work, attack, or defend itself better.

But not all cultural entities are beneficial to the biological fitness of their hosts in the short run. Even though cultural change occurs much faster than genetic change, for an innovative cultural item to generally be adopted may take generations. So we must explain the evolution of culture without this even flexible link to biological fitness, which amounts to individual agents maximizing their options of survival and reproduction. The Dawkinsian theory of cultural evolution provides us an alternative explanatory principle. The meme, the unit of selection proposed by this theory, has its own fitness, quite autonomous of the genetic fitness of the host.

I will explain it with an example. While we are walking in the country, we see an ant climbing up a stalk of grass, falling, then climbing up again and falling again. Why is it trying to climb up that stalk, what is at the top, or what in its actions is beneficial for the ant? The answer is nothing, we know of no benefit at all for the ant to climb that stalk. Why then does the ant climb? A fluke, a tiny parasite, has invaded its brain. This parasite needs to get into the stomach of a sheep or a cow in order to reproduce. To achieve that goal, it infects the ant's brain and drives it up the grass stalk, improving its chances of being ingested by a passing cow and enter the cow's stomach. This is an undeliberate but brilliant strategy, occurring in nature, to exploit the ant's brain to the fluke's benefit. The fluke commits a sort of kidnapping, in that the parasite invades the ant's brain to make it behave in a suicidal way, against the selective pressure of its own species.

We can think of memes as parasitic ideas invading our brains, exploiting us even as we remain oblivious of our best biological interest. The United States' state of New Hampshire has a motto, boasted on all its license plates, "Live Free or Die." We find plenty of ideas to die for: freedom, truth, justice, communism, Catholicism, Islam. All of them are contagious, commandeering their hosts to spread them and to infect other people. This phenomenon is unique to our species on this planet: no other species can subordinate its genetic interests to other interests or values.

Put in this way—parasites invading our brains, driving us to behave as we do—the concept sounds terrifying: But this process allows us to entertain new perspectives that can change our values. It constitutes us as persons, instances of a new type of biological entity which pursue goals other than merely reproduction for survival of the species.

I am a philosopher, and philosophers are supposed to disclose the meaning of life. Some journalism student always asks me, "Please Professor, tell me the outcome of all your philosophical wisdom, extract the essence of your philosophy and the meaning of life." I say, "Find something more important than yourself and dedicate your life to it."

This wisdom may sound obvious. But as long as our ideas remain alien to genetic or biological fitness, as long as we remain enslaved by them, we can be taught to be unselfish and prone to an evolution uniquely human.

Notes

1. *Bajo la Piel del Conflicto*, (*Getting under Conflict's Skin*), DVD, artistic director and co-author, H. Carmona, scientific director and co-writer, O. Vilarroya (Valencia, Spain: Universitat de Valencia, 2004).

2. Eytan Avital and Eva Jablonka, *Animal Traditions: Behavioural Inheritance in Evolution* (New York: Cambridge University Press, 2000).

3. Charles Darwin, *On the Origin of Species by Means of Natural Selection*, facsimile ed. (Cambridge, Mass.: Harvard Univ. Press, 1981 [1859]), pp. 30–40).

4. Francis Crick, personal communication with the author, circa 1995.

5. Richard Dawkins, *The Selfish Gene* (Oxford: Oxford University Press, 1976), p. 66.

Three

LEARNING IN A BIO-CULTURAL DEVELOPMENTAL PERSPECTIVE

Katherine Nelson

"Can we teach people to be unselfish?" is the theme of this session, and the excellent overview of brain systems involved in learning and memory presented by Núria Sebastián Gallés provides us a basic understanding of the biological background. I will address the question from a developmental perspective that emphasizes the social, cultural, and biological contributions to development. The phrasing of today's theme led me to raise four critical questions related to some of the assumptions about learning social values implied in the session theme and more generally in the theme of the social brain. For example, the wording of the question suggests that people are born selfish and that we need to teach people to be unselfish. This phrasing assumes a conflict between nature and nurture, in that we view nurture (teaching) to work against the nature of individuals (their genetic heritage). Contemporary work in biology, anthropology, and psychology indicates that the "natural" state of selfish behavior is much more complex than this. Unselfish behavior is observable in some circumstances among many animals and among all human beings, for whom cooperative behavior is as critical to survival as is competition. Also questionable is the implication that learning may be simply achieved through teaching.

From a bio-social-cultural approach to psychological development, these assumptions reflect a misunderstanding of human development, especially in their focus on individual brain processes as the center of learning. In many animal species, individual learning is under the control of evolved brain structures adapted for designated environments. Without denying the necessity of this base for human beings as well, the perspective of bio-cultural developmental psychology takes for granted that human cognition and its development are more complex. My response to today's theme is that we cannot understand the role of the "social brain" in human learning, especially learning of social values, unless we understand the role of social and cultural transactions among the learners. To elaborate on this position I raise the following questions in this chapter: Where is learning? Does age matter? Does language matter? What is the role of a teacher?

1. Where Is Learning?

Brain science proceeds under the implicit assumption that the mechanisms of the brain—molecules, neurons, synapses—are the locations of learning. These mechanisms are involved in learning and memory processes, but they are not the whole process and cannot constitute a whole explanation. Embodied aspects of the learner, prior knowledge and learning, and the social and cultural conditions and activities of the learning situation all enter into the process. Whether and how the brain may process learning by an individual acting alone in the environment or as the result of social or cultural interaction, symbolic or non-symbolic, and how these ways may differ, are critical issues for any explanation of learning.

The interactions of the learner with the environment are not situated in the brain but in active transactions at the interface of an organism-environment system. We need theories of the interface, and models of the brain, body, and of the environment, especially the social and cultural environment. Only then can we understand the different kinds of learning and memory involved in producing conflict, cooperation, and unselfishness. We can view implicit and explicit learning as distinct kinds of experience that may result in the preservation of distinctive aspects of that experience.

Experience begins for infants centered in social and cultural ecological niches, places where infants and young children receive care and are nursed and comforted by adults and perhaps older siblings. Later, children begin to take an active part in the routines and activities of the community. At all ages, these daily activities result in a variety of experiences that may produce learning. Implicit experience is absorbed unconsciously from activities carried out in the world for varying purposes (for example, looking, crawling, and sucking by an infant). Infants and young children learn through implicit experience the sound structure of the language (phonemes, prosody), familiar faces, speech characteristics, body language, and a myriad of ways of acting and behaving in our communities.

Explicit experience is that to which we consciously attend, or that called into consciousness after the experience has been preserved in memory. Experience becomes explicit when it is involved in making sense, for example, in the initial learning of routine scripts of how to carry out a new activity (such as learning the routines of a new job), interacting with new people and things, learning the meaning of words, hearing and interpreting stories or explanations, solving tasks, or playing games. The distinction between what is explicit and what is implicit does not reside in the brain but in activities seen in relation to interests and intentions of the individual learner based on the history of experience and knowledge of the individual and its perceived meaning.

Learning in social interactions, learning from others, whether facts or how-to knowledge, is different from, and more complex than, individual learning. Merlin Donald identified mimesis, a key version of social learning, as uniquely human.[1] According to Michael Tomasello, cultural learning involves a still higher level of interactions concerning conventions and collaborations.[2] Working during the 1920s and 1930s, Russian psychologist Lev Semenovich Vygotsky coined the term scaffolding, which involves a teacher collaborating with the learner, providing hints or constructing steps that enable moving ahead, without direct didactic instruction.[3] Donald's emergent levels of narrative and theory are higher level modes of cognition that depend on language and cultural learning.

Terrance William Deacon argues that human beings are pre-eminently the "symbolic species." Identifiable brain centers have evolved to support the abstractions involved in symbolic processes, primarily, but not exclusively for natural language (for example, mathematics).[4] Brains must be capable of working at different symbolic and non-symbolic (implicit, mimetic) levels, but brains alone do not determine the level involved in any given occasion of learning. The brain serves the learning activities of the person; the learning activities do not serve the brain.

2. Does Age or Developmental State Determine Learning?

Sebastián Gallés emphasizes the maturation of the brain, especially its plasticity, during the early years, even into adolescence. She implies that some kinds of learning have sensitive periods for optimum learning potential. We observe a strong positive correlation between stages of brain development and how children learn, or can learn things. But age is only a measure of time; what we need to understand is what happens during time and how development changes brain processes.

Development conditions learning in many ways. Embodiment, the way the physical body relates to mind and cognition, changes greatly over the first two decades. Physical growth, mobility, and dexterity enable new kinds of learning that were impossible previously. The history of learning determines what we can learn from any new experience. Prior knowledge constrains the acquisition of new knowledge in either negative or positive ways. How the social conditions change over time is equally significant.

From the developmental perspective, the brain is "social" because of the social conditions of human life, especially those involving the social and cultural contexts of human infancy. During the past forty years, we have seen an explosion of research on infant cognition, most of it focused on how infants perceive and conceive of objects. This research has told us a lot, but not much about what most interest infants: people. Even Jean Piaget failed to recognize the crucial point in this regard: he treated the infant's recognition of the breast as its first object scheme instead of its first social relationship.

Socio-biologist Sarah Hrdy emphasized that the premier interest of newborns is to establish an attachment with one or more parent figures; their survival depends upon it.[5] Compared with other primates and mammals, human infants are dependent on caretakers to an extraordinary degree and over an exceptionally long period. For much of the first year, they remain virtually immobile, unable even to change body positions independently. During this period, many crucial brain developments take place, although development continues for years thereafter. So too does the child's dependency on parental figures. Neural networks and pathways, many dependent upon experiential input for their development (including language centers), are established in the context of this intimate social dependency of infancy and childhood.

Consequently, children establish the potential for both implicit and explicit learning with others during this dependency period. Among the most important of these developments is the acquisition of language during the first four years of life, beginning with the acquisition of words, a process that continues throughout life. Infants imbibe the sound systems of their language (phonemes, prosody, grammatical phrasing) as they hear and attend to the language of parents and others close to them, even while still *in utero*. This is not to suggest that their brains are not prepared for this kind of learning; they are. But the conditions of learning involve the interest of another person talking with and to the infant. The contrast in effectiveness for learning a new language between interactive talk and that overheard on television, as reported in Sebastian's paper, illustrates this concept.

The acquisition of language is one of the most important developments of childhood, beginning with the learning of words and their meanings during the second year of life. Language is crucial to the infant because of its role in communication, even before the infant is able to understand the referential meaning of the words of the language. The sounds of language are part of the social intimacy of infancy, becoming part of the infant's implicit recognition of security. These conditions do not obtain during later life when a person has already established language. A plausible hypothesis is that the sensitive period for language results from the social conditions of infancy and childhood, not from any special cognitive or brain mechanisms that vanish in later life.

Many developmental psychologists believe that children acquire language to be able to express ideas or concepts.[6] Language makes a difference only in what we can express, not in what we can think. A strong bias exists against the idea that language might modify those ideas. All agree that children are able to learn new things through language, but not on how learning through language takes place.

My work, and that of others, challenges this perspective on language learning, especially the relation of concepts and words. Learning experiments with object words bolster the idea that words map, but not change, concepts. Observational research in natural contexts shows that children learn their first words in more varied and complex ways than laboratory experiments on object words can reveal, and that children's learning varies with their cultural and linguistic environment. Research with young learners suggests that their interests influence which words they learn, but so does the scaffolding efforts of parents, and the characteristic interactions, activities, communicative styles, and language that form the context of learning. Contrary to common assumption, instead of only object words, beginning learners master a variety of linguistic forms, many of which lack concrete referents, for example, "help" or "give."

Research with abstract words reveals more about how children may learn the concept of "selfish" from experience with the word. Studies of the acquisition of abstract language terms by preschool children reveal the power of a combination of implicit learning and constructive processing taking place over months, and sometimes years, that eventually yields meanings for words that are *first* used pragmatically, in appropriate contexts, but without conventional, or any, meaning. Examples from our studies include causal ("because," "so"), temporal ("before," "after"), and mental state words ("know" and "think"). Children first hear these words used informally in conversations. Over time, they acquire meanings in terms of the underlying abstract concepts that the words represent.

Both the acquisition of conceptual content from discourse context and the extended period required for the process of establishing meaning from use are crucial. The process involved includes identifying the word form and noting its application. The delicate part is identifying the criteria for use of the word, as Ludwig Wittgenstein proposed. In the case of the word "unselfish," instances of behavior to which we refer when using the word as a modifier, serve as the basis for a construction of meaning. But the crucial aspects of the meaning may remain obscure to the child for a long time, as many related research studies have indicated. The process of learning words and concepts through use is a general one applicable to much of the cultural knowledge that adults tend to take for granted. Children who do not yet speak the same language cannot share this cultural knowledge.

As Esther N. Goody stated:

Once a lexicon has been established, a speaker hears the same word as does his listener [which] may [be] the crucial factor in escaping from the private worlds of thought into the shared social world of spoken language.[7]

3. What Difference Does Language Make to Learning?

I am constantly amazed that psychologists appear capable of overlooking the significance of language in human learning and cognition, subsuming it under the rubric of social or cultural learning. As Anna Wierzbicka stated, "Mainstream modern psychology . . . at times seems to behave as if language is irrelevant to the study of mind."[8] This attitude is perhaps less surprising in the case of those studying adult cognition, who often work under the assumption that language is a sort of transparent delivery system for transmitting messages from one person to another. I am more startled to discover the attitude among developmental psychologists whose subjects range from early life when infants have not yet acquired language to the time when children have begun to master it.

Vygotsky considered language to be the main tool of human thinking, distinguishing it from the nonverbal communication and thinking of young children and animals. He viewed it as a cultural tool in addition to a tool of thought, recognizing that it reflected the history of the culture. Individuals within a culture might have greater or lesser access to a language's more advanced levels of knowledge. Vygotsky's view of the fundamental importance of language to human learning and thinking implies a revolution in learning and memory taking place within an individual during the years the individual is first acquiring language. This revolution eventuates in what I have termed "entering the community of minds," a notion in line with Wittgenstein's aphorism, "To learn a language is to enter a form of life."[9]

In addition to the study of word learning, we have been able to examine the ways that children learn both implicit and explicit aspects of knowledge through their interactions in emerging conversations with parents during their first years of language use. Analysis of transcripts of conversations and monologic narratives by children and their parents reveals the ways in which young children gradually acquire the forms of narrative and the practice of retelling (and preserving) their memories of experienced events. For example, investigators tape-recorded the bedtime monologues of a single child Emily, two years of age, over a period of sixteen months. Analysis of her talk while she was alone showed her early sensitivity to the rhythms of story telling in speech, including ways of simulating the voice of another actor. Not until months later did she master the temporal and causal sequential form of retelling, and still later, she included times, settings, motivational, and emotional states in her narratives. Through implicit processes by listening to both personal and fictional stories, she acquired the formats—prosody and voice register appropriate to the narratives that she was not yet competent to compose in conventional forms.[10] Children learn not only the formats; reciprocally, the formats support learning the meanings.

4. What Is the Role of the Teacher?

Can we teach social values like unselfishness or cooperation? Does learning of social values require a teacher? Individuals, children or adults, might acquire such values in the same way they acquire language: through interactive use in social situations, without a didactic teacher. For example, no teacher guided Emily's acquisition of narrative structure, although she experienced exposure to role models for the conversational displays. In terms of the content of what is included in memorized retelling, we have observed scaffolding by parents. Robyn Fivush and I have documented that parents engage their children in talk about the past and the future from about two years of age, sometimes younger. Typically, children begin to contribute to this kind of talk by mentioning a detail or two on which the mother may elaborate to compose a story about the past in collaboration with the child.[11] These efforts have long-term effects: children whose mothers provide more elaborative scaffolding produce increasingly extensive memories later in their childhood. They become capable of telling a coherent memory narrative by five years of age. The questions that parents ask in relation to the child's memory scaffold abstract patterns of how to tell a memory narrative.

One of the most striking outcomes of early childhood is the emerging sense of self and of conventional ideas of time, both centered within narratives of memory casually exchanged in talk about the past. As Fivush's work has shown, issues of values such as selfishness and emotional displays are other aspects highlighted in these exchanges. The question we have been addressing is how children learn these concepts. The frequency of such conversations, the timing of the emergence of autobiographical memory, and the construction of concepts of self and time, all vary across cultures in their timing and contents. Observations of learning the narrative format and content of memory recounting by young children indicate a kind of cultural learning dependent upon and emerging as the narrative discourse genre, the format that Donald and others have identified as the basic cultural mode of human life. Children rely heavily on this mode to support their movement into the cultural community—the community of minds. In the process, they become practiced in the ways of the community; they learn social values implicitly as they learn to tell their stories and to listen to the stories of others.

5. Conclusion

Children learn much of what they know about the world through their lived experience, including their experience in monitoring the behavior and language of others, employing implicit and explicit processes, symbolic and non-symbolic. In the process, they absorb the cultural knowledge and values of those they monitor, without necessarily depending on explicit teaching. Unselfishness is a value of most human societies, although its applications and appropriate contexts may vary. To understand how children become part of the "community of minds" of their societies, we need to account for the following aspects of the developmental process:

(1) Learning takes place in transaction: the individual-environment interface, supported by brain mechanisms adapted to social learning;

(2) Developmental state of brain, body, and experiential knowledge affects the process of learning and the possibility of achieving the learning of values such as unselfishness;

(3) Language is critical to becoming a cultural learner where the culture is the model for the learner and language is its major mode. This is especially the case for abstract concepts such as 'selfishness' or 'unselfish' that require symbolic form (language) for clarifying applications of values across contexts;

(4) Learning without a teacher takes place as social values are displayed in the ubiquitous social-cultural milieu and made available for implicit "taking"; and

(5) Teaching values through scaffolding may take place in informal contexts of story telling and conversations, beginning with the child's own starting point and building toward a higher level of understanding of a concept.

I conclude that the answer to the theme question—Can we teach people to be unselfish?—is a conditional yes, provided we modify the answer by the conditions I have discussed here. The people we might wish to teach—children or adults—are always at a particular point in a developmental and cultural matrix, one not primarily determined by biology or the state of brain, but by the prior history of experience. Learning of values, like any learning, is a history-dependent process.

Notes

1. Merlin Donald, *Origins of the Modern Mind: Three Stages in the Evolution of Culture and Cognition* (Cambridge, Mass:: Harvard University Press, 1991).

2. M. Tomasello, A. C. Kruger, and H. H. Ratner, "Cultural Learning," *Behavioral and Brain Sciences*, 16 (1993), pp. 495—552.

3. Lev Semyonovich Vygotsky, *Thought and Language* (Cambridge Mass.: MIT Press, 1986).

4. Terrence William Deacon, *The Symbolic Species: The Co-Evolution of Language and the Brain* (New York: W. W. Norton, 1997).

5. Sarah Hrdy, *Mother Nature: A History of Mothers, Infants, and Natural Selection* (New York: Pantheon Books, 1999).

6. Lois Bloom, "The Intentionality Model of Word Learning: How to Learn a Word, Any Word," *Becoming a Word Learner: A Debate on Lexical Acquisition*, ed. Roberta M Golinkoff (New York: Oxford University Press, 2000), pp. 19–50; and Paul Bloom, *How Children Learn the Meanings of Words* (Cambridge, Mass.: MIT Press, 2000).

7. Esther N. Goody, "Social Intelligence and Language: Another Rubicon," *Machiavellian Intelligence 2: Extensions and Evaluations*, eds. Andrew Whiten and Richard W. Byrne (Cambridge, UK: Cambridge University Press, 1997), pp. 365—377.

8. Anna Wierzbicka, "Cognitive Domains and the Structure of the Lexicon: The Case of the Emotions," *Mapping the Mind: Domain Specificity in Cognition and Culture*, eds. Lawrence A. Hirschfeld and Susan A. Gelman (New York: Cambridge University Press, 1994), pp.431–452.

9. Ludwig Wittgenstein, *Philosophical Investigations* (New York: Macmillan, 1953).

10. Katherine Nelson, and Robyn Fivush, "The Emergence of Autobiographical Memory: A Social Cultural Developmental Theory," *Psychological Review*, 111:2 (2004), pp. 486—511.

11. Ibid.

Four

WHEN IS ETHICAL LEARNING?

Eric Bredo

In this series of discussions, we have been asked to consider the biological basis of human behavior with particular emphasis on social conflict and cooperation. The present session focuses on learning and on whether unselfishness can be taught. Since every parent believes that ethical conduct can be taught and hopefully has evidence of the fact in the behavior of their children, we could just answer "yes" and go home. But, the question appears to be a shorthand way of referring to an ancient problem that is not so easily resolved.

A long tradition of thought suggests that an inherent division exists between the realities of human nature and human social ideals. Plato was among those introducing a strong split between mind and body, depicting the mind as the source of "higher" things, such as the idea of justice, and the body as the source of "lower" impulses, such as the emotions and appetites. Since reason enabled people to understand the essence of the good, the good society should be ruled by philosopher kings in whose souls reason dominated. Early Christians, like Augustine of Hippo, adopted this division, viewing human beings as torn between ideals, which come from God, and bodily impulses, which have a profane origin. The Christian conception of original sin suggested that human nature is inherently corrupt relative to the ideal. This dualistic tradition continued with René Descartes, who viewed mind and body as two as different substances, one natural, the other supernatural. While these dichotomies may appear obsolete today, a similar contrast often occurs in current discussion of the relation between nature and culture, or science and the humanities.

Considered in the context of this long tradition of dualistic thinking, we can regard the question whether unselfishness can be taught as a version of the ancient question of the relation between human nature and ethical ideals, reconsidered in the light of modern biology. Instead of approaching this question in terms of opposing categories, however, we might rephrase it in more practical terms, by asking, "How can we foster a good social life given what we know about human biological limitations and possibilities?" Because we cannot answer "yes" or "no" to this question, I would suggest we remain and consider it in more detail.

In what follows, I address these issues primarily as a philosopher and educator. As a philosopher, I am concerned with whether common ways of thinking about these issues are good ones. As an educator, I am concerned with how we can foster ethical conduct in practice, and how it can be learned or taught. I begin by considering two areas of conceptual difficulty that come up in discussions of this topic: the relationship between "is" and "ought," and the relationship between explanatory accounts at different levels of analysis.

1. Is and Ought

The revised question of how we can foster ethical conduct, given human limitations and possibilities, requires answers to three sub-questions. First, what are the limitations and possibilities of human nature? Second, what conception of a good person or a good society are we aiming for? Third, how can we get from the biologically given to the ethically desirable? The first is about means, the second about ends, and the third about how to relate the two.

While the problems of determining ends and means, or "ought" and "is," appear obviously interrelated, common practice treats these two issues as though the answer to one unilaterally determined the answer to the other, or as though the two issues are entirely separate. The naturalist Edward O. Wilson, for example, recently claimed that the ethical "ought" can be derived from the biological "is." He argued that innate "epigenetic rules" bias human perception, learning, and mental development in directions that animate and channel the acquisition of culture.[1] Fear of snakes, for example, derives (he suggests) from an innate predisposition to note and be afraid of crawly things without legs. Wilson used this notion of "epigenetic rules" or innate predispositions to some kinds of learning, to arrive at a conception of human nature: "What is human nature? . . . It is the epigenetic rules, the hereditary regularities of mental development that bias cultural evolution . . . and thus connect genes to culture."[2] In effect, Wilson viewed culture as derived from, or shaped by, genetic predispositions. He also used this conception of innate predispositions to argue that since some social norms are more natural than others are, more in line with the innate tendencies of human nature, they should be the preferred to other less natural ones.

Others reverse the equation and attempt to determine the biological "is" on the basis of a previously accepted ethical "ought." The Soviets attempted this when Trofim Denisovich Lysenko promoted a party line about the infinite malleability of human nature that was congenial to Stalinist orthodoxy. Modern-day fundamentalists do much the same when they reject the Darwinian conception of evolution because it does not square with their preexisting ethical ideals and related beliefs about God.

A third attitude is evident in attempts to isolate "is" and "ought" and treat each as largely irrelevant to the other. The logical positivists, for example, developed a conception of science that separated it largely from matters of value or ethics. They viewed anything not verifiable by elementary physical observations as not meaningful, or "without sense," concluding that only science has any claim to knowledge. In so doing, they rejected the notion that ethics involves testable knowledge, by arguing that while ethical statements like "Killing is bad" sound like factual claims they actually constitute imperatives, commands to follow a rule. Since such commands are not statements of fact, ethical claims are "without sense."[3]

Each of these approaches has difficulties. Wilson's attempt to derive ethical imperatives from biological facts fails, like all attempts to derive "ought" from "is," because being *able* to do something is not a good or sufficient reason for doing it. Just because you *can* jump in a swamp is not a good reason to do so. Still, the tendency to argue in this way is widespread. In educational circles, for example, many people claim that "brain science" tells us how to teach. We should make it clear to them that science, when genuine, can only tell us what is possible, not what is desirable.

The attempt to determine scientific beliefs based on previously accepted ethical ideals or convictions also has obvious failings. Just because you want something to behave in a particular way does not make it do so, no matter how strong your desire, although strong desire may lead someone to overlook evidence to the contrary.

The problem with the third strategy is trickier. Science and ethics are intrinsically related because the concepts a scientist uses have evaluative significance. A given set of concepts, like any tool, is good for some purposes and bad for others. As a result, the way we approach a subject expresses an attitude toward it, just as gripping a hammer suggests that the person is on the lookout for a nail. Often scientific attitudes are so esoteric as to have little obvious everyday significance, but the great historical interplay between scientific and everyday attitudes and values suggests that the two are not isolatable.

Just as science sometimes has more ethics, or value, built into it than we recognize, ethics may be more scientific than we commonly believe[4] We commonly make ethical judgments with future consequences in mind. We sanction an individual, for example, with an eye to how this will influence the future behavior of that individual and others in the community. This expected result is an empirical hypothesis that we can test, making ethical judgment in some respects not so different from scientific judgment.

When we think of the relationship between is and ought, or biology and morality, we should not approach it in a one-sided manner. We cannot derive ethical ideals from biological findings, and we cannot determine what is scientifically believable based on previously accepted ethical norms or ideals. Scientists should not be telling ethicists what to conclude, nor should ethicists be telling scientists what to believe. Finding out how things work (science) and where we should go (ethics) are different questions; neither one is reducible to, or fully separable from, the other. Instead of treating them as completely independent, or trying to dictate the answer to one from an answer to the other, we should approach the relationship between them as though they were parts of a division of labor in which each has a distinctive job to do that should be coordinated with the other. I will return to the implications of this suggestion more fully later. For the moment, I hope these considerations might dissuade us from trying to jump too rapidly from biological findings to ethical conclusions.

2. Reductionism and Holism

A second problem concerns the relationship between analyses based on the behavior of entities at different levels of organization. Several of the papers in this dialogue describe life as having a nested hierarchical organization, like Chinese boxes or Russian dolls. Molecules such as DNA make up cells. Cells such as neurons make up organs. Organs, like the brain, make up organisms. And groups of interacting organisms make up societies. Núria Sebastián Gallés, for example, used such distinctions to discuss what we know about learning at molecular, cellular, organ, and whole-organism levels of analysis.

Such hierarchies complicate the task of relating biology to social behavior and ethics because they raise problems about the proper level of analysis to adopt. Should we look at things from a gene's eye view? An individual's? A society's? (Or a neuron's or brain's?). If we adopt a perspective based on entities at one level of analysis, how can we relate it to the behavior of entities at other levels? How do we similarly relate findings from different disciplines such as biology, psychology, and sociology?

This issue is central to present discussion like that stimulated by the study of the Social Brain. Biology has come back into the consideration of social and ethical life largely because of a shift in perspective to a new level of analysis. In the older debate about the relation between biology and social behavior, the individual was taken to be the basic unit of analysis.[5] This was consistent with the Darwinian view that conceived of evolution in terms of variation and selection among individuals. The molecular revolution in biology has led some, like Richard Dawkins, to propose a shift to a gene's eye view as a way of throwing new light on old problems.[6] This shift in viewpoint provides a way of understanding behavior whose "rationality" is incomprehensible from an individual-centered point of view. From an individual standpoint, for example, to give up your life for others appears irrational, since then you lose everything of value. But from a genetic point of view, giving up your life may be "rational" if it aids the survival of our genes sufficiently, such as by protecting many close kin. This paradoxical result, which suggests why "selfish" genes may result in unselfish individual behavior, has opened up a completely new line of discussion.

While a "gene's eye view" has challenged, the older focus on the individual organism, others have adopted the social group or culture as the basic unit of analysis. Social constructivist and post-modernist conceptions of culture, for example, suggest that human nature is largely a product of the way cultural norms and concepts are institutionalized, creating facts consistent with the original assumptions. What we take to be "natural" may be a cultural artifact. Notions of human development that depict women as falling behind men in formal rationality or moral reasoning, for example, may be the product of observations based on male norms and ideals.[7]

When one group defines the rules of the game and the measures of performance to suit them, we should not be surprised that others do not score so well. While scientific research seeks to discover the nature of human nature, social studies of science suggest that both human "nature" and science itself are socially and culturally constructed.[8]

As this brief discussion suggests, competing ways of thinking based on lower (genetic) and higher (socio-cultural) units of analysis have challenged the older focus on the individual, common to older psychological and evolutionary thought. A debate in which biologists attempt to explain culture genetically, and cultural scholars attempt to explain biology culturally, has replaced the older debate about the extent to which variation in individual traits, like IQ scores, is due to nature or nurture. Today, each side appears to want to swallow the other whole instead of merely explaining more of the variance. These debates tend to get heated because they resonate with wider political conflict over social norms. Conservatives trying to impose more normative constraints, and liberals trying to make a wider range of behavior acceptable, add greatly to the heat of the discussion.

While scientists may focus on entities at any level of analysis, problems arise when they view entities at their preferred level as the basic or ultimate units. When this is the case, we lose sensitivity to the interplay of processes at different levels of analysis that are not reducible to, or absorbable by, others. A fuller discussion of work favoring some of these differing levels of analysis may elucidate the point.

3. Selfish Individuals

The older debate about the relation between biology and social or ethical conduct adopted the individual as the basic unit of analysis. Darwin argued that individual intellectual and moral sensibilities are, in part, heritable.[9] His cousin, Francis Galton, pushed this idea further in is work on heritable genius in prominent British families. In *The Bell Curve*, Charles Murray and Richard Hernstein recently resurrected the argument for a relation between human nature and the good society, based on the notion of selfish individualism. They argued that since IQ is highly heritable and statistically exhibit a normal distribution (the plotted scores forming a bell curve), and society increasingly stratified on the basis of IQ, due to selective hiring and intermarriage, we should accept this fact and adopt laissez faire social policies allowing each person to reach or sink to its natural level. In short, they used psychological research on IQ to bolster modern-day Social Darwinism as state policy.[10]

Two biological "facts" were central to reaching this ethical conclusion. First, they took individual "intelligence" to be largely innate and fixed, since studies of identical twins found the heritability coefficient to be quite high. Second, they took the "bell curve" distribution of IQ's in the population to be a stable and unchangeable fact. But both of these "facts" present difficulties. As Richard C. Lewontin noted, the size of the heritability coefficient tells us nothing about whether IQ scores can be causally altered by changing people's environments.[11] If diverse individuals are placed in identical environments, the heritability coefficient would be a perfect 1.0, since the only differences among people would be their initial genetic differences. With no environmental variation, environmental factors drop out entirely as *predictors* of difference. Yet this says nothing about whether putting these individuals in different environments would affect their IQ scores. The heritability coefficient tells us about the correlation between differences among individuals and environments, and some outcome, like IQ, in a given population, not about causation.

    The claim that the bell curve distribution of IQ's is a stable fact of nature also has problems. An IQ score is inherently comparative. A score of 115 means a person is one standard deviation above the mean, for example, while a score of 85 means they are one standard deviation below. If the average raw score for the population rises, as it has in Sweden,[12] then IQ scores are corrected to take this into account by subtracting enough from each raw score so that the average always remains 100. If the raw scores become more equal, as evidence indicates they have in the United States, IQ's are corrected by multiplying raw score differences from the mean by a factor such that the standard deviation remains the same. In effect, the ruler is moved and stretched as needed so that the mean and the standard deviation always remain the same despite changes in task performance in the population. The bell curve distribution of IQ will always be with us because test developers manipulate the measure to make it so.

    In both of these cases, the "facts" supporting a Social Darwinist moral conclusion are artifacts of a way of thinking about the problem in the first place. An inherently "selfish," or zero-sum conception of intelligence apparently leads to the conclusion that Social Darwinist social policies are appropriate or necessary. But we need not think of intelligence in this way. If we think of acting intelligently as selecting means with due regard to their likely consequences in a situation, as William James did, then we find no reason that my becoming more intelligent must result in your becoming less so. [13] Everyone can become a more intelligent reader, musician, or car mechanic in the sense of becoming better able to anticipate and respond to contingencies in these activities, without reducing the intelligence of others.

    The apparently fixed biological "fact" that human mental abilities are normally distributed with a fixed mean and standard deviation is a construct, a hypothetical idea inferred from the available data. Recent research on the size of the heritability coefficient suggests that the environment may also play a stronger role in predicting differences when we take into account a wider range of environments (less limited to the middle class) and study interaction effects between individuals and environments. (A supportive environment may have stronger effects on the IQ of some children than on others). As this example suggests, some authors use an approach based on "selfish individualism," which takes the individual as the penultimate unit of analysis to sneak in unwarranted ethical conclusions.

4. Selfish Genes

Work based on the notion of selfish genes has also led to both factual and conceptual problems. In this case, biology has been used to argue for something like "old time family values" instead of laissez faire individualism, as in the prior example. But the speciousness of the jump from "is" to "ought" is the same.

In his recent book, *Consilience*, biologist Edward O. Wilson argues that some forms of social behavior have a natural genetic basis. [15] These include altruistic behavior towards near kin, preference for a division of labor in which men hunt and women stay at home, and, possibly, differences in mathematical ability between men and women. Wilson advocates a reductive approach to explaining such behavior by first exploring the putative effects of genes on individual behavior and then extrapolating to the social or cultural level by considering the distribution of genes in a population, and using this distribution to explain aggregate social behavior. While Wilson admits that culture may affect genes, he focuses nearly all of his attention in the other direction, hypothesizing about the causal effects of genes on social and cultural phenomena. As he puts it, "culture is ultimately a biological product."[16] In another place he says, "Culture has arisen from the genes and forever bears their stamp."[17]

Wilson's analysis suffers both factual and logical problems. Perhaps the most glaring problem comes from the way he underplays social contingencies by viewing social norms as derived from genetic influences. If it is true that we are strongly programmed to propagate our genes then why is one of the strongest demographic trends in the world today for people to delay or forego childbearing? Wilson's claim does not seem to fit the facts. Wilson also argues that forms of social behavior universal across all peoples are likely to be genetically determined, citing incest taboos as an example. But this conclusion does not follow, as Daniel Dennett argues:

> Showing that a particular type of human behavior is ubiquitous or nearly ubiquitous in widely separated human cultures goes *no way at all* towards showing that there is a genetic predisposition for that particular behavior. So far as I know, in every culture . . . the hunters throw their spears point-end first, but this obviously doesn't establish that there is a pointy-end-first gene. . . .[18]

The incest taboo is not universal, despite Wilson's claim. We need only think of Egyptian or European royalty, who experienced strong social pressures to marry near kin, to see that social or political considerations such as a desire to consolidate authority, sometimes lead to other norms.

The problem in this case comes not from considering the influence of genes, but from becoming overly fixated on their unilateral influence. In some cases, a single gene, or a limited number, may determine the behavior of individuals in virtually any environment. But as the biologists Peter McGuffin, Brien Riley and Robert Plomin put it recently:

> single genes do not determine most human behaviors. Only certain rare disorders such as Huntington's disease have a simple mode of transmission in which a specific mutation confers certainty of developing the disorder. Most types of behavior have no such clear-cut pattern and depend on an interplay of environmental factors and multiple genes.[19]

Other studies find that factors in the social environment turn some genes affecting social behavior on or off. The social behavior of other honeybees, for example, triggers a given bee's physiological transformation from hive worker to external forager, thereby changing their role in the hive's division of labor.[20] Therefore, the social behavior that genes enable may be both highly variable (when multiple genes and gene-gene interactions are involved) and contingent on the social environment, instead of being uniquely and directly determined.

5. Selfish Cultures

Perhaps we should focus on the needs or aims of social groups, then, instead of on selfish individuals or selfish genes. Social constructivism views language and culture as defining, constituting, or socially "constructing" objects, much as Immanuel Kant viewed the basic categories of the mind as shaping the sensory flux into perceived objects. Adopting a group or culture-centered view tends to lead to depicting individuals as having socially constructed minds and identities. Social activities even modify the bodies of individuals, just as participating in different kinds of social activities alter the brain and other tissues.

Taking group life as the starting point has the advantage of making the origins of individual reflective intelligence and the self more understandable than when we start from an individual or genetic viewpoint, since we can understand both as learned social functions.[21] A genetic view may be subject to similar decentering when we begin consideration from a socio-cultural perspective. The argument for group selection in biology, for example, suggests that social contingencies may have shaped people's genetic heritages, some of which affected population genetics. If so, the contingencies of social life may have shaped the human species, instead of the reverse. This position is controversial, and I would not want to argue for one-way causation at any level, but the argument deserves its due.

I find difficulties in this approach as well, which I cannot discuss at any length here. A colleague, Daniel Ortiz, calls this conception of community "categorical community." He points out that many post-modern thinkers, who question the notion of the essentialized individual, fail to apply the same criticism to the notion of the essentialized community.[22] Focusing on the needs or aims of a group, understood categorically or selfishly as a bounded entity, can lead to internal intolerance and external hostility, even while it legitimizes group rights and claims for autonomy. As their opponents, the adherents of the group-centered view also appear to smuggle ethical conclusions in the way they conceptualize things at the beginning.

6. From Levels to Situations

The main point I have been trying to make is that an approach based on the needs or aims of any of these neatly bounded units, that ignores interactions among its internal elements and other units in its environment, fails to provide either a good understanding of social behavior or a good basis for a social ethic. It fails in part because "is" does not determine "ought." It also fails because focusing on the "aims" of a given level of "agent" neglects those of others internal or external to that agent. If we regard ethical consideration as the attempt to harmonize, in the broadest and most long run way, all of the interests actively at stake in a situation, then none of these strategies is likely to result in ethical conduct. Each draws overly neat lines that trip us up, since each is blind to the side effects of its way of conceptualizing the situation.

But where does this leave us? Do we have to look at things from all levels? If so, are we caught between having too few perspectives and too many? One way to avoid this dilemma is to focus on functions or activities instead of on entities. Things like the "mind" or the "self" have appeared so mysterious in the past because, by referring to them with nouns, we took them to be entities. Once one thinks of either as an entity it is tempting to try to find its location. Yet the location of mind or self turns out to be hard to identify, even today with brain scanning techniques. As hard as you look, you can never find an idea of a chair in the brain. Difficulty finding a physical location for mind led to people viewing it as a supernatural entity, the soul, which is presumably located in some other, non-natural space. This led, in turn, to the whole mind/body dualism in Western thought and the mystery of how to relate mind and body when the two exist in separate realms, one supernatural, the other natural. But the root of this problem was to think of mind or self as an entity in the first place.

Viewed as a function instead of as a thing, acting mindfully means acting in a way sensitive to means-ends relations in the situation, like "minding" the low doorway when entering a room. Mind has no identifiable physical location, just as your "health" is not located in some definable place in your body, because it is a functional relationship, not a thing.

If we adopt a functional or activity-based perspective, then we can see that ethical problems emerge when a function breaks down or interferes with others. When you and I cannot coordinate our actions resulting in our interfering with one another's activity, we have an ethical problem in miniature. We do not know *a priori* which structures, at which level of organization, interacting with which features of the environment, may have caused the problem. Instead of presupposing that the problem has its origin in an entity at a given level of analysis, we can begin by looking for the source of the functional difficulty in context. When we look at functioning in context, as opposed to beginning with a bounded entity, we shift our perspective from a "selfish" to a potentially more collaborative view.

I do not have space to discuss this shift from entities to situations more fully, but will briefly suggest some implications for ethical conduct and learning. The principal consequence of a shift to a functional or interactional perspective is that the question changes from "Where is learning?" (or ethical conduct) to "When is learning?" (or ethical conduct). We often look for learning or ethical conduct inside of some entity. We look for it in the genes, neurons, brain, individual, or society. But if we view learning or ethical conduct as always involving a dynamic relation of person and environment, then it is not inside the person or the brain or the neuron. Necessary structures exist there, but ethical conduct is not a product of inner structures or environmental conditions alone. Organisms affect their environments, which affect them in return (and similarly for units at every other level of analysis). This is why we have norms, laws, and mechanisms for enforcing conformity to them, thereby altering the environment in which conduct occurs. We make environments that help us behave as we wish we did. Instead of trying to find *where* ethical behavior, minds or selves are located, we would do better to focus on *when* these functions occur successfully, and why. This is the reason that the title of my talk is *when* is ethical learning, instead of *where*.

7. When Is Ethical Learning?

So when *is* ethical conduct or learning? If we approach ethics interactionally, focusing on situations instead of on entities, then every situation has its unique good.[23] We cannot derive what is good or right from social norms, individual needs, or genetic propensities. Although these may play a role in our deliberation, we need to consider what a concrete situation presents in the way of difficulties and possible improvements. We need to consider the interplay of the behavior of the parties in a relationship and the possible unintended side effects of their activities on one another, as well as on those external to their interaction. This suggests that to be an ethical person, I need to do more than behave well myself. I must also consider how to foster an environment in which other people will also behave well. I need to help create conditions in which cooperation can spread.[24]

The best way to foster the development of the sort of ethical person and society implied by this view would appear to be to give people experience in addressing ethical dilemmas, as partners with the others, beginning with those within their joint capability. Japanese elementary schools appear to be excellent at doing this. They allow students considerable latitude in learning how to deal with their interactional difficulties without adult intervention. We need to learn to address difficult social problems with others, hear the full range of views of those affected, enact possible solutions in practice, experience and note the consequences of these hypothetical solutions, including their side effects on others, and alter the situation again as needed.

But is this sort of activity "learning"? Many authors define learning as improvement in performance by the same person over repeated trials of the same task or class of tasks.[25] What remains ambiguous in this definition is who defines the task. Whose task is it? If learning means getting better at someone else's task, as is often the case at school, then traditional teaching is not a good way to foster ethical "learning" because it merely trains students to comply with externally approved norms, which is equivalent to training a servant instead of educating a future partner.

Ethical *education*, on the other hand, occurs when we work together to address social difficulties, admitting that how we should view the problem in the first place forms part of the question. It is a form of education based on an experience in collaboratively and openly working out mutual problems, and in discussion without violence or threat of violence. The result of such ethical education can be the formation of partners who can work with one another to foster a continually improving form of life. In considering how to foster ethical learning, then, we should not begin with lines too neatly drawn around "selfish" entities at any level for part of what needs to be considered is how best to define ourselves in relation to one another.

8. Relating the Real and Ideal

Let me return, finally, to whether a basic or essential conflict between ethical ideals and human nature, or between ethics and biology, exists. I would suggest that the notion that an essential conflict exists between the two is a product of an overly rigid and unilateral approach based on given entities.

If we begin with the needs of a given unit, considered in the abstract, conflicts with the needs of units at other levels will always exist, virtually by definition. We will be caught between biological and psychological needs, or psychological and social needs. Focusing on situations instead of entities helps avoid this kind of dilemma, which is created more by our way of thinking than by real practical difficulties. If we focus on the concrete difficulties and opportunities in the situation at hand, then we can relate ideals and reals, ends and means, more easily and flexibly. In hiring someone or buying a house or car, people often start with abstract criteria. It may not hurt to think in this way for a while, but I am impressed that we do not make good practical choices in this way. Better to relate your ideals to what is realizable and then look for what idealizable in apparent realities. A practical ethics looks at what is idealizable and realistic in a concrete situation given relevant constraints and possibilities of human nature. Belief in a necessary and irresolvable conflict between the needs of different level entities, such as a conflict between human nature and ethics, is the product of entitative thinking that dissolves once we adopt a more practical, situational perspective.

What, then, is the biology of ethical learning or education? To think about this is to take quite a leap, but I imagine that ethical conduct must involve a balance between different psychological functions, much like the balance between the legislative, executive, and judicial branches of democratic governments.[26] In a well balanced person, affect and cognition will have to work well with one another. Cognition should be open and responsive to feeling, instead of closed, stubborn, or insensitive. Affect must be similarly responsive to cognition, so that new beliefs about objects in the environment lead to new feelings for their personal significance. Affect and cognition must also eventuate in practical commitment to actions sensitive to them, whose consequences affect these processes in return. In short, in a well-balanced personality that both contributes to and is a product of wider patterns of ethical conduct, different psychological functions work probably well with one another in a division of labor. A biological substrate of such functioning must obviously exist, although apparently we have no reason to think that it will be unique. Many different structural arrangements could perform the same functions in differing environments. Considered in this way, Plato was wrong about the need for reason to dominate other the functions of the psyche, such as emotion and appetite. Reason must work well with these other functions, instead of dominating them. But then, Plato was no democrat.

Acknowledgments

Presented in a dialogue on "The Social Brain," part of "Forum Barcelona 2004," Barcelona, Spain, 17 July 2004. I am grateful to the city and people of Barcelona, the event's sponsors, and Oscar Vilarroya for inviting me and for organizing and supporting this dialogue.

Notes

1. Edward O. Wilson, *Consilience: The Unity of Knowledge* (New York: Alfred A. Knopf, 1998), p. 157.

2. Ibid., p. 16.

3. Rudolf Carnap, "The Rejection of Metaphysics," *20th-Century Philosophy: The Analytic Tradition*, ed, M. Weitz (New York: Free Press, 1966 [1935]).

4. John Dewey, *Reconstruction in Philosophy* (New York: Henry Holt, 1920).

5. A. R. Jensen, "How Much Can We Boost IQ and Scholastic Achievement? *Harvard Educational Review*, 39:1 (1969), pp. 1–123.

6. Richard Dawkins, *The Selfish Gene* (Oxford: Oxford University Press, 1976).

7. Carol Gilligan, *In a Different Voice: Psychological Theory and Women's Development* (Cambridge, Mass.: Harvard University Press, 1982).

8. Bruno Latour and Stephen Woolgar, *Laboratory Life: The Social Construction of Scientific Facts* (Beverly Hills, Calif.: Sage, 1979).

9. Charles Darwin, *The Descent of Man and Selection in Relation to Sex* (Princeton, N.J.: Princeton University Press, 1981 [1871]).

10. Charles Murray and Richard Herrnstein, *The Bell Curve* (New York: The Free Press, 1974).

11. Richard C. Lewontin, "The Analysis of Variance and the Analysis of Causes," *The IQ Controversy: Critical Readings*, ed. Ned Joel Block and Gerald Dworkin (New York: Random House, 1976).

12. Christopher Hurn, *The Limits and Possibilities of Schooling* (Boston: Allyn and Bacon, 1993).

13. William James, *The Principles of Psychology*, 2. vol. (New York: Dover Publications, 1950 [1890]).

14. Richard E. Snow, Lyn Corno, and Lee J. Cronbach, *Remaking the Concept of Aptitude: Extending the Legacy of Richard E. Snow* (Mahwah, N.J.: Erlbaum, 2002).

15. Wilson, *Consilience*.

16. Edward O. Wilson, *In Search of Nature* (Washington, DC: Island Press, 1996), pp. 82, 92, 110, 113; quote from p. 107).

17. Wilson, *Consilience*, p. 163.

18. Daniel C. Dennett, *Darwin's Dangerous Idea: Evolution and the Meanings of Life* (New York: Simon and Schuster, 1995), p. 486.

19. Peter McGuffin, Brien Riley, and Robert Plomin, "Toward Behavioral Genomics," *Science*, 291: 5507 (2001), pp. 1232–1249.

20. Y. Ben-Shahar, A. Robichon, M. B. Sokolowski, and G. E. Robinson, "Influence of Gene Action across Different Time Scales on Behavior," *Science*, 296:5568 (2002), pp. 741–744.

21. George Herbert Mead, *Mind, Self, and Society: From the Standpoint of a Social Behaviorist*, 1st ed (Chicago, Ill.: University of Chicago Press, 1934); Lev Semyonovich Vygotsky, *Mind in Society: The Development of Higher Psychological Processes* (Cambridge, Mass.: Harvard University Press, 1978).

22. Daniel R. Ortiz, "Categorical Community," *Stanford Law Review*, 51 (1999), pp. 769–806.

23. Dewey, *Reconstruction in Philosophy*.

24. Robert Axelrod, *The Evolution of Cooperation* (New York: Basic Books, 1984).

25. Eric Bredo, "The Social Construction of Learning," *Handbook of Academic Learning: The Construction of Knowledge*, ed. Gary D. Phye (New Cork: Academia Press, 1997).

26. William James, "Reflex Action and Theism," *The Will to Believe and Other Essays in Popular Philosophy* (New York: Dover, 1956 [1896]).

Five

PERSPECTIVELESS CERTAINTY IN SOCIO-CULTURAL-POLITICAL BELIEFS

Emily A. Parker and Lawrence W. Barsalou

Despite being ubiquitous, conflict is not inevitable. In any given dispute, other outcomes are possible. Why then does conflict grip us repeatedly despite the horrors that war veterans, movies, television, and history books promise? Undoubtedly, many factors related to the time and place of a conflict are ultimately responsible for its occurrence. Here we explore one factor that may contribute to the amazing energy that people exert in pursuing their interests, and in denying those of others.

Our premise is that perceptions of certainty are central to selfishness and conflict, and to their resolution. We first distinguish two ways that people can perceive certainty: perspectiveless certainty (C), and perspectival certainty (C_P). We then describe two domains where perceptions of certainty apply: the basic perceptual domain (BP), and the socio-cultural-political domain (SCP). After introducing these distinctions in certainty and domain, we explore two possible relations between them: covariance and independence. We suggest that people tend to adopt C independent of domain, with one outcome being selfishness and conflict in the SCP domain. We then explore two possible reasons for independence: (1) the grounding of higher cognition in the brain's perceptual systems, and (2) the social process of in-group bonding. Finally, we explore ways to induce greater C_P in the SCP domain.

1. Perspectiveless Certainty and Perspectival Certainty

By *certainty* we mean strength of belief, or what is often called *truth*. As described shortly, we avoid the use of truth, given its ontological and epistemological implications. Instead, we focus on the psychological construct of certainty and explore two forms it can take: perspectiveless certainty (C) and perspectival certainty (C_P). We use C and C_P to convey the idea that perspectiveless certainty does not entail a perspective (C alone), and that perspectival certainty does (C with a $_P$).

Perspectiveless Certainty (C). Perspectiveless certainty is the idea that a belief is "true" or "the way things are" from no perspective. Consider the belief that "the world is flat." Adopting C means viewing this belief as not dependent on perspective. Even if no person existed to perceive the Earth's surface, we view this statement as "true." Even when people exist who perceive the Earth as flat, certainty about this belief does not depend on their perspective. We are using certainty here as a description of people's psychological states—not as a philosophical or scientific claim about truth. People can view a scientifically false belief such as "the Earth is flat" with C, believing it to be true, independent of perspective.

In the preceding discussion, the word "true" is in quotation marks because historically it has been used to mean C: Things that are "true" are "true" independent of perspective. Often, claims about truth amount to claiming, with absolute authority, perspectiveless certainty about a state-of-affairs, even in the face of legitimate antithetical claims.

This notion of C has traveled under different names for millennia, including *objectivity, realism,* and *rationality.* Until the twentieth century, a primary goal of philosophy has been to address the nature of "objective truth." Since the foundational contributions of sixteenth to eighteenth century rationalist and empiricist epistemologists, many philosophers have remained concerned with C. How do we arrive at C? How we can demonstrate that we have arrived at it?

The sciences have also reflected similar assumptions about C. In frameworks such as logical positivism, scientific discoveries are viewed as capturing C about the natural world. Perspective has often found its way into scientific thinking, as in Albert Einstein's theory of relativity and the Heisenberg uncertainty principle. Modern scientists are highly aware that any observation is theory dependent, and that many possible theories explain any finding.

Perspectival Certainty (C_P). Perspectival certainty is the idea that the certainty of a belief reflects the perspective of the person holding it. Even when beliefs are held with high certainty, the importance of perspective is appreciated. Today, when we believe that "the Earth is round," we may still appreciate that this belief reflects our current perspective, perhaps because people have previously thought otherwise. We could view "The Earth is round" with C. Alternatively, people can realize that this belief reflects their personal, historical, and cultural perspective. As a result, people can appreciate that others having a different perspective could hold a different belief with equally high certainty.

Western philosophy since the nineteenth century has increasingly acknowledged the dependence of certainty on perspective. Many philosophers, notably Frederich Nietzsche,[1] John Dewey,[2] Maurice Merleau-Ponty,[3] and Martin Heidegger[4] have raised fundamental questions about C and the aspiration to it. Feminist theorists have extended this work.[5] For these thinkers, certainty about anything is always a function of perspective, where perspective includes personal history, cultural context, bodily experience, time, location, and many other factors. According to these views, establishing knowledge free of perspective is an impossible task, given that knowledge always reflects the perspective used to produce it. Further, these views argue that attempting to develop perspectiveless knowledge reflects a philosophical perspective that assumes this is possible.

2. Two Domains Where Beliefs about Certainty Apply

We could explore perceptions of certainty in a wide variety of domains. Here we focus on two that appear relevant to exploring how certainty contributes to selfishness and conflict: the basic perceptual domain and the socio-cultural-political domain.

The BP domain (BP). People have powerful perceptual systems that provide them with information about their environments and internal states. Sensory systems for vision, audition, touch, taste, and smell tell us about the external world, whereas introspective systems for emotion, motivation, and cognition tell us about the internal world. In neither case do these systems provide complete accounts. Sensory systems are only sensitive to designated ranges of stimulation, and introspective systems are notoriously limited in their access to our internal workings.

As much scientific research has shown, these systems produce basic forms of perceptual experience. The visual system produces experiences of shape, color, and motion. The auditory system produces experiences of pitch, volume, and timbre. Although the experience of fundamental perceptual properties reflects experience to some extent,[6] these experiences are largely universal across cultures, reflecting a common human biology. Any person having normal vision, who looks at a round red object, would see and believe that something of that color and shape exists in the world. Training and education are not necessary for the development of BP systems and the low-level beliefs that they produce. As long as these systems receive normal input during development, they largely develop independently of individual experience and culture.

Our discussion of the BP domain focuses on *early* perceptual processing. We do *not* include late perception, which is subject to conceptual influences. Our later discussions of certainty depend on the relative absence vs. presence of conceptual processes. To disentangle conceptual influences from sensory processing can be difficult, if not impossible, given that higher cognitive systems reach far into early perception.[7] In general, though, early perceptual systems appear less influenced by individual-specific and culture-specific learning factors than are late perceptual systems.

The SCP domain. In contrast, we assume that the SCP domain is influenced heavily by individual-specific learning factors. Each person's developmental, social, and cultural history fundamentally shapes his or her social knowledge about stereotypes, relationships, and ambitions. These same factors also have tremendous impact on a person's cultural knowledge about conventions, rituals, explanatory systems, and myths, and also on their political knowledge about rights, responsibilities, laws, individuals, governments, and countries.

Whereas our beliefs in the BP domain primarily reflect biological constraints, our beliefs in the SCP domain primarily reflect experience (although biological factors also contribute). Knowledge acquired from experience determines how we operate in the SCP domain. People's knowledge about the

SCP domain varies widely. Depending on a person's history, different knowledge develops, causing differences in how people perceive, comprehend, and act in the SCP domain. Notably, this is the opposite of the BP domain, which exhibits a much more universal pattern.

3. Possible Relations between Certainty and Domain

We next explore two possible relations between certainty and domain: covariance vs. independence.

Covariance. As Figure 1 illustrates, covariance occurs when people experience C about the BP domain, but experience C_P about the SCP domain. In the BP domain, people intuitively adopt C. If they see an object visually, they believe with high certainty that an object is actually there. Further, they believe that anyone else who looked would also believe it is there, and that it would be there even if no one perceived it.

	C	C_P
BP	x	
SCP		x

Figure 1. One form of covariance between certainty and domain.

We do *not* assume that everyone *categorizes* perceived entities the same way, given that categorization depends on conceptual systems. Instead, we only assume that C in the BP domain applies to *early perceptual experience*. When people perceive something, they believe that something is present, and that its presence exists independent of perspective.

We *not* suggesting that early perception is actually perspectiveless. Early perception is heavily perspective-dependent. For example, the different sensory systems of different species produce different perceptual experiences. Similarly, context has profound effects on perception. Our claim is that people *act* as if early perception is perspectiveless. When early perceptual systems detect something, people believe it to be present with a high degree of C.

This intuitive naiveté may serve people well. Given that, most human beings share the same BP systems, if one person senses something in a setting, other people are likely to sense it as well. On sensing something, it may be socially useful to conclude with certainty that the sensed entity exists independent of perspective. By making this inference, a perceiver is likely to make further correct inferences about what other people in the same setting experience.

As Figure 1 further illustrates, the covariance hypothesis proposes that people adopt a different view toward certainty in the SCP domain. Here they recognize that their beliefs reflect their perspective. They further recognize that other people's perspectives may cause them to see the SCP domain differently, but to be no less certain about their beliefs.

The covariance hypothesis assumes that people perceive certainty as increasingly perspective-dependent as the domain becomes increasingly less tangible. For the tangible world of perceptual experience, people view the certainty they experience as relatively perspective-free. For the less tangible world of SCP relations, people view their certainty as increasingly dependent on perspective.

Independence. Figure 2 illustrates the form of independence between certainty and domain of focal interest here. In this form, people experience C not just about the BP domain but also about the SCP domain. Instead of realizing that their certainty about a SCP belief reflects their perspective, people believe that their certainty is perspective free—this is "the way it is." As a result, people's SCP reality takes on the same perspective-free certainty as their BP reality. Examples include the beliefs that only one God can confer salvation and that a true marriage can only be heterosexual.

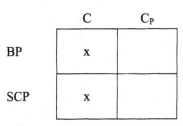

Figure 2. One form of independence between certainty and domain.

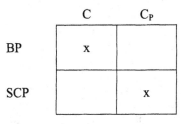

Figure 3. A second form of independence between certainty and domain.

We see this perspective-free stance toward the SCP domain everywhere: in politics, churches, mosques, synagogues, schools, gangs, academic circles, and families. We believe that this stance contributes considerably to selfishness and conflict. Not seeing the perspective-dependence of our SCP views prevents us from appreciating the validity of different views. Conflict ensues when people attempt to impose what they mistakenly see as perspective-free views on other people. Notably, this problem does not generally arise in the BP domain. Again, it generally appears useful that people perceive the environment similarly and view it as perspective free. Notably, selfishness and conflict do not arise here.

Figure 3 illustrates a second possible form of independence, one that strikes us as even more sophisticated than covariance. Here, people recognize that beliefs across all domains depend on perspective. This view may largely result when people scrutinize their experience and beliefs carefully. Persons becoming aware of how their body and brain influence perception may be critical.

4. Possible Reasons for Adopting C in the SCP Domain

Here we focus first on a cognitive mechanism that may produce C in the SCP domain, and then on a social mechanism.

Grounding of the conceptual system in perceptual systems. Increasing empirical research indicates that knowledge heavily utilizes perceptual systems for representational purposes. When representing knowledge about an entity, event, or mental state, people appear to use *simulations* of their perceptual experience with these entities. For example, when people represent knowledge about *apples*, they imagine apples look, feel, and taste. Notably, the same perceptual systems that operate in the BP domain represent these simulations. Some even make arguments for the importance of simulation in abstract concepts.[8]

Knowledge involves much more than simulations of prior experience.[9] It also relies heavily on the use of the same mechanisms that operate in the BP domain. In general, higher cognition appears to rely on the brain's modality-specific systems. We can find considerable amounts of evidence for this conclusion in cognitive and social psychology, and in cognitive neuroscience.[10]

This conclusion leads to our first speculation about why people adopt C in the SCP domain. We suggest that people intuitively generalize C about experience in the BP domain to the SCP domain via the common perceptual systems that construct representations in both domains. We make the following argument:

Premise 1. C is associated with BP experience.
Premise 2. BP mechanisms are used to represent SCP beliefs
Conclusion. C becomes associated with SCP beliefs.

Because BP systems implicitly and automatically engender C, they also engender C during the representation of SCP beliefs. SCP beliefs are less abstract and more concrete than we might have imagined. As a result, though, we fail to see how perspective-dependant they are.

An intriguing finding reviewed by Marcia K. Johnson supports this proposal.[11] She found that the amount of perceptual and contextual detail accompanying a memory tends to correlate positively with the certainty that the event actually occurred. BP information in a memory increases its certainty, consistent with our proposal.

In-group bonding. A second factor may also produce C in the SCP domain: the social mechanism of in-group bonding. Much research on social psychology has shown that belonging to a social group induces powerful cognitive forces in individuals.[12] For example, members in the same group see other members more positively than they see the members of "out" groups. Similarly, in-group members tend to treat each other better than they treat out-group members.

We propose that groups induce C about shared SCP beliefs. A group's members do not agree on everything. Yet often they share many fundamental SCP beliefs, such as beliefs in deities, authority relations, and marriage practices. Most importantly, adopting C about a group's SCP beliefs strengthens both the group and its individuals.

Groups become powerful and effective when their members adopt C about shared SCP beliefs. When members believe that the group's beliefs have C, they are less likely to question them. Further, strong conviction in these beliefs may often give individuals a sense of power that is highly motivating and that causes them to act, and even sacrifice, for the sake of the group. If individuals adopted C_P toward these beliefs, they might be more likely to diverge from them, and be less likely to act on them on behalf of the group.

Conversely, individuals also benefit from adopting C towards SCP beliefs. Doing so signals an individual's commitment to the group. In return, the group may become committed to the individual, doing its best to ensure the individual's safety, needs, and ambitions. Because "going it alone" in the world can be dangerous, affiliating with a group can be beneficial to survival and success. Adopting C towards SCP may be one key step towards establishing this bond. The cost, though, is loss of the ability to appreciate the certainty that individuals in other groups feel towards their SCP beliefs. In turn, this may make it easier to initiate aggression and produce conflict.

Group formation may be a fundamental organizing principle in many animal species because of the evolutionary advantages it confers on survival, resource gathering, and reproduction. Powerful biological factors may be at play in the group processes that induce C in SCP.

5. Possible Ways to Induce C_P

To the extent that the mechanisms producing C are under genetic control, most individuals possess them, and they operate relatively automatically and implicitly. But reining them in and operating on the basis of C_P appears possible, given its presence in some individuals and groups. Here we explore several possible ways of inducing greater C_P.

Correlational analyses of C vs C_P. What is it about some individuals that make them adopt either C or C_P towards SCP? Do some biological, developmental, and personality factors play a role? What about education, lifestyle, and occupation? Similar studies could be performed of groups that exhibit either C or C_P toward SCP, including religions, cultures, and institutions. Do some historical factors, belief systems, practices, and organizational structures predispose a group towards C vs. C_P?

Developing interventions. Once we have some sense of the factors that produce CP in SCP, developing interventions that recreate those factors in individuals and groups who exhibit C might be possible. Conversely, once we have some sense of the factors that produce C about SCP, developing interventions that weaken those factors might also be possible.

Cognitive interventions could aim at helping individuals recognize that their SCP beliefs inherently reflect C_P. Similarly, social interventions, especially in areas of conflict, could aim to engender increasing awareness that C contributes to conflict and that adopting C_P could reduce it. Obviously, everyone knows this, and putting it to work effectively is difficult. To develop new, more powerful forms of this intervention appears essential.

One good example is The Ulster Project. This organization invites Roman Catholic and Protestant youths from Northern Ireland on international trips to unfamiliar settings. There, they get to know each other personally, away from the backdrop of their familiar social struggle, and they discuss their perspectives. Seeing how C_P can apply to SCP beliefs appears to be a crucial component of successful conflict resolution.

In conclusion, we believe that the only appropriate certainty in the SCP domain is one that minimizes selfishness and conflict. The aspiration to C in the SCP domain is a contributor to these problems. Such aspirations yield inappropriate declarations of "how things are" in domains where tremendous diversity does and should exist. We contend that human beings have an ethical responsibility to adopt C_P in the SCP domain out of respect for life. Out of this respect will grow the world in which we would all like to live.

Acknowledgment

Research supported by National Science Foundation Grant BCS-0212134 to Lawrence Barsalou.

Notes

1. Friedrich Nietzsche, *On the Genealogy of Morals*, trans. Walter Kaufmann (New York: Vintage Books, 1989); *Beyond Good and Evil*, trans. Walter Kaufmann (New York: Vintage Books, 1989.)

2. John Dewey, *The Later Works, 1925–1953*: vol. 1, 1925, ed. Jo Ann Boydston (Carbondale, Ill.: Southern Illinois University, 1981).

3. Maurice Merleau-Ponty, *Phenomenology of Perception*, trans. Colin Smith (New York: Routledge Classics, 1962).

4. Martin Heidegger, *Being and Time*, trans. John Macquarrie and Edward Robinson (Oxford: Oxford University Press, 1967.)

5. Lorraine Code, *What Can She Know? Feminist Theory and the Construction of Knowledge* (Ithaca, N.Y.: Cornell University Press, 1991); Sandra G. Harding, *Whose Science? Whose Knowledge?: Thinking from Women's Lives* (Ithaca, N.Y.: Cornell University Press, 1991); Evelyn Fox Keller, *Reflections on Gender and Science* (New Haven, Conn.: Yale University Press, 1985); Helen E. Longino, *Science as Social Knowledge: Values and Objectivity in Scientific Inquiry* (Princeton, N.J.: Princeton University Press, 1990); and A. Wylie, "Rethinking Objectivity: Nozick's Neglected Third Option," *International Studies in the Philosophy of Science*, 14 (2000), pp. 5–10.

6. Jeffrey L. Elman, *Rethinking Innateness: A Connectionist Perspective on Development* (Cambridge, Mass.: MIT Press, 1996).

7. R. E. Crist, W. Li, and C. D. Gilbert, "Learning to See: Experience and Attention in Primary Visual Cortex," *Nature Neuroscience*, 4 (2001), pp. 519–525; and A. G. Samuel, "Lexical Activation Produces Potent Phonemic Percepts," *Cognitive Psychology*, 32 (1997), pp. 97–127.

8. Lawrence W. Barsalou and K. Wiemer-Hastings, "Situating Abstract Concepts," *Grounding Cognition: The Role of Perception and Action in Memory, Language, and Thought*, eds. Diane Pecher and Rolf Zwaan (New York: Cambridge University Press, 2005), pp. 129–163; and George Lakoff and Mark Johnson, *Metaphors We Live By* (Chicago, Ill.: University of Chicago Press, 1980).

9. Lawrence W. Barsalou, "Perceptual Symbol Systems," *Behavioral and Brain Sciences*, 22 (1999), pp. 577–600; and "Abstraction in Perceptual Symbol Systems," *Philosophical Transactions of the Royal Society of London: Biological Sciences*, 358 (2003), pp. 1177–1187.

10. Lawrence W. Barsalou, "Situated Simulation in the Human Conceptual System," *Language and Cognitive Processes,* 18 (2003), pp. 513–562; Lawrence W. Barsalou, P. M. Niedenthal, A. K. Barbey, and J. A. Ruppert, "Social Embodiment," *The Psychology of Learning and Motivation*, vol.43, ed. B. H. Ross (San Diego, Calif.: Academic Press, 2003); and A. Martin, "Functional Neuroimaging of Semantic Memory," *Handbook of Functional Neuroimaging of Cognition*, eds. R. Cabeza and A. Kingstone (Cambridge, Mass.: MIT Press, 2001), pp. 153-186.

11. M. K. Johnson, "Individual and Cultural Reality Monitoring," *The Annals of the American Academy of Political and Social Science,* 560 (1998), pp. 179–193.

12. Michael A. Hogg and R. Scott Tindale, *Blackwell Handbook of Social Psychology: Group Processes* (Boston, Mass.: Blackwell, 2002).

Six

SPARE ME THE COMPLEMENTS: AN IMMODERATE PROPOSAL FOR ELIMINATING THE "WE/THEY" CATEGORY BOUNDARY

Stevan Harnad

1. The We/They Category Boundary

Some biological facts are undeniable: Any creature born with a tendency to ignore the calls of nature—not to eat when hungry, not to copulate when sexually aroused, not to flee when in harm's way—would not pass on that unfortunate tendency. Such a creature would instead be the first in a long line of extinct descendents. Natural selection eliminates maladaptive traits from the gene pool by the sheer definition of what it means to be maladaptive.

An indifference to survival of the self is such a maladaptive trait. Even daredevils, heroes, and saints differ from the mean by only a bit: They still thrash for breath if deprived of air and trample their fellows to escape encroaching flames.

So in seeking unselfishness and cooperation, do not aim too high. We need basic creature-needs satisfied before we can talk about sharing or sacrifice. Exceptions exist. We all know about "inclusive fitness" ("I will lay down my life for two brothers, four cousins"), but that is all in the family, so although the rule may be "every gene for him or herself," between genes are causal dependencies, sometimes even when they are in different bodies. A mother is better off feeding and sometimes even sacrificing herself for her babies, instead of eating them if she is to pass on that tendency—or any tendency at all.

Then, besides selfish genes helping their closest in kin, we have the question of kin detection itself. We are not equipped with genetic kin detectors. We must *learn* who our kin are. The main way we learn this is from early exposure. We imprint on those with whom we live and those we see quite often from birth, favoring them for sharing and disfavoring them for mating. (Sibling competition for goods is another matter, one in which assertive egoism—kept in check by older kin—is probably more adaptive in the earliest years of life than lackadaisical sharing.)

But once you open the door to learning, you have already let in non-kin, for "kin" becomes defined by experience, not by genetics. The most probable primary caregivers are genetic parents, but not necessarily; and the probability shrinks as you move beyond the nuclear family. Locally, no great risk exists because even those who are not our kin are still our kind, with shared experiences, goods, interests, and, most importantly, shared enemies. Cooperation does not end, and conflict begin, at the boundary of the gene, the organism, the kin line, or the local kind, but at the frontier with the enemy kind.

Still, frontiers shift and enmity comes in degrees: In some cases, the enemy of my enemy becomes my friend. Common interests create strategic alliances; enemy may even become kin-in-law. But always some boundary is present, always a current "we" versus a "they," an "in" versus an "out." Does any way to eliminate those boundaries exist, too?

We may find an answer in category-learning theory: Learning who are our kin and our kind are just special cases of the learning of categories (kinds) in general. Animal and plant species are kinds; so are many natural objects and artifacts; so are many actions, events, and states (running, walking, thunderstorms, droughts, days, nights) including feeling-states (fear, fondness, longing, loathing). To pick out a category, all we need is a sample of what is in the category and what is not in the category.

A dichotomy is the simplest form of category (for example, male/female), but most categories have more than two possibilities: Many kinds of animals exist, not just zebras or giraffes. But whether a category is dichotomous or polychotomous, something basically binary—categorical—is inherent in categorizing. With every category, a particular instance is either *in* that category or *not in* it. This characteristic explains why so many English nouns and adjectives have a "non-" or "un-" version: "member/non-member," "athletic/unathletic," or "white/ nonwhite." The "un-" refers to the complement of the category. Every well-defined category needs a complement—the set of things *not* in the category. For if a "category" has no complement (or you do not know what its complement is), then "it" is not a category (or not a category that you yet know).

The complement of a category is significant because the *invariant features* of members of a category determine what is and is not a member of that category. The only way for a cognitive system to find out what the definitive characteristics of a category are is to sample from the category and its complement, to learn to detect which features will reliably differentiate them. The cognitive system must detect the invariance in the variation between members and non-members.

For some categories, the invariant-feature detectors are innate: We probably do not have to learn the difference between a friendly and a threatening face, and we definitely do not have to learn the difference between being hungry and nonhungry, or between pain and pleasure, (though learning may modulate the boundaries in some cases). Color categories (red, green, blue) are probably innate as well, although room for some modulation by experience may be possible.

But most categories we have to learn from experience: Open a dictionary and you will find mostly content-words (nouns, adjectives, verbs, adverbs) that signify names of categories, most of them learned, not innate categories. How did we learn them? By sampling positive and negative instances (members and non-members of the category) and getting corrective feedback (whether we have categorized them correctly or incorrectly), we learn and refine the categories. A good example would be learning which kinds of mushrooms are edible and inedible. The corrective feedback could come from an instructor guiding our selection or from our digestive systems as we either get sick or not as we taste sample bits of our selection.

Finding a better way to learn to categorize things, such as learning from instruction or from role modeling, is plainly more adaptive than trial-and-error sorting (such as tasting potentially lethal mushrooms to categorize them), with its natural consequences. Trial-and-error learning with corrective feedback is not only time-consuming, but also risky. We would be better served if an instructor already competent to detect the critical features could spare us the tasting and stomach-aches, or, better still, could tell us explicitly, in words, what the distinguishing features are.

To learn from others who use words to convey experience vicariously to spare us the need for direct learning by experience, we had to evolve natural language, whose most basic function is to allow us to learn new categories from explicit verbal descriptions instead of just from implicit feature learning guided by feedback from trial-and-error sampling of members and non-members.

Members and non-members must exist, in any case, otherwise no distinguishing features can be discerned, hence, no category. If we are to learn the category from a description instead of direct experience, the distinguishing features must not only exist, but also be known to the describer, who must be able to put them into words.

So what if a category had only positive instances? Would we have any way to learn it, either from direct experience or from a verbal description? What would constitute an example of such a category? For such a category to be possible, the only thing we can sample must be *in* the category, not what is not in it. Its complement must be either unreachable for some reason, or empty.

Let us consider the unreachable case first: Recall that some feeling-categories are innate: We do not need to learn the features of pain vs. pleasure because we are born able to detect them (and approach/avoid accordingly). Let us now consider other feeling-categories. What does being a bachelor feel like? Can any bachelor who has never experienced being married know? He may guess, filling in the missing complement that he has not experienced, either by analogy and extrapolation from approximations to the married state that he has already experienced, or by imagination. He guess correctly; he may correctly guess the critical features that distinguish what being a bachelor feels like vs. what be married feels like. But he might be wrong, so that if and when he does marry, he might say, "this not what I thought being married feels like, so only now do I truly know what being a bachelor feels like.

But the married state is not a feeling category unreachable in principle, just one that may not be reached by some, in their experiential lifetimes. Perhaps a few words of wisdom from someone who knows what being married feels like would have done the trick too, conveying the distinguishing features. But to get an idea of what dealing with a truly uncomplemented category is like, we have to consider other feeling categories:

What does being awake feel like? You might believe that you know, that this is a perfectly well defined category, but is it? You have sampled different degrees of alertness and drowsiness, but those differences are differences in *degrees* of wakefulness. They do not define the boundary between being awake and being unawake. You have also experienced the onset of being awake. You know what being awake feels like when you are unable to remember feeling anything immediately before. That is still just another example of what being awake feels like. To say that you know what being unawake feels like is self-contradictory, because, by definition, when you are unawake you are not feeling anything at all.

With that said, we are not too handicapped because we do not have the category "what it feels like to be awake." The relevant distinctions—the differences that make a difference in our lives, like the difference between an edible and inedible mushroom—are differences in degrees of wakefulness ("I am too tired to drive," "I need to get some sleep"), and not differences based on what being awake feels like. The category awake/asleep is determined on an objective, not a subjective basis. I do not know what to be asleep *feels like* (I am omitting dreaming, which is a special form of wakefulness.) I am speaking here of dreamless sleep, when you are gone, and no one is there, feeling anything. We can make the awake/asleep distinction in objective, behavioral, third person terms. Everyone knows the difference between a moving, responsive person and a snoring, unresponsive one. The rest is what it feels like transition from the unfelt to the felt state.

You may be wondering what all this has to do with unselfishness and cooperation. I ask for just a little more patience. Consider just one more case, this time not a subjective but an objective one: the category, *something that exists*. Philosophers have always had problems with that category. Talking about things that you can and cannot see in the street is easy: You can sometimes see zebras, but never unicorns. A zebra is a horse with stripes; those kinds exist. A unicorn is a horse with a horn; those kinds do not exist. That is a perfectly well complemented category. We all know what a horse, stripes, and horns look like, and what you do and do not see in the street.

But what about a drawing or animation of a unicorn, that horse with a horn that I have no trouble imagining, even though I will never see a live one in the street? What do I mean by saying "that" does not exist, when I have just finished talking about "it" and imagining "it" in my mind (or drawing it on paper)? The feature "never appears in the street" is a perfectly adequate feature for distinguishing kinds of things that do and do not appear in the street. But "nonexistent" is more than just that: Can I say of anything that I can imagine and talk about it yet describe that it does not exist? Or, does everything I can imagine and talk about exist, so that the rest is just about what *other* features it has, besides existing? "Existing" is a feature shared by the members of all categories, fictional and nonfictional, visible and invisible, but all alike—conceivable.

Last exercise, before we return to conflict and cooperation: What if I tell you that that thing over there (a zebra) is a "laylek"? That too—a drawing of a unicorn. So is running, walking, red, green, pain, pleasure, friend, foe, and what it feels like to be a bachelor, or married, or awake: All of those are members of the category "laylek." Open a dictionary and pick any content word, any object, property, action, event, relation or state, abstract or concrete—I tell you they are all members of the category "laylek." Anything and everything is a laylek. Now do you know what a laylek is? Do you have any idea of where the boundary lies between a laylek and a nonlaylek? Can you say what the distinguishing features of a laylek are?

Having some way to make people just as oblivious to the boundary between "kin/kind" and "other's kin/kind," between "we" and "they" would be nice, no—some means of making "us" into an uncomplemented category like laylek, for all of us—would be nice, no?

We are speaking here about the first person plural, not the first person singular. What we are contemplating here is not some mystical dissolution of the boundary between "self" and "other," for that would take us down a biologically maladaptive path, which, as noted earlier, leads to a dead end. My pain/pleasure must continue to be mine, felt by me, not blending into some nebulous shared collective consciousness. So we are not talking about "I" but about "we."

Who or what are "we"? Like every category, the answer to this question changes with context: In a room that has women and men, "we" might be the men vs. the women, or, in a room containing children and adults, age groups might be the way identifications and allegiances align. If we then redistribute the same people in a bigger population, say, mostly quite aged people, the adults and children might all coalesce into the single category "we, the young," even though age]had initially divided them in the first context. Ethnic kind, nationality, and local neighborhood work this way, too, generating ever-changing groupings, depending on which distinctive feature you use to sort (any feature would demonstrate this principle).

But the original we/they sorting was the local kin group—parents, children, grandparents, aunts, uncles, siblings, cousins—versus non-kin. The infant does not need to learn the boundary between itself and the outer-world, but it does need to learn who "kin" are and who are not kin. I put "kin" in scare-quotes not only because the distinction does not depend on genetic screening, but also because the distinction is so circumstantial and context-dependent. The infant imprints on its early caregivers and familiars. While early caregivers and familiars are not only the ones that the child will thereafter perceive as kin, that early interaction, which occurs in a finite critical period in early infancy and childhood, then becomes the model for all later we/they distinctions.

A child deprived of affectionate early caregivers is a child susceptible to all sorts of later social and psychological problems. So let us not even contemplate depriving children of this crucial early human contact. How can we finesse the we/they distinction?

We must return to category learning. We learn to categorize learning mechanisms are present in our brains—perhaps kinds of neural nets— adept at analyzing sensory input to detect *invariants*. Recall that the simplest category is a dichotomy: The members of the category are the positive instances; the non-members (the members of the category's complement) are the negative instances. What the brain's invariance detectors learn to do—under the guidance of corrective feedback from the consequences of categorizing (for example, eating an edible or an inedible mushroom)—is filter out all the variation from instance to instance not correlated with being a member or non-member and extract only the features correlated with being a positive, not a negative instance.

These are the distinguishing features of the category, the features impossible for us to extract in the case of feeling awake or knowing what a laylek is, because all instances were positive. Nothing distinguishes what being awake feels like—or what a laylek is—from what not being awake feels like—or what a non-laylek is. What it feels like to be awake has instance-to-instance differences, but those are just variations among positive instances, exactly the features that an invariance-detector learns to *ignore*, as it learns to distinguish the positive instances from the negative. The same is true with all the things that are layleks: Everything is a laylek, every instance is positive. So we have no way to extract an invariance from all that variation. The issue is not that things may not have features in common. Things may have many features in common. An invariance must not only be present in the members of a category, but also it must be absent in non-members. An uncomplemented category has no non-members.

So if we are agreed that we should not deprive an infant of its caregivers, how can we deprive it of the we/they distinction? I suggest a simple way exists, though it may sound shocking, perhaps even Orwellian or worse. Throughout their critical period, we could rear children in aggregates-in-flux instead of in an invariant nuclear family. An aggregate-in-flux is a population of caregivers and age-mates into which an infant "rotates," from the time of its birth until the critical period for imprinting, and formation of the we/they distinction, is over. The optimal number of caregivers and age-mates is to be determined empirically—one male and one female, plus a few age-mates being the default option. The interval between each "rotation" (perhaps a few days, perhaps a week or two, but not longer) and the end of the critical period (perhaps puberty, perhaps later, perhaps earlier) is determined empirically also.

During that critical period, in normal child rearing, the child not only imprints upon and forms life-long attachments to particular people (mostly kin), but the distinction between kin and non-kin becomes the model for later we/they distinctions, distinctions that always involve a discrimination in favor or some (we), and against others (they). But in the aggregates-in-flux, on what could a child to imprint? The invariants are there: affectionate caregivers, age-mates, but all the other particulars keep varying. The only invariant that exists in all this variance on which the child can imprint is that all these changing caregivers and age-mates are all human beings. But being a human being is an invariant that all people share, so is the category "human being" is uncomplemented (or the only boundary it marks is human/nonhuman— not quite optimal for vegetarians like me!)

Apart from the problem about the species boundary, some doubt remains about whether and when the "window" for attachment closes. Is the critical period for attachment ever quite over? When can the flux stop and ordinary life begin? We can make female rats lactate throughout adult life by constantly giving them new pups to suckle, but could we find a way to make grownups keep on living in aggregates-in-flux, considering people's proclivity to become constant and recurrent at some point? If the attachment window is still open at that time, the we/they boundary could still erupt. We go on forming categories all of our lives; but perhaps later attachments are not as fiercely partisan as early ones.

Would rearing children in aggregates-in-flux during their critical period for kin attachment succeed in eliminating the we/they boundary? We will never know, because our selfish genes bias us against even trying such an immoderate proposal. Parents want to keep and form attachments to their children— naturally enough, we are inclined to say, but here we are contemplating whether we can improve upon nature, in view of some of its less admirable outcomes.

Perhaps some less radical approximations to aggregates-in-flux are possible during the critical period, but I have a difficult time envisioning what those might be. Orphanages are unhappy places, serial foster homes are probably too small, change too slow, and the contrasts with normal family life too intrusive, while kibbutzim are merely bigger families. None of these settings provides the requisite unrelenting flux I propose; all of these still allow imprinting on invariant individuals.

Even if the We category is bound to be complemented in natural life, thought experiments such as this one might give us a little more insight into how and why the We is an invariant of social life, and whether Charles Darwin might have found a better, kinder way.

2. Evan

Evan had always been aloof, cerebral. He was forever creating theoretical systems—not practical ones that people could build and use, but completely abstract ones, usually social and ethical ones, that people could only contemplate hypothetically. They were "abstract inventions," such as a "tit-for-tat" society in which people were forced to behave in accordance with the Golden Rule because whatever they did to others was done to them in return—not in some remote afterlife, but almost immediately. Or, a communicative system that would teach everyone to express every thought succinctly, because no one would be permitted do anything for themselves. Each person had to convey every wish—even the most mundane—through "Chinese whispers," in which the wisher tells it to someone else, who then goes away and tells it to someone else, and so on, through chains of no fewer than six others. Only the last person in the chain would implement the wisher's wish, and the result depended on each person in the chain communicating unambiguously enough for the message to survive transmission through the chain.

"Why are you so obsessed with people theoretically, Evan? They are all around you and you hardly notice them as you build your utopian castles."

Although he was not unattractive, either physically or mentally, Evan tended to remain aloof from others. Although people enjoyed listening to him, they had to coax him to open up about his thought experiments.

Evan suffered extremely poor eyesight. His eyes, which always appeared quite shrunken behind his thick lenses, magnified and took on a dreamy and distant look quite like the characteristics of his abstractions. So people—older women especially—wished, sometimes silently, often aloud, that he were not so aloof and cerebral, that he would forget a little about his "systems" and look at them, look into their eyes, to feel something. They all believed that they could teach him how to feel, if only . . .

If only what? What element was missing? Did people think Evan was deliberately holding himself back from something? Was he arrogant, snobbish, or disdainful? Not at all. Obviously, he was far too lost in his abstractions to feel such earthly pettiness. Was he afraid then, embarrassed, or shy? Some felt that was closer to the truth. After all, he easily blushed and lost his train of thought (sometimes it would be something someone else said, sometimes it would be something that he said or thought). In moments of confusion, he would appear lost, unsure whether to continue with what he had been saying, or to apologize, or to give up. Some kinds of mild criticism had the same effect on him, but because most of his interlocutors were sympathetic, they quickly learned not to say things that hurt his feelings in that way.

So his aloofness was due neither to lack of feelings nor pride. Was it obsession? Was "aloofness" the right word to describe it at all? We do not (to pick an overdramatic example) say that schizophrenic persons are "aloof" or "cerebral" when they are listening to their inner voices. Then why should Evan be so described when he is building or describing his systems?

Still, few people could get close to Evan. His mother, Freda, was very much like him, though less single-mindedly so. She had managed to raise three children, Evan's older sisters were not at all aloof. Her devotion to Evan's father, Theodore—bed-ridden and on a dialysis machine since almost the day they had met as newly graduated law clerks, both clerking for the American Civil Liberties Union (ACLU) in Brooklyn—could hardly be described by anyone as aloof. But she, too, had her moments of abstraction and reverie. Perhaps the ACLU was an outgrowth of one of them and linking her fate with a young, brilliant man suffering from an old man's kidney ailment was another.

So, Evan was close to his mother, and to his father, with whom he had been having intense conversations ever since Evan had been old enough to speak or listen. Sadly, Theodor's increasing debilitation as his disease progressed (and as kidney transplants failed) caused his side of their bedside conversations to become increasingly incoherent. Theodor progressively repeated himself more, and over time, he made increasingly less sense. Evan still sat by his father's bedside (he still lived at home), listening more than speaking, just as he always had. But silence would often be two-sided now, with Evan lost in a system he was contemplating and Theodor lost wherever high Blood Urea Nitrogen levels transported his mind.

Evan's sisters were long married, having hastened out of what they found to be an increasingly less hospitable—because increasingly more hospital-like—atmosphere of the household, as the dialyses increased from monthly, to weekly, to daily, the abstractions of their mother and brother grew ever more remote, the thoughts of their father grew less and less rational.

Some thought this medical/mentational atmosphere kept Evan distant. Freida, a fellow-student, a few years ahead of Evan in law school, thought it was something else. She thought his abstractions were not all destined to remain mere distractions. Soon seconded by Freda, she became increasingly convinced that some of Evan's ideas were feasible. One that Evan had told her about early in their relationship (they had become lovers) was something he called "aggregates-in-flux." This experiment, a new way of rearing children, was inspired partly by the Kibbutz experiments in Israel, partly by Evan's ruminations when he had studied divorce and child custody law, and partly by some things he had read about newborn ducklings and Temple rhesus monkeys. His idea was that human selfishness and favoritism—ultimately racism and xenophobia—all originated from early imprinting. He hypothesized that children attach to their family members, and that due to this attachment they would favor them, invariably at the expense of others, who are not family members: In this way, a "We versus They" categorization scheme is ingrained.

The Kibbutz had tried to enlarge this "we," but that was all: A bigger we against "they." What Evan believed to be needed was a child-rearing system that would never allow the boundary to be formed separating the "we" from the "they" at all. According to his plan, children—all children, so there would be no stigma or sense of loss—would be reared in different families, on a monthly, weekly, or even a daily cycle, if necessary. This way, the only thing they could "imprint" on was what was invariant in all that flux, namely, that these were all human beings.

When Evan described this system to outsiders, they were shocked. "It would be like putting everyone in foster care! And we all know how damaging that is to the foster children." "It would be fascistic to take children away from their parents and force them to be reared by constantly changing strangers."

Evan had always dropped the topic when people said such things, not because he did not believe in the idea or could not think of a reply to the objections, but because he found their expressions of disapproval distressing.

For her part, Freida did not disapprove. After a while, neither did Freda. Together, they focused on this system more than they had focused on others. They worked out more of its ramifications and considered how they could implement such a system. They conjectured about its potential long-term effects on society. They concluded that it was feasible only in a closed system: An entire society, out of touch with any other society, would be required, so no contrast cases would exist that could give birth to a we/they boundary, or any sense of stigma, deprivation, or abnormality. Their prediction was that these children would mature into an altruistic society where everyone would share everything and prefer no one to any other: a society that socialists had previously hoped a mere change in political system could effect. They believed that to accomplish their goal, society would have to modify human nature, not genetically, by rearranging our selfish genes, and not through behavioral engineering, by rescheduling our rewards and punishments, but by reshaping our brains through universal early experience.

After considerable contemplation about these matters, an series of events transpired, more serendipitous than planned, which put Evan's system into action. Freida had no special genius to implement this system. Although chance that had thrown her together with a population of disaffected ACLU lawyers and clerks, she singled out a subset of them who were unmarried, childless, and not in committed relationships. She conducted seminars and expounded Evan's to this growing circle, some of whom came from quite prosperous families. Before long, they believed that they had reached a critical mass and determined that they were ready to establish a colony that would implement the "aggregates-in-flux." They pooled funds and conducted negotiations with a slightly dotty English Lord who owned an offshore island near the UK that had legal independent-nation status.

Before meeting Freida and Evan, this Lord had not had much of an agenda for his little country. He had populated it with his household servants and hangers-on, but he owned many other properties and was prepared to decamp in favor of this Utopian experiment that went far beyond his expectations (and far beyond his ability to understand abstractions). He gave them, without charge, leasehold for 100 years for the Republic of Huma, as they decided to call it.

The initial population of Huma was mostly American, but recruits also came from many other countries. They were mostly intellectuals, but with a reasonable blend of subsistence skills among them. They numbered approximately 10,000 individuals, childless, of breeding age, with approximately 50 percent of each gender. All agreed that, just as they would rear their progeny in constant flux, their mating and pairing would be in constant flux, too. Freida and Evan joined them. Like the others, they bade farewell to their families, explaining that their experiment depended critically on making sure that Huma was a closed system, with no outside influences.

At first blush, the implementation proved successful. They had selected the 10,000 members of the founder population well. By temperament and ideology, and even by their previous practices, they were all well attuned to this new system. They were comfortable with constantly changing partners, and they were ready to give up their biological offspring, including any knowledge or trace of the connection. No one tried to trace connections between children and birth parents because no one—not the parents who had opted for the system or the children who knew no other reality because of their aggregates-in-flux background—cared. The children grew into exactly the kind of humanists that Evan had predicted they would become.

What became of Evan and Freida? Soon after they arrived, as was everyone else, they were required to split up to form other bonds, and they did. Or, I should say, they tried. Freida succeeded. Contacting previous partners was not strictly forbidden as contacting biological children was, but it was strongly discouraged. Organizers assumed that the Huma population was large enough to minimize lifetime re-couplings if the average coupling duration lasted only a few months, weeks, or even days. Accordingly, Evan and Freida ran across one another occasionally, but when Evan proposed their third re-coupling, Freida said she did not think it would be a good idea.

Evan did not protest Freida's refusal, but he found that he was not as able to detach from his previous relationship, as others appeared to be. He found that when he chose, or was chosen by, or assigned to, new partners, he continued to think of Freida. He lost sexual interest in new partners quite quickly, sometimes before he had sexual contact at all. He lost interest in other things as well. He assumed that among the growing ranks of Human youngsters were some children of his. He obsessively scrutinized children he encountered to see whether he could detect any family resemblance—he sometimes thought he could—but children would just look at him with the same bland, friendly look, so he gave up.

Against accepted practice, Evan kept contacting Freida. He asked her whether she was having any of these kinds of feelings that plagued him. She was surprised, because he had never appeared interested in such matters before, even during their pre-Human days. She replied, honestly, no. She thought more about how, now that the experiment had proven so successful, they could spread it to the rest of the world. She suggested that Evan, as the originator of the theory, might now turn his intellectual skills to that task. She suggested that planning might get his mind off these other uncomfortable distractions.

Although Humans tended to detach themselves from their accomplishments in the same way, they detached themselves from their partners and their progeny, Freida proposed informing the Humans that Evan was their founder. She hoped that acknowledgment and acclaim might lift Evan's spirits encourage him to recommit to his brainchild. Evan acquiesced, but only to please Freida. He fixed his hopes more on Freida's feelings for him than on any social acclaim for his contribution. He remained pained by Freida's distance and her preoccupation with enlarging the experiment that he perceived as having failed.

When the Aggregate-Counsel convened, to which Freida would Evan as the Founder, he found himself feeling worse. He felt he did not understand these Humans. They appeared so distant from him and from one another, so aloof, so cerebral.

Evan contemplated leaving Huma, but all he wanted was Freida, and he knew that if nothing could bring her closer, his leaving could only drive her farther away. He tried to think of an abstract solution, but abstraction failed him. He found he could not even recall what had been the system-building's obsessive appeal for all those ears. Everything he called to mind appeared meaningless, empty, and hopeless.

Huma had some medical facilities. After his breakdown following the Counsel, Freida arranged Evan's admission for psychiatric help. A routine blood test identified significantly elevated BUN levels. X-rays showed that one kidney had already failed and the other was enlarged and near collapse. There was no dialysis unit on Huma, so the doctors shipped him to mainland United Kingdom and hospitalized him in the Chalybeate hospital. When his two sisters flew to see him, they found that his conversation had already become incoherent.

Part Two

THE NEUROBIOLOGY AND/OR
PSYCHOLOGY OF MORAL THOUGHT

Seven

BENUMBING AND MORAL EXALTATION IN DEADLY MARTYRS: A VIEW FROM NEUROSCIENCE

Adolf Tobeña

Of all the differences between man and the lower animals, the moral sense or conscience is by far the most important. This sense has a rightful supremacy over every other principle of human action; it is summed up in that short but imperious word ought, so full of high significance. It is the most noble of all the attributes of man, leading him without a moment's hesitation to risk his life for that of a fellow creature; or after due deliberation, impelled simply by the deep feeling of right or duty, to sacrifice it in some great cause.[1]

Suicide attacks, through their unpredictability and devastating potential, have become one of the most disturbing weapons of our day. Since their tremendously lethal nature was demonstrated in the attacks of 11 September 2001 on New York City and Washington, D. C., we have had no shortage of volunteers eager to emulate such deeds—as was only to be expected that the vulnerability of the North American giant was demonstrated. The tactic of suicide attacks has since become widespread and all too common in several of the world's hotspots. Despite the efforts invested in preventing this type of attack, they have also—occasionally but with ominous consequences—been carried out in more peaceful parts of the planet. Nowadays, the possibility that weapons of mass destruction might fall into the hands of an organization capable of harboring suicide bombers is a major concern for security services around the world. We live under a threat that, in the end, hangs on the determination and nerve of a handful of individuals: the combative cell that provides a home for the phenomenon of suicide terrorism.[2] Given that suicide attacks depend, ultimately, on conviction—on events that occur in the brain of an individual—it may be useful to consider such behavior from the perspective of neuroscience. Remember, suicide for non-combative purposes has been and continues to be a compulsory area of study for clinicians—although this form of self-destruction has little to do with the behavior of interest here. Recent advances in the neurobiology of morality may help to shed some light on the exceptional behavior of these deadly martyrs.

Among the most bewildering aspects of the behavior of deadly martyrs, one is especially striking, namely, the moral boundaries established by those who carry out suicide attacks. They usually share these boundaries with mem-

bers of their cell or group and with a sector of the society in which the phenomenon is bred.[3] Kamikazes do not only plan and carry out horrific massacres
with the utter conviction that they are doing good, but also act in accordance
with values and beliefs associated with what they regard as the greatest good.[4]
They kill in the name of supreme justice and duty. They exterminate in obedience to infinite and impartial Providence, or having given themselves up to
the orders of their just and discerning guides. Deadly martyrs are the most
spectacular examples of an impregnable morality towards a person's group,
which co-exists, without any apparent contradiction, alongside a radical amorality towards members of another group. The inter-group barrier delimits the
domain of moral behavior. Their fellow community members regard suicide
killers as heroes and hail them as paragons of virtue, while their targets regard
them as cold-hearted butchers.

Treating the "other" as an object is a necessary condition for this intimate
relationship between deadliness and virtue to be established.[5] Strategists know
that teaching soldiers to suppress empathy for adversaries is expedient in military confrontations. Training to suppress empathy has undoubtedly been a factor
in the long history of deadly hostilities between human groups. In the age of
smart weapons that enable selective strikes with exquisite accuracy from great
distances without face-to-face confrontation, suppressing empathy remains
part of the training of frontline forces and, more often than not, the indoctri-
nating propaganda of the populations who stand behind them. To be effective in
combat, the closer soldiers get to such predatory urges the better. When we view
our opponent as vermin suitable for capture or extermination, empathy or other
inhibitions typically induced by learning to respect others counts for nothing.

These suicide martyrs who attack take an additional step in this paradoxical combination of moral and amoral tendencies, namely, a total disdain
for existence per se—the irremissible squandering of individual interests in
the pursuit of communal justice. Such waste has lately taken on an obscene
form in the explosive self-dismemberment of suicide bombers. In this way,
the immediate family of the martyr may be ennobled and have honors or advantages bestowed upon them, yet those who sacrifice themselves have no firm
guarantees that this will be the case, even when they act under contract. The
only sure thing is their contribution without recompense to group interests.
Consequently, an especially challenging area of enquiry into moral convictions
faces us.

1. The Origins of Morality

In addressing this issue from a biological perspective, we must begin by referring to Charles Darwin, who believed that human morality was usually restricted to the confines of the group.[6] Despite being the author of the eloquent
statement with which I began this text, a few pages later in the same essay, he
offers a host of examples through which he proclaims insistently that the
moral sense of human beings is not extended to all their fellows. Tribal limits

usually mark out the territory of confrontation where the ties of sympathy, affection, and the exchange of favors which sustain moral inclinations and obligations are rudely extinguished. He was the first to discern that frequent wars between neighboring groups could induce the selection of the most demanding loyalties in many individuals—a conjecture that has regained favor in recent decades despite having been overlooked for most of the twentieth century.[7]

Yet long before he addressed this issue, Darwin had already sought to bring down the lofty pretensions of that most moral of animals, proposing connections with the behavior of other social animals and putting forward different conjectures as to why the peculiar obligations towards our fellows that we call morality should arise. In his words:

> Any animal whatever, endowed with well-marked social instincts, the parental and filial affections being here included, would inevitably acquire a moral sense or conscience, as soon as its intellectual powers had become as well, or nearly as well developed, as in man. For, firstly, the social instincts lead an animal to take pleasure in the society of its fellows, to feel a certain amount of sympathy with them, and to perform various services for them. . . . Secondly, as soon as the mental faculties had become highly developed, images of all past actions and motives would be incessantly passing through the brain of each individual. . . . Thirdly, after the power of language had been acquired, and the wishes of the community could be expressed, the common opinion how each member ought to act for the public good would naturally become in a paramount degree the guide to action. . . . Lastly, habit in the individual would ultimately play a very important part in guiding the conduct of each member; for the social instinct, together with sympathy, is, like any other instinct, greatly strengthened by habit, and so consequently would be obedience to the wishes and judgment of the community.[8]

This passage provides us with a well-developed working hypothesis with which to enquire into the origins of moral behavior. Darwin equated the foundations of human morality to the following sum of factors: sociability + recognition of emotions in fellows + regular exchange of services + obedience to the wishes of the community. These attributes depend on a brain developed enough to make them viable, a brain with sufficient neurocomputational power to enable these mechanisms to work and achieve the necessary subtle balances during private self-scrutiny (conscience), those which we perceive in the form of scruples, inclinations and obligations.

Table 1 shows the pioneering conjectures of Darwin alongside the mechanisms of biological selection that have since been demonstrated, both in terms of ultimate functionality (adaptive strategies) and the ordinary operations, that support it (behavior and its neural mechanisms). We can see that Darwin's view was correct. Bear in mind that the aim of convincingly elucidating the origins of altruism became a fundamental problem in evolutionary thought because explaining the genesis of cooperative behavior at the expense of individual interests, including pro-group sacrifice, was necessary. Although debate about most of the mechanisms shown in Table 1 has tended to diminish as we have gathered new evidence, controversy continues to rage over the viability of pro-group altruism.[9]

Table 1. Human Moral Behavior

Definition: By human behavior is meant behavior, attitudes, desires and beliefs that take into account the interests of fellow human beings.	
In animals with social instincts, and whose intellectual powers are developed enough to enable them to contemplate the result of interactions with their fellows, cooperative tendencies and moral conscience should come about through selection.[10]	
Darwinian Conjectures	**Biological Selection**
Origin of Moral Conscience	*Demonsrated Mechanisms*
Parental/filial affection	Nepotism (kin selection)
Exchange of services/fulfilling obligations	Direct reciprocity (reciprocal altruism)
Reputation in the group/community	Indirect reciprocity
Obedience to social norms	Altruism induced by punishment
Loyalty/pro-group sacrifice	Group selection
Abstract moral principles	???
Neural Pre-Requisites	
Recognition of fellows and markers of identity	
Detection/expression of social emotions (affection, empathy, guilt)	
Operational memory for comparing/weighing up and predicting the results of social interactions	
Traits of temperament (loyalty, obedience, credulity)	

The main body of results from studies of animal behavior, computer simulations of evolutionary contests, and experiments with human beings indicates that forms of altruism which are non-nepotistic and not based on direct reciprocity do exist;[11] some propensities toward establishing cooperative relationships go beyond biological filiations, the exchange of favors, and the weighing up of returns. Non-restricted altruism exists and is perpetuated because different mechanisms maintain it: the generation of reputation, intra-group size and signaling, moralizing punishment, and unconditional trust.[12] Altruism at a price and without guaranteed returns occurs because it tends to promote gains in biological revenues, not only for the recipients of help but also for the givers. This principle does not apply in cases (like our object of study here) where the givers perish too soon as a result of their exaggerated investments, yet these strategies of cooperation at a price do prove worthwhile for those givers who stay around.

So we must take into account the trait of altruism and be able to measure, reliably, individual differences in it.[13] This should be our starting point. For the existence of this trait implies that among all populations will be pockets of extreme altruists willing to make high-cost investments of trust in others, investments that involve great personal risk. Until recently, the prevailing models in biology and economics were determined to discard this supposition because in all populations are systematic egoists able to take advantage of the propensity toward innocence and sacrifice of genuine givers. Despite these quite unflattering views regarding the place of extravagant generosity in the process of evolution, mechanisms exist that geared nature toward fostering and maintaining it.[14]

2. A Neuroimage of Moral Decisions

When an awareness of "duty" and "sacrifice" accompanies behavior, a uniquely human form of some attributes faces us. This has firm adaptive foundations and reflects selective forces operating at different levels. Neurobiological research ignored this conscious state of moral inclinations for many years, due, among other things, to a lack of procedures for carrying out reliable empirical investigations in the area. For too long, the work of evolutionary biologists, aimed at outlining the adaptive means required to explain variability in altruism, remained disconnected from that of psychologists and neurobiologists, who sought to describe the mechanisms behind behavior and social cognition. In recent years, the situation has taken a radical turn and the area of research known as the cognitive neuroscience of morality is now a hive of activity.[15] The first stimuli for this shift came from the renewed interest in neurological patients with selective deficits or anomalies in moral decision making,[16] and from there, attention switched to the exploration of pro-social and moral inclinations in many different areas. Research teams brought together neurologists, radiologists, philosophers, engineers, and other professional fields with an interest in these unsolved enigmas.

In recent decades, researchers have designed several procedures to obtain quantitative measures of moral decisions. One of the most useful methods in developing this kind of "experimental ethics" poses moral dilemmas, problems whose possible solutions affect the interests of other people and where subjects are asked to make a decision, which they can not retract. By introducing variations into these dilemmas, or by presenting different versions sequentially, we can analyze response trends and individual differences. As some of these problems are simple and can be presented in the form of brief texts on a screen, the process of moral decision making has become a topic of study within the field of neuroimaging. A team of researchers from Princeton University first carried out this type of enquiry in a study comparing two dilemmas, which have proved to be a headache for philosophers concerned with the origin of ethical values.[17]

The first of these, known as the trolley dilemma, is formulated as follows: a runaway trolley will kill five people on the track ahead if it continues on its course. The only way to avoid this is by hitting a switch, inside the trolley or at the control center that will turn the trolley onto a side track where it

will kill one person who happens to be crossing at that moment. Nobody in
the trolley will be injured in either scenario. The dilemma is whether to hit the
switch and change the course of the trolley is a right action. Most people respond by saying that, under these circumstances, to sacrifice the life of one
person to save the other five is acceptable. Many possible variations on the
dilemma have been formulated: changing the number of people, changing the
relationship to, or familiarity with, the people to be saved or sacrificed, or
introducing different degrees of chance (instead of a passerby crossing the
road at just the wrong moment, a man could be working on the overhead
power lines), among other variables, able to add interest to the dilemma. We
are concerned here with the results of the basic situation where most people
opt to deliberately sacrifice one person to save the lives of the other five about
to be run over by the tram.

The second problem, known as the footbridge dilemma, derives from
the first: a runaway trolley will kill five people before it hits the buffers at the
end of the line. No way to avoid the event is possible. You are standing on a
footbridge over the tracks and realize what will happen. You then notice that
next to you is a large stranger leaning over the rail to see what's going on below. If you push the stranger onto the tracks, killing him, his bulky body will
stop the trolley from reaching the others, saving five lives. Nobody in the trolley will be injured in either alternative. Do you push the stranger onto the
tracks to save five lives? Under these circumstances, most people change their
mind and judge it not right to use the life of one person to save five others.
These results pose a puzzling enigma: human beings tend to consider it acceptable to sacrifice deliberately the life of one person in exchange for five
when all it requires is the flick of a switch, but not when it would involve a
direct act to sacrifice an actual person.

Given that the costs and benefits are the same in both situations, what
produces this radical switch in most people's moral criterion? Apparently, we
cannot explain the evidence by recourse to ethical theories. The team of
neurobiologists at Princeton hypothesized that the second dilemma leads to
greater emotional involvement than the first due to the proximity of, and contact with, the victim, thereby changing most people's moral criterion. To test
this hypothesis, they decided to use functional magnetic resonance imaging
(fMRI) to scan subjects while they were resolving the dilemmas.

Their first experiment involved nine university students (five men and
four women) who gave their informed consent to participate in the sessions.
Investigators presented each of them with sixty dilemmas, which appeared on
a screen visible from inside the fMRI tube. Each dilemma involved three
screen stages: the statement, the question, and, on the final screen, the words
"appropriate" and "inappropriate." All the dilemmas lasted a maximum of
forty-five seconds; they measured reaction times in each case, along with
whole and regional brain activity during the decision-making period.

They presented the sixty dilemmas at random, but each belonged to one
of three conditions comprised of twenty dilemmas in each: Group 1: per-

sonal/close (with greater emotional involvement), comprising variations of the footbridge dilemma and equivalents; Group 2: impersonal/distant (variations on the trolley dilemma and equivalents) with less emotional charge; and Group 3: non-moral dilemmas (harmless choices, such as taking the subway instead of the bus into town, or having dinner at a Chinese instead of a Thai restaurant). The results indicated that Group 1 dilemmas significantly increased brain activity in areas associated with emotional regulation: the medial frontal gyrus, the posterior cingulate gyrus, and the angular gyrus. In contrast, Group 2 produced increased brain activity in areas concerned with working memory, but with no appreciable increases in areas of emotional regulation. All these results were compared with baseline activation levels in harmless dilemmas (Group 3).

A second experiment performed with nine new subjects replicated the data in terms of regional brain activation, lending further support to the findings. The researchers also studied the relationship between reaction times and the type of response to the dilemmas presented. In personal/close dilemmas subjects found it much more difficult (a delay of around one second more) to give the response "appropriate" instead of "inappropriate," while they observed the opposite trend with impersonal/distant dilemmas. Those subjects who opted to give the fateful push in the footbridge dilemma took longer to reach this decision, as did those who considered it inappropriate to hit a switch and change the course of the trolley in the first dilemma. These data lend support to the initial assumption that the emotional charge associated with a situation interferes with, and modulates, moral decisions. Through additional control studies using much more demanding dilemmas (involving the sacrifice of a parent's child) the authors demonstrated that the results obtained were not due to majority or minority bias. This research opens a door to the analysis of the neural mechanisms underlying moral values. In what follows, we will consider other ways to approach the questions.

3. The Neuroradiology of Cooperative Interactions

The ultimatum game is one of the experimental situations used by economists to study egoistic or altruistic choices in social interactions. It is a one-time and non-negotiable game that consists in a "take it or leave it" offer. The simplicity of the approach has led researchers to use neuroimaging techniques with subjects in order to monitor their brain activity while they are making decisions.[18]

In the ultimatum game, participants receive a sum of money which they can keep on the condition that they offer a fraction of it to another participant to whom the participant has just been introduced immediately prior to commencing the experiment. Both the first (the Proposer) and the second player (the Responder) will have carefully read the rules of the game: these are that if the Responder freely accepts the Proposer's offer, then they both keep the share agreed. If the Responder rejects the offer, neither of them gets anything and the experimenter keeps the money. No negotiation or opportunity to change your mind is allowed. Players are situated in separate cubicles and make their responses via a computer terminal. Several rounds are usually played, but always with different subjects to respect the rules of the game. The supposed rationality that people use in optimizing costs and benefits and on which economic theory is based would predict that Responders should accept any offer because something is always better than nothing is. Likewise, Proposers, assuming such rationality in the Responder, should propose a deal favorable to them, as they alone decide how to distribute shares of the money.

Such studies of experimental economics have found that these predictions are not borne out by reality. A majority of Responders prefer to do without a cash gift if this prevents a stranger from keeping the lion's share in a deal regarded as unfair: offers giving 20 percent of the total to the Responder have a 50 percent chance of being rejected, while for those offering less than 20 percent the rejection rate rises sharply and may exceed 70 percent. Put in another way, under these circumstances, over 50 percent of subjects punished a fellow human being even at the expense of personal loss. This situation is a glaring example of altruistic punishment: a palpable cost with no benefit other than having defeated the plans of another whom they deemed to be taking unfair advantage. [19]

Proposers, in reality, anticipate such behavior and tend to make offers close to an equal share; this has proved to be the case in most experiments carried out in different parts of the world, although we observe some variations depending on culture and relationships to money. Feedback from participants given after the experiments suggests a sense of indignation leads to the altruistic punishment: any interest in making a quick buck is abandoned in favor of a desire to reject a share regarded as unfair. This is an illustration of circumstances in which participants resolve a genuine dilemma where emotional reactions (spite, envy, scorn) modulate the opportunity for financial gain.

The neuroimaging studies consisted in exploring the brain activity of nineteen subjects who received ultimatum proposals from ten Proposers whom they had met briefly just prior to the brain scans being carried out. [20] Once inside the fMRI scanner, they received, via a screen and in a sequence identical for each round, the offers to be accepted or rejected. They made selections by pushing a button situated within hand's reach. After twelve seconds of preparation, the photograph and name of one of the ten Proposers appeared, for seconds, on the screen. The proposed share then appeared and the Responder, from inside the magnet, had six seconds to reach a decision. Once they accepted or rejected the offer, the winnings of each player (or loss of the gift) was shown on the screen. This procedure was repeated in consecutive rounds with the different Proposers were interspersed at random with both analogous offers made by a computer program (in this case the screen showed the image of a laptop acting as the Proposer) and control runs where Responders tried to win the amount shown on the screen by responding as quickly as indicated (no dilemma was present in these cases). Each scanned subject underwent thirty sequences in all, the handouts coming from an initial pot of ten dollars per round provided by the experimenters. The accumulated amounts at the end of each session were sufficient recompense for the participants.

In terms of the decisions subjects made, the results were consistent with previous research, and in this sense, the brain scan equipment did not prove to be a constraint. Equal offers (five dollars for each player) were accepted without hesitation, whatever their source, while those giving seven dollars to the Proposer and three dollars to the Responder produced the excellent acceptance rate of 90 percent. Offers of eight dollars for the Proposer and two dollars for the Responder were only accepted half the time (50 percent rejection), while those giving nine dollars to the Proposer and just one dollar to the Responder produced a rejection rate of 70 percent. These results confirm the tendency to punish unfair offers even when this means losing money. A good number of Responders decided to apply an analogous criterion of altruistic punishment, albeit weaker, to some of the offers made by the computer: 20 percent of subjects decided against keeping the two dollars offered by the program when the computer was going to keep eight dollars for itself, and almost half chose to reject the single dollar if the computer kept nine dollars. These results confirm the unique power of the drift toward a sense of equal justice shown by many human beings. This drift is not solely a human prerogative, as some primates also reject unfair deals in circumstances where they obtain a reward for little or no effort.[21] These rejections include primates doing without tasty food when their companion in the interaction has been rewarded ostentatiously with something better.

Returning to the ultimatum experiment, the brain areas showing increased activity in the face of unfair offers were the dorsolateral prefrontal cortex, the anterior cingulate gyrus, and the anterior insula. Increased neural activity in the first two areas probably corresponds to the cognitive effort involved in weighing up complex options (prefrontal circuits) in a conflictive dilemma situation (cingulate circuits): unfair offers meet these requirements because, when subjects contemplate rejection, they involve the loss of a gift out of consideration for moral compensation.

Previous studies of the functions of these brain areas support this assumption. The most interesting result is without doubt the bilateral activation of the anterior insula. Research has associated these areas with the processing of physical disgust, unpleasant reactions to olfactory or taste stimuli that, ordinarily, people find disgusting or repugnant.[22] If these results are confirmed in subsequent studies of economic games, it will demonstrate that the neural circuits involved in producing feelings of disgust at the sight or consumption of food, or in response to unpleasant body odors, are the same as those used to process feelings of indignation at the unfair behavior of another human being. This makes perfect sense in terms of saving neural resources. Studies such as these are opening up the field of neuroeconomics,[23] one which has already produced strong evidence relating the development of trust between individuals in financial interactions to the selective activation of pleasure areas in the brain and the secretion of neurohormones that modulate responses such as attachment and affective proximity.[24]

4. The Neuroimagery of Amorality

The possibility of working with normative individuals to study moral decision making constitutes a significant advance, because until recently, research into the biology of human morality depended heavily on data obtained from people with mental disorders or those with lesions in designated brain areas. This long tradition of studies in people with selective brain lesions has been significant in providing useful clues. The combination of clinical and anatomical evidence from patients with singularly conflictive behavior and measurable neural anomalies has enabled different brain systems to be identified as substrates for the crystallization of moral values.[25] The appearance of reasoning and normative moral reactions depends necessarily on particular brain areas and circuits being intact; if they are damaged in some way, striking deficits in moral behavior, hard to remedy, arise—even though the ability to perceive the content, meaning, and value of social conventions and ethical norms remains unimpaired. Lesions in designated areas of the brain leave fully intact motor, sensory, and perceptive functions, such as memory, language, and most aspects of cognitive acuity, but produce deficits in or the absence of moral behavior.

These results are especially evident in children who have suffered lesions in designated areas of the prefrontal cortex (in the more anterior, medial, and basal regions of the cerebral hemispheres) at extremely early ages. When such lesions occur in an already developed brain, patients conserve their memory of norms and may agree entirely with other people when asked about moral limits in different situations, even though this is often not borne out by their behavior. We should conclude, therefore, that in these patients, the learning of moral boundaries has been able to occur and take root, despite the subsequent lesion resulting in repeated transgressions of such inhibitory boundaries. In the few children studied in similar conditions and over their development into adults, not even awareness of norms appears to have been properly implanted.[26] Not only do they regularly transgress ordinary moral boundaries but also they show signs of never having learned them and an absence of guilt or remorse over their behavior. In any case, despite the power of these results, this type of lesion probably produces gross or indirect alterations in the circuits responsible, in intact brains, for moral decision-making processes. These results open the door for studies using ordinary subjects of the neural correlates of that particular set of attitudes and decisions, which we term moral behavior and to studies of amoral behavior and propensities.

The area of emotions may again prove relevant, just as we saw with the studies involving dilemmas. Ordinary people changed their moral criterion according to the degree of empathy invoked by the situation: in terms of the disaster about to be caused by the runaway trolley, the emotional closeness or distance from the person to be sacrificed modified subjects' reaction to the suffering of others and their subsequent choice of action. Empathy is a crucial emotion in defining moral and amoral reactions because it is part of the basis of sociability. This capability to tune into the happiness or suffering of others was, for Darwin, the first requisite of well-founded social instincts. We now have a substantial body of research concerning the neural mechanisms underlying empathic attributes in both animals and human beings.[27] Alongside empathy a wide range of moral emotions (disdain, indignation, guilt, remorse, shame) may be evoked by positive and negative interactions with others, by the obligations established during these interactions, and by the contrast between expectations and outcomes—emotions increasingly beginning to be addressed by researchers.[28] Like empathy, these emotions also influence moral decisions, especially in interactions that imply key commitments between those involved, is reasonable. Under such circumstances, the role of pretense and lying is crucial, and neural-based methods for detecting this are already beginning to bear fruit.[29]

In the future, we are likely to see a proliferation of studies that put normative individuals in different frames of mind involving moral emotions and decisions while simultaneously scanning their brain activity with sufficiently powerful neuroimaging and computer equipment. Some researchers have used a procedure in which they present subjects with vignettes showing conflictive interactions between different people (abusers and abused, or executioners and their victims) and then ask them to evaluate the scenarios on specially designed scales. The results of studies conducted with children and adolescents have already served to establish quantitative degrees of morality.[30] Such approaches are easily applied even with neuroimaging equipment and some preliminary findings have already been reported.[31] Research must also address situations that more closely reflect real personal involvement and the conditions of everyday life because a sizeable body of data evinces substantial differences between subjects' responses to abstract dilemmas and vignettes as opposed to circumstances that touch upon their real lives.[32] The degree of suffering caused by temporary social rejection in video games designed for entertainment purposes, in which different players take part, has also been studied using neuroimaging equipment,[33] suggesting that even the recourse to ostracism as a form of social punishment can be investigated using such apparatus. The door is wide open and I hope that research in this field focuses on adolescents and young people as they are usually at the forefront of combative cells fostering harmful tactics.

5. Moral Deficiency, Hypermorality, and Fanaticism

We can now return to our objective of shedding light on the origins of deadly martyrs. The passionate belief in a doctrine widens the gap between groups, a gap which, as a matter of course, already serves to limit cooperative behavior and feelings of solidarity. This form of combative fervor, fanatical sectarianism, usually takes root within tiny pockets of society, but occasionally, and with an all-encompassing vigor, it colors the beliefs of large communities. The sectarian creed governs so strongly inside the bubble of its associated doctrine that the propensities and decisions produced therein are often incomprehensible to those who contemplate the process from the outside. This can lead to a state of moral deficiency, for not only is irreparable damage done to those who remain outside the realm of "undisputed virtue" (the exo-group) but outrages are also committed against those suspected of dissidence within the confines of "virtue"—barbarities that may even come to affect members of the same family or the local neighborhood. Indoctrination can result in people's inclinations going beyond the most basic social instincts, the tendencies that serve to build the most peremptory links in the chain of morality (for example, cases of young-mother suicide bombers in Palestine whose actions irreparably condemn their children to be orphans). Indoctrination can modify people's moral inclinations and obligations to such an extent that it leads to behavior patterns comparable to those observed in people with personality disorders.

The notion of "moral deficiency" underlies the first attempts to describe those singular variants on human temperament termed psychopathy.[34] The core characteristic of this type of personality is precisely the striking lack of moral emotions. Although psychopaths are peculiar people, they do not stand distinctly apart from the profuse variety of human character. Their highly special temperament has yet to be associated with ostensible brain lesions, despite their having been subjected to detailed studies in the search for them.

Much evidence has recently been reported about possible disorders of functioning and connectivity in the same neural circuits that, when damaged, produce amoral behavior.[35] Although these data are obviously meaningful, we should not presently regard them as definitive because the methods used to access these subtle aspects of brain functioning still lack the necessary degree of resolution. In contrast, studies of emotional reactions in individuals with a psychopathic temperament do provide consistent profiles. Such research suggests these subjects to be people perfectly capable of developing intense desires and of feeling joy, boredom, or rage, to give some examples of everyday emotions, but who find it difficult to experience guilt, remorse, or shame in a genuine way: they struggle with the shades of emotion normally associated with interactions in which somebody, usually someone from the immediate environment, is hurt. Lack of empathy with, or sympathy for others' suffering, and a radical absence of fear accompany all of this. These two attributes are likely the most important, because the memory traces generated by empathic reactions, together with the outcomes of interactions with others, enable moral emotions of greater depth and scope to be crystallized than is the case through more fleeting connections. The lack of fear prevents such people from developing a sense of anticipatory caution with regard to social punishment. As individuals, they are decidedly unable to make powerful commitments (loyalties) and are not bothered by their lack of compliance or transgression. Their engaging in predatory or shameless behavior is highly likely, giving rise to the term, "moral deficiency." Such people engage in behavior that entails not only great risk to others but also, in the event that they are caught, to themselves.[36] We find some are capable of combining these unique emotional profiles with a gift for persuasion and an ability to lie so astute and assured that they avoid being reprimanded in any way and end up holding influential positions in society.

The moral deficits of deadly martyrs are strictly unilateral. They only share with psychopaths one side or aspect of predatory behavior, limits of which are marked out by doctrine. The benumbing or annulment of empathic responses is applied only to those on the other side of the gap, which separates them from the world of virtue, to members of the exo-group. Inside the realm of doctrine, their behavior is the exact opposite and becomes exemplary, even hypermoral. Their fellow believers can expect to witness a commitment to the most tenacious and costly acts, which may culminate in self-sacrifice. Those drawn to martyrdom are readily exploited by those who preserve, under all circumstances, selfish interests. As a rule, psychopaths do not usually squander their personal choices on group commitments. On the contrary, exploitive others use their gift for simulating altruism for individual gain without any other kind of consideration. Potential martyrs, on the other hand, are, by definition squanderers. Although they share with psychopaths some aspects of moral benumbing, the two phenomena are quite distinct.[37] Whereas psychopaths are dangerous predators or pure villains by nature, martyrs tend to be gullible souls with a "beneficent" predisposition that fails to prevent—in such cases it does just the opposite—them from leaving a host of victims in their wake upon offering themselves up as weapons of sectarian combat. We are dealing here with a form of deadly altruism, a collateral and highly damaging drift away from the cooperative tendencies of human beings, one that requires a detailed understanding.

6. Work Suggestions

We have characterized the phenomenon of the deadly martyr as a peculiar aspect of moral behavior. If this is a suitable approach, then the detailed description of brain mechanisms associated with morality may prove crucial. We have seen that areas and systems are present in the human brain responsible for processing moral sensibility. These neural areas present a progressively demarcated functional specificity. Therefore, Darwin's criterion for the development of a moral sense and conscience in animals with well-founded social instincts is met, namely, a brain sufficiently developed to enable individuals to recognize their fellows, read their fellows' emotions, and to remember and weigh up the outcomes of interactions. Consequently, we have already taken the first step.

We now have available procedures that offer a tentative way into that remote area of conscious self-scrutiny concerned with scruples and moral obligations. The complex road ahead involves teasing apart the subtleties of moral sensibility and its connections with neural mechanisms. To monitor the stages of moral sensibility during human development and to study patterns of individual variability will be especially key.

In the future, we will likely see research conducted on evaluating moral discernment and its concomitant brain functioning in people selected for their heightened doctrinaire leanings (for traits such as loyalty, credulity, radicalism, or sectarianism). By this, I mean that we must develop an experimental program to address the paradoxical co-existence of benumbing and moral exaltation characteristic of those prepared to sacrifice themselves for the good of the group. We require data, for example, on empathic perception with regard to the suffering of members of the exo-group, comparing normative with sectarian individuals. Likewise, we must further our understanding of the links between biologically-rooted markers of group identity and mechanisms of neurocognitive biases, as doctrinal creeds usually exploit this interdependence to widen the gap between one group and another.[38] This kind of evidence should serve to support, much more strongly, the approach suggested in this chapter. Suffice it to say that this is a real possibility.

In sum, I believe we should take seriously the contributions of neuroscience in a field traditionally reserved for the social sciences, because our lack of knowledge about the forces which mold deadly martyrs and those who encourage them is proving far too costly.[39]

Acknowledgment

This paper was the original source of material analyzed at length in Adolf Tobeña, *Mártires Mortíferos: Biologia del Altruismo Letal* (*Deadly Martyrs: The Biology of Lethal Altruism*) (Valencia, Spain: Bromera Publish.-Valencia University Press, 2004).

Notes

1. Charles Darwin, *The Descent of Man, and Selection in Relation to Sex* (Princeton, N.J.: Princeton University Press, 1981[1871]).

2. Scott Atran, "Genesis of Suicide Terrorism," *Science*, 299 (2003), pp. 1534–1539; and Paul C. Stern, "Why Do People Sacrifice for their Nations?" *Perspectives on Nationalism and War*, eds, John L. Comaroff and Paul C. Stern (Amsterdam: Gordon and Breach, 1997).

3. Atran, "Genesis of Suicide Terrorism"; and A. Merari, *Terrorismo Suicida* (*Suicide Terrorism*), Proceedings of the Conference: *Violencia, Mente y Cerebro* (Violence, Mind and Brain) (Valencia: Reina Sofía Centre for the Study of Violence, 2002), pp. 157–169.

4. Raphael Israeli, *Islamikaze: Manifestations of Islamic Martyrology* (New York: Frak Croos, 2003).

5. Steven R. Quartz and Terrence J. Sejnowski, *Liars, Lovers and Heroes: What the New Brain Science Reveals about How We Become Who We Are* (New York: William Morrow-Harper Collins, 2002); Matt Ridley, *The Origins of Virtue* (London: Viking, 1997); and Elliott Sober and David Sloan Wilson, *Unto Others: The*

Evolution and Psychology of Unselfish Behavior (Cambridge, Mass.: Harvard University Press, 1998).

6. Darwin, *The Descent of Man.*

7. Richard D. Alexander, *The Biology of Moral Systems* (New York: Aldine de Gruyter, 1987); Jane Goodall, *The Chimpanzees of Gombe: Patterns of Behavior* (Cambridge, Mass.: Harvard University Press, 1986); D. L. Krebs, "The Evolution of Moral Dispositions in the Human Species," *Evolutionary Perspectives on Human Reproductive Behavior*, Annals of the New York Academy of Sciences, eds. Dory Le-Croy and Peter Moller, 907 (2000), pp. 132–148; R. Paul Shaw and Yuwa Wong, *Genetic Seeds of Warfare: Evolution, Nationalism, and Patriotism* (Boston, Mass.: Unwin Hyman, 1989); Stern, "Why Do People Sacrifice for their Nations?"; and Richard W. Wrangham and Dale Peterson, *Demonic Males: Apes and the Origins of Human Violence* (New York: Houghton Mifflin, 1997).

8. Darwin, *The Descent of Man.*

9. Robert Boyd and Joan B. Silk, *How Humans Evolved* (New York: Norton, 2000); Richard Dawkins, *The Selfish Gene* (New York: Oxford University Press, 1976); E. Fehr and U. Fischbacher, "The Nature of Human Altruism," *Nature*, 425 (2003), pp. 785–791; Ridley, *The Origins of Virtue*; J. K. Rilling, D. A. Gutman, T. R. Zeh, G. Pagnoni, G. S. Berns, and C. D. Kilts, "A Neural Basis for Social Cooperation," *Neuron*, 35 (2002), pp. 395–405; S. W. West, I. Pen, A. S. Griffin, "Cooperation and Competition between Relatives," *Science*, 296 (2002), pp. 72–75; and Robert Wright, *The Moral Animal*: Evolutionary *Psychology and Everyday Life* (New York: Pantheon Books, 1994).

10. Darwin, *The Descent of Man.*

11. T. Clutton-Brock,"Breeding Together: Kin Selection and Mutualism in Co-operative Vertebrates," *Science*, 296 (2002), pp. 69–72; R. Heinshon and C. Parker, "Complex Cooperative Strategies in Group-Territorial African Lions," *Science*, 269 (1995), pp. 1260–1262; D. C. Queller, E. Ponte, S. Bozzaro, and J. E. Strassmann, "Single-Gene Greenbeard Effects in the Social Amoeba Dictyostelium Discoideum," *Science*, 299 (2003), pp. 105–106; T. Singer, B.Seymour, J. O'Doherty, H. Kaube, R. J. Dolan, and C. D. Frith, "Empathy for Pain Involves the Affective but not the Sensory Components of Pain," *Science*, 303 (2004), pp. 1157–62; and D. W. Stephens, C. M. McLinn, and J. R. Stevens, "Discounting and Reciprocity in an Iterated Prisoner's Dilemma," *Science*, 298 (2002), pp. 2216–2218.

12. R. Boyd and P. J. Richerson, "Punishment Allows the Evolution of Cooperation (or Anything Else) in Sizable Groups," *Ethology and Sociobiology*, 13 (1992), pp. 171–195; E. Fehr and S. Gachter, "Altruistic Punishment in Humans," *Nature*, 415 (2002), pp. 137–140; E. Fehr and B. Rockenbach, "Detrimental Effects of Sanctions on Human Altruism," *Nature*, 422 (2003), pp. 137–140; M. Millinski, D. Semmann and H. J. Krambeck, "Reputation Helps Solve the "Tragedy of the Commons," *Nature*, 415 (2002), pp. 424–426; M. A. Nowak and K. Sigmund, "Evolution of Indirect Reciprocity by Image Scoring," *Nature*, 393 (1998), pp. 573–577; R. L. Riolo, M. D. Cohen, and R. Axelrod, "Evolution of Cooperation without Reciprocity," *Nature*, 414 (2001), pp. 441–443; and Christopher Wilson, *Darwin's Cathedral: Evolution, Religion, and the Nature of Society* (Chicago, Ill.: Chicago University Press, 2002).

13. T. J. Bouchard, D. T. Lykken, M. McGue, N. Segal, and A. Tellegen, "Sources of Human Psychological Differences: The Minnesota Study of Twins Reared Apart," *Science*, 250 (1990), pp. 223–250; M. H. Davis, C. Luce, C. and S. J. Kraus, "The Heritability of Characteristics Associated with Dispositional Empathy," *Journal of Personality*, 62 (1994), pp. 369–391; and K. McCourt, T. J. Bouchard, D. T. Lykken, N. Tellegen, and M. Keyes, "Authoritarianism Revisited: Genetic and Environ-

mental Influences Examined in Twins Reared Apart and Together," *Personality and Individual Differences*, 27 (1999), pp. 985–1014.

14. Fehr and Fischbacher, "The Nature of Human Altruism"; A. Navarro, "Conflict and Cooperation in Human Affairs," Paper presented to the Universal Forum of Cultures, The Social Brain: Biology of Conflict and Cooperation, Barcelona, Spain, June 2004, see this volume chap. 14; and Sober and Sloan, *Unto Others*.

15. R. Adolphs, "Cognitive Neuroscience of Human Social Behavior," *Nature Reviews Neuroscience*, 4 (2003), pp. 165–177; and J. Haidt, "The Moral Emotions," *Handbook of Affective Sciences*, eds. Richard J. Davidson, Klaus R. Scherer and H. Hill Goldsmith (New York: Oxford University Press, 2002), pp. 852–870.

16. S. W. Anderson, A. Bechara, H. Damasio, D. Tranel, and A, Damasio, "Impairment of Social and Moral Behavior Related to Early Damage in Human Prefrontal Cortex," *Nature Neuroscience*, 2:11 (1999), pp. 1032–1037; and Adolf Tobeña, *Anatomía de la Agresividad Humana* (*Anatomy of Human Aggressiveness*) (Barcelona: Galaxia Gutenberg, 2001).

17. J. D. Greene, R. B. Sommerville, L. E. Nystrom, J. M. Darley, and J. D. Cohen, "An fMRI Investigation of Emotional Engagement in Moral Judgment," *Science*, 293 (2001), pp. 2105–2108.

18. Paul W. Glimsher, *Decisions, Uncertainty and the Brain: The Science of Neuroeconomics* (Cambridge, Mass.: The MIT Press, 2003).

19. Fehr and Gachter, "Altruistic Punishment in Humans."

20. A. G. Sanfey, J. K. Rilling, J. A. Aronson, L. E. Nystrom, and J. D. Cohen, "The Neural Basis of Economic Decision Making in the Ultimatum Game," *Science*, 300 (2003), pp.1755–1758.

21. S. F. Brosnan, and F. B. De Waal, "Monkeys Reject Unequal Pay," *Nature*, 425 (2003), pp. 297–299.

22. M. L. Phillips, A. W. Young, C. Senior, M. Brammer, C. Andrew, A. J. Calder, E. T. Bullmore, D. I. Perret, D. Rowland, S. C. R. Williams, J. A. Gray, and A. S. Davids, "A Specific Neural Substrate for Perceiving Facial Expressions of Disgust," *Nature*, 389 (1997), pp. 495–498.

23. C. F. Camerer, "Strategizing in the Brain," *Science*, 300 (2003), pp. 1673–1675; and Glimsher, *Decisions, Uncertainty and the Brain.*

24. Rilling, et al., "A Neural Basis for Social Cooperation."

25. Anderson, et al., "Impairment of Social and Moral Behavior"; and Tobeña, *Anatomía de la Agresividad Humana.*

26. Anderson, et al., "Impairment of Social and Moral Behavior."

27. Frans B. M. De Waal and Fieke Lakmaker, *Good Natured: The Origins of Right and Wrong in Humans and Other Animals* (Cambridge, Mass.: Harvard University Press, 1996); S. D. Preston and F. B. M. De Waal, "Empathy: Its Ultimate and Proximate Bases," *Behavioral and Brain Sciences*, 25:1 (2002), pp. 1–72; and Singer, et al., "Empathy for Pain Involves the Affective but not the Sensory Components of Pain."

28. Haidt, "The Moral Emotions."

29. V. E. Stone, L. Cosmides, J. Tooby, N. Kroll, and R. T. Knight," Selective Impairment of Reasoning about Social Exchange in a Patient with Bilateral Limbic System Damage, *Proceedings of the National Academy of Science*, 99:17 (2002), pp. 11531–11536.

30. R. J. R. Blair, "Moral Reasoning and the Child with Psychopathic Tendencies," *Personality and Individual Differences*, 22:5 (1997), pp. 731–739.

31. J. Moll, R. De Oliveira-Souza, P. J. Eslinger, I. E. Bramati, J. Mourao-Miranda, P. A. Andreioulo, and L. Pessoa, "The Neural Correlates of Moral Sensitiv-

ity: A Functional Magnetic Resonance Imaging Investigation of Basic and Moral Emotions," *Journal of Neuroscience*, 22 (2002), pp. 2730–36.

32. Krebs, "The Evolution of Moral Dispositions in the Human Species."

33. N. I. Eisenberger, M. D. Lieberman, and K. D. Williams, "Does Rejection Hurt? An fMRI Study of Social Exclusion," *Science*, 302 (2003), pp. 290–292.

34. Robert D. Hare, *Without Conscience: The Disturbing World of Psychopaths among Us* (London: Warner Books, 1994).

35. K. A. Kiehl, A. M. Smith, R. D. Hare, A, Mendrek, B. B. Forster, J. Brink, and P. F. Liddle, "Limbic Abnormalities in Affective Processing by Criminal Psychopaths as Revealed by Functional Magnetic Resonance Imaging," *Biological Psychiatry*, 50 (2001), pp. 677–684; and A. Raine, T. Leucz, S. Bihrle, L. Lacasse, and P. Polleti, "Reduced Prefrontal Gray Matter Volume and Reduced Autonomic Activity in Antisocial Personality Disorders," *Archives of General Psychiatry*, 57 (2000), pp. 745–751.

36. Tobeña, *Anatomía de la Agresividad Humana*.

37. R. F. Krueger,B. M. Hicks, and M. McGue, "Altruism and Antisocial Behavior: Independent Tendencies, Unique Personality Correlates, Distinct Etiologies," *Psychological Science*, 12 (2001), pp. 397–402; A. Tobeña, "Individual Factors in Suicidal Attacks," *Science*, 304:5667 (2004), p. 47; A. Tobeña, *Mártires Mortíferos: Biologia del Altruismo Letal (Deadly Martyrs: The Biology of Lethal Altruism)* (Barcelona, Spain: Tusquets Ed., forthcoming, 2004); and C. Tudge, "Natural Born Killers," *New Scientist*, 2342 (11 May 2002), pp. 36–39.

38. B. Sinervo, and J. Clobert, J. "Morphs, Dispersal Behavior, Genetic Similarity, and the Evolution of Cooperation," *Science*, 300 (2003), pp. 1949–1951; A. Tobeña, I. M. Marks, and R. Dar, "Advantages of Bias and Prejudice: An Exploration of Their Neurocognitive Templates," *Neuroscience and Biobehavioral Reviews*, 23 (1999), pp.1047–1058; and Tobeña, *Mártires Mortíferos*.

39. Atran, "Genesis of Suicide Terrorism"; Merari, *Terrorismo Suicida*; Richard E. Nisbett, and Dov Cohen, *Culture of Honor: The Psychology of Violence in the South* (New York: Harper and Collins, 1996); and Tobeña, *Mártires Mortíferos*.

Eight

RELIGION, SUICIDE, TERRORISM, AND THE MORAL FOUNDATION OF THE WORLD

Scott Atran

1. Introduction: The Religious Basis of Moral Commitment

Every society has:

(1) widespread counterfactual and counterintuitive belief in supernatural agents (gods, ghosts, goblins);

(2) hard-to-fake public expressions of costly material commitments to supernatural agents: offering and sacrifice (goods, property, time, life);

(3) mastering by supernatural agents of people's existential anxieties (death, deception, disease, catastrophe, pain, loneliness, injustice, want, loss); and

(4) ritualized, rhythmic sensory coordination of bodies (1), (2) and (3): communion (congregation, intimate fellowship), which almost always involves dance or sway and chant or music,[1] and displays of social hierarchy and submission typical of primates and other social mammals (outstretched limbs baring throat and chest or genitals, genuflection, bowing, prostration).

In this work, I make no conceptual distinction between "culture" and "society" or between "mind" and "brain."

All societies evince an evolutionary canalization and convergence of (1), (2), (3), and (4) that tends towards what I call "religion." By religion, I mean passionate communal displays of costly commitments to counterintuitive worlds governed by supernatural agents.[2] Although these facets of religion emerge in all known cultures and animate the majority of individual human beings in the world, considerable individual and cultural differences exist in the degree of religious commitment.

Religion is not defective science. As American anthropologist Roy Rappaport pointed out, the constant danger of replacement by other possible moral worlds does not primarily concern the everyday physical world of substances and species, locomotion and lakes, hawks and handsaws.[3] We can point to independent commonsense grounds for discovery and validation of knowledge about natural kinds and relations in the everyday physical world. This occurs through routine processes of perceptual verification conceptually allied to inference programs (sometimes rigidly via mental modules). These verification and inferential processes do not (and often cannot) appreciably change the nature of the entity or relation scrutinized. (I am obviously not talking about the phenomena of quantum physics). No such grounds exist for independent discovery and evaluation of the truth about socially constituted relationships and human kinds, such as reciprocity and responsibility, honor and humility, good and evil, or who should be beggar and who should be king.

Supernatural agents contribute to maintaining the cooperative trust of actors and the trustworthiness of communication by sanctifying the actual order of mutual understandings and social relations as the only morally and cosmically possible one. The causal scope of supernatural agents subsumes both the physical and social elements of the environment under a sanctified moral order. Whatever certainty, coherence, or verifiability attached to physical understanding becomes solid inductive evidence for corresponding certainty, coherence, and verifiability with respect to the social and cosmic order governed by supernatural agents.

Unlike (but not necessarily in opposition to) science, religion does not have factual knowledge as its principal occupation. In religion, factual knowledge plays only a supporting role. Only in the last decade has the Roman Catholic Church reluctantly come to acknowledge the factual plausibility of theories described by Nicolaus Copernicus, Galileo Galilei, and Charles Darwin. Earlier rejection of their theories stemmed from the challenges posed to a cosmic order unifying the moral and material worlds. Separating out the core of the material world would be like draining the pond where a water lily grows. A long lag time was necessary to refurbish and remake the moral and material connections in such a way that would permit faith in a unified cosmology to survive. Religion survives science as it does secular ideology not for its being prior to, or more primitive than, science or secular reasoning, but because of what it affectively and collectively secures for people. According to French philosopher Jean-Paul Sartre, science cannot tell us what we *ought* to do, only what we *can* do.

Religious sacrifice generally runs counter to calculations of immediate utility, such that future promises are not discounted in favor of present rewards.[4] As the world's richest man, Microsoft founder Bill Gates noted, "Just in terms of allocation of time resources, religion is not very efficient. There's a lot more I could be doing on a Sunday morning."[5] In some cases, sacrifice is extreme. Although such cases tend to be rare, society often views them as religiously ideal, for example, sacrificing one's life or nearest kin. As the Danish religious philosopher, Sören Kierkegaard, insisted, the greater the sacrifice for the factually absurd—as in Abraham offering to slit the throat of his beloved son on the orders of a God only he could hear—the more others trust the religious commitment of the person willing to make the sacrifice.[6] The more others trust a person's religious commitment, noted German economist Max Weber, the more others trust that person generally.[7] Even atheists in the United States are more likely to vote for a religious presidential candidate than for a nonbeliever.[8]

Researchers sometimes take extreme religious sacrifice as prima facie evidence of "true" (nonkin) social altruism,[9] or group selection, wherein individual fitness decreases so that overall group fitness can increase (relative to the overall fitness of other, competing groups).[10] But this may be an illusion. A telling example is contemporary suicide terrorism.[11] Consider the "Oath to Jihad" taken by recruits to Harkat ul-Mujahedeen, a Pakistani affiliate of the World Islamic Front for Jihad against the Jews and Crusaders, the umbrella organization formed by Osama Bin Laden in 1998. The oath affirms that by their sacrifice, members help secure the future of their family of fictive kin: "Each [martyr] has a special place—among them are brothers, just as there are sons and those even more dear."[12] In the case of religiously-inspired suicide terrorism, these sentiments are purposely manipulated by organizational leaders, recruiters, and trainers to the advantage of the manipulating elites instead of the individual (much as the fast food or pornography industries manipulate innate desires for naturally scarce commodities like fatty foods, sugar, and sex to ends that reduce personal fitness but benefit the manipulating institution). No "group selection" is involved, only cognitive and emotional manipulation of the genetic kin altruism of some individuals by the persuasive utility-maximizing powers of others.

Previous neuro-biological studies of religion have focused on tracking participant's neuro-physiological responses during episodes of religious experience and recording individual patterns of trance, vision, revelation and the like. This has favored comparison of religious experience with temporal lobe brain-wave patterns during epileptic seizures and acute schizophrenic episodes.[13] Cognitive structures of the human mind/brain in general, and cognitions of agency in particular, are usually represented in these studies (often under the trendy banner of "neuro-theology") in simple-minded terms (binary oppositions, holistic vs. analytical tensions, and hierarchical organization). Such conceptualizations have little input from, or pertinence to, recent findings of cognitive and developmental psychology.[14] Perhaps, as Adolf Tobeña suggests, more telling is recent work on the role of the prefrontal cortices in processing concepts of agency and self and in cognitive mediation of relevant emotions originating in (what was once called) "the limbic system."[15]

For the most part, relatively few individuals in our society have intensely arousing mystical experiences, although the overwhelming majority of individuals consider themselves to be religious believers (polls over the last thirty years consistently show that well over 90 percent of Americans profess religious convictions). Neither do we find any evidence that more mundane religious experiences have a characteristic temporal lobe signature, or any other specific type of brain-activity pattern. The neurophysiological bases that commit the bulk of humanity into the care of supernatural agents remain a complete mystery.

The same appears to be the case even among suicide bombers who cite religious devotion as their most important incitement to action, insofar as I can tell from debriefings of captured and would-be suicide bombers and their recruiters. Suicide bombers appear to be quite normal individuals, with no discernible pattern of psychopathology, economic or educational disadvantage, or social estrangement. They are not "morally deficient," but morally hypersensitized to the apparent grievances and needs of their own group. True, they utterly disregard and dehumanize the different yearnings of their enemies. Yet as Darwin rightly noted, such wanton disregard and hatred of competing outgroups may well be the default condition of our species.[16]

"Humanity," after all, is the relatively recent invention of monotheism. Earlier societies considered killing, violating, or otherwise harming members of other groups by denying them the status of members of the same moral category, similar to—with only some constraints—how they treated animals. Only since the Enlightenment has the modern world's major movements—the big "isms" of recent history—given themselves the moral mission of saving "all of humanity" by making it the moral equivalent of their humanity. Modernism is the industrial legacy of monotheism (however atheist in appearance), secularized and scientifically applied. No non-monotheistic society (except perhaps Buddhism) ever considered that all people are, or should be, essentially of a kind or morally equal to one's own kind. The trouble with missionary modernism—colonialism, anarchism, fascism, socialism, communism, democratic liberalism, or jihadism—is that those people not viewed as falling into one's own camp—say, "The House of Islam" or "The House of Democracy"—automatically belong to "The House of War" and "Evil." That means that a great chunk of residual humanity remains destined to have dominant groups despise and war upon them.

Even after 11 September 2001, many people have scant recognition that unforeseen events of history perpetually transform or destroy the best-laid plans for historical engineering. The catastrophic wars and revolutions of the modern era teach us that the more uncompromising the design and the more self-assured the designer, the harder both will fall.

2. Misconceiving Root Causes of Suicide Terrorism

A common notion held by the President George W. Bush administration and evinced by media spin on the war against terrorism is that suicide attackers are evil, deluded, or homicidal misfits who thrive in poverty, ignorance, and anarchy. "These killers don't have values," Bush declared in response to the spreading insurgency in Iraq. He continued "these people hate freedom. And we love freedom. And that's where the clash is." Secretary of State Colin

Powell previously told a World Economic Forum that "Terrorism really flourishes in areas of poverty, despair, and hopelessness."[17]

This portrayal lends a sense of hopelessness to any attempt to address root causes because some individuals will always be desperate or deranged enough to conduct suicide attacks. But as logical as the poverty-breeds-terrorism argument may seem, study after study shows that suicide attackers and their supporters are rarely ignorant or impoverished. Nor are they crazed, cowardly, apathetic or asocial. The common misconception underestimates the central role that organizational factors play in the appeal of terrorist networks. A better understanding of such causes reveals that the challenge is actually manageable: the key is not to profile and target the most despairing or deranged individual but to understand and undermine the organizational and institutional appeal of terrorists' motivations and networks.

The United States *National Strategy for Combating Terrorism* highlights the "War of Ideas" and "War on Poverty" as adjunct programs to reduce terrorism's pool of support and recruitment.[18] The war of ideas is based on the premise that terrorists and their supporters "hate our freedoms," a sentiment Bush has expressed both with regard to al-Qaeda and to the Iraqi resistance.[19] Yet survey data reliably show that most Muslims who support suicide terrorism and trust bin Laden favor elected government, personal liberty, educational opportunity, and economic choice.[20]

Mark Tessler, who coordinates long-term surveys of Muslim societies from the University of Michigan's Institute for Social Research, finds that Arab attitudes toward American culture are most favorable among young adults, regardless of their religious orientation. This is the same population that terrorist recruiters single out. Khalil Shikaki, Director of the Palestinian Center for Policy and Survey Research, consistently finds that a majority of Palestinians has a favorable impression of United States (and Israeli) forms of government, education, economy, and even literature and art, even though nearly three-fourths of the population supports suicide attack.[22]

In sum, we find no evidence that most people who support suicide actions hate Americans' internal cultural freedoms. Instead, we have every indication that they oppose United States foreign policies, especially regarding the Middle East. After the 1996 suicide attack against United States military housing at Khobar Towers in Saudi Arabia, a Defense Department Science Board report stated, "Historical data show a strong correlation between United States involvement in international situations and an increase in terrorist attacks against the United States."[23] United States intervention in Iraq is but the most recent example. A United Nations report indicated that as soon as the United States began building up for the Iraq invasion, al Qaeda recruitment picked up in thirty to forty countries.[24] Recruiters for groups sponsoring terrorist acts were telling researchers that volunteers were beating down the doors to join.

Similarly, the war on poverty is based on the premise that impoverishment, lack of education, and social estrangement spawn terrorism. Economist

Gary Becker advances the theory that the greater the amount of human capital (including income and education) a person accumulates, the less likely that person is to commit a crime.[25] He reasons that the greater a person's human capital, the more that person is aware of losing out on substantial future gains if captured or killed. Similar thinking applies to suicide terror: the less promising individuals' futures are, the greater the probability that they might choose to end their lives. Almost all current United States foreign aid programs related to terrorism pivot on such assumptions, now generally accepted by the mainstream of both United States political parties, but although the theory has proven useful in combating blue-collar crime, no evidence indicates its bearing on terror.

Studies by Princeton economist Alan Krueger and others find no correlation between a nation's per capita income and terrorism,[26] but do find a correlation between a lack of civil liberties, defined by Freedom House,[27] and terrorism. A recent National Research Council report, *Discouraging Terrorism*, finds:

> Terrorism and its supporting audiences appear to be fostered by policies of extreme political repression and discouraged by policies of incorporating both dissident and moderate groups responsibly into civil society and the political process.[28]

United States backing of weak, failed, and corrupt states generates animosity and terrorism against the United States There appears to be a direct correlation between United States military aid to politically corroded or ethnically divided states,[29] human rights abuses by those regimes,[30] and rise in terrorism,[31] as initially moderate opposition is pushed into common cause with more radical elements.

Despite these realities, the meager United States monies available for non-military foreign aid are far too concentrated in poverty reduction and literacy enhancement. In Pakistan, literacy and dislike for the United States have increased while the number of Islamist *madrassa* schools grew from 3,000 to nearly 40,000 since 1978. According to the United States' Department of State report, "Hope is an Answer to Terror," development aid is based "on the belief that poverty provides a breeding ground for terrorism. The terrorist attacks of September 11 reaffirmed this conviction."[32] In 2002, Bush declared at a United Nations conference on poor nations, International Conference on Financing for Development, in Monterrey, Mexico: "We fight against poverty because hope is an answer to terror."[33] Yet study after study demonstrates that suicide terrorists and their supporters are not abjectly poor, illiterate, or socially estranged.[34]

Another misconception that implicitly drives current national security policy is that suicide terrorists have no rational political agenda and that terrorists are not sane. According to General Wesley Clark, unlike nineteenth-century Russian terrorists who wanted to depose the czar, current Islamic terrorists are simply retrograde and nihilist: "They want the destruction of Western civilization and the return to seventh-century Islam."[35] In 2002, Senator John Warner testified that a new security doctrine of preemption was necessary because "those who would commit suicide in their assaults on the free world are not rational."[36] According to Vice President Richard Bruce "Dick" Cheney, the 11 September 2001 plotters and other like-minded terrorists "have no sense of morality."[37]

In truth, suicide terrorists generally have no appreciable psychopathology and are often wholly committed to what they believe to be devout moral principles. The report, *The Sociology and Psychology of Terrorism*, used by the Central and Defense Intelligence Agencies (CIA and DIA) finds "no psychological attribute or personality distinctive of terrorists."[38] Recruits are generally well adjusted in their families and liked by peers, and often more educated and economically better off than their surrounding population. Researchers Basel Saleh and Claude Berrebi independently find that the majority of Palestinian suicide bombers have a college education (versus 15 percent of the population of comparable age) and that less than 15 percent come from poor families (although about one-third of the population lives in poverty). DIA sources who have interrogated al Qaeda detainees at Guantanamo note that Saudi-born operatives, especially those in leadership positions, are often "educated above reasonable employment level, a surprising number have graduate degrees and come from high-status families."[39] The general pattern was captured in a Singapore Parliamentary report on prisoners from Jemaah Islamiyah, an ally of al-Qaeda:

> These men were not ignorant, destitute or disenfranchised. Like many of their counterparts in militant Islamic organizations in the region, they held normal, respectable jobs. Most detainees regarded religion as their most important personal value.[40]

Except for being mostly young, unattached males, suicide attackers differ from members of violent racist organizations to whom they are often compared, such as American white supremacist groups.[41] Overall, suicide terrorists exhibit no socially dysfunctional attributes (fatherless, friendless, jobless) or suicidal symptoms. Inconsistent with economic theories of criminal behavior, they do not kill themselves simply out of hopelessness or a sense of having nothing to lose. Muslim clerics countenance killing oneself for martyrdom in the name of God but curse personal suicide. "He who commits suicide kills himself for his own benefit," warned Sheikh Yussuf Al-Qaradhawi (a spiritual leader of the Muslim Brotherhood), but "he who commits martyrdom sacrifices himself for the sake of his religion and his nation . . . the Mujahed[een] is full of hope."[42]

Another reason that personal despair or derangement may not be a significant factor in suicide terrorism is that the cultures of the Middle East, Africa, and Asia, where suicide terrorism thrives, tend to be less individualistic than our Western culture more attuned to the environmental and organizational relationships that shape behavior, and less tolerant of individuals acting independently from a group context.[43] Terrorists in these societies also would be more likely to be seeking group, or collective, sense of belonging and justification for their actions.

A group struggling to gain power and resources against materially better-endowed enemies must attract able and committed recruits—not loaners—willing to give up their lives for a cause. At the same time, the group must prevent uncommitted elements in the population from simply free-riding on the backs of committed fighters, sharing in the fighters' rewards and successes without taking the risks or paying the costs of fighting. Insurgent groups manage this by offering potential recruits the promise of great future rewards as opposed to immediate gain, such as freedom for future generations or eternal bliss in Paradise. Only individuals committed to delayed gratification are then liable to volunteer. Insurgent groups also tend to seek individuals with better education and economic prospects, because they view a persons' investment of resources in education and training for a better economic future as indication of willingness to sacrifice today's satisfactions for tomorrow's rewards and as ability to make commitments. For this reason, relative level of education and economic status is often higher among insurgent groups that recruit primarily on the basis of promises for the future than among traditional armies that rely more on short-term incentives.[44]

3. Relative Deprivation and Religious Redemption

The connection between suicide, terrorists, and religion might be explained by the role that religious ethnic groups can play. Ethnic groups offer a good foundation for sustaining resource-deficient insurgencies because they provide a social structure that can underpin the maintenance of reputations and the efficient gathering of information about recruits. But ethnicity alone may not be enough; religion may also be needed to cement commitment. A comparison of ethnic Palestinians with ethnic Bosnian Muslims (matched for age, income, education, and exposure to violence) shows that the Palestinians are much more liable to use religious sentiments to confidently express hope for the future by their willingness to die for the group, whereas the Bosnians do not express religious sentiments, hope, or willingness to die.[45] Martyrdom, which involves "pure" commitment to promise over payoff, and unconditional sacrifice for fictive "brothers," will more likely endure in religious ethnic groups.

None of this denies that popular support for terrorism is sustained, in part, by economic factors, such as explosive population growth and underemployment, coupled with the failure of rigidly authoritarian governments to provide youth outlets for political and economic advancement. Middle Eastern and more broadly most Muslim societies, whose populations double within one generation or less, have age pyramids with broad bases: each younger age group has substantially more people than the next older generation. Even within states that allow for a modicum of political expression or economic employment, society's structure of opportunities can have trouble keeping pace with population.

Regional governments are increasingly unable to provide these opportunities, enhancing the attractiveness of religious organizations able to recruit tomorrow's suicide terrorists. Weak and increasingly corrupt and corroded nationalist regimes in Muslim countries have sought to eliminate all secular opposition. To subdue popular discontent in the post-colonial era, the Ba'athist socialist dictators of Syria and Iraq, the authoritarian prime ministers of Pakistan and Malaysia, the monarchs of Morocco and Jordan, and the imperial presidents of Egypt, Algeria, the Philippines, and Indonesia all initially supported militant Islamic groups. To maintain their bloated bureaucracies and armies, these "failed states"—all poor imitations of Western models with no organic history in the Arab and Muslim world— readily delegated responsibility for the social welfare of their peoples to activist Islamic groups eager to take charge. These groups provided schooling and health services more efficiently and extensively than governments were able to, offering a "desecularized" path to fulfill modernity's universal mission to improve humanity. Radical Islam finally vented political aspirations beginning with the 1965 "Islamic Manifesto," *Milestones,* written in prison by the Muslim Brotherhood's Sayyid Qutb just before he was hanged for sedition by Egyptian leader Colonel Gamal Abdul Nasser. Once begun, popular support proved too deep and widespread to extinguish.

Although we can identify the process of rising aspirations followed by dwindling expectations that generates terror, disentangling the relative significance of political and economic factors in the Muslim world is difficult and perhaps even impossible. During the 1990s, momentous political developments in Algeria (multiparty elections, including Islamic groups in 1992), Palestine (Oslo Peace Accords in 1993), Chechnya (dissolution of the Soviet Union and the end of communist control), Indonesia (Haji Mohammad Suharto's resignation in 1998 and the end of dictatorship), and elsewhere fanned rising aspirations among Muslim peoples for political freedom and economic advancement. In each case, economic stagnation or decline followed as political aspirations were thwarted (the Algerian Army cancelled elections, the Israel-Palestine Camp David negotiations broke down, Russia cracked down on Chechnya's bid for autonomy, and Suharto army loyalists and paramilitary groups fomented interethnic strife and political disaccord).

Support and recruitment for suicide terrorism occur not under conditions of political repression, poverty, and unemployment or illiteracy as such, but when converging political, economic, and social trends produce diminishing opportunities relative to expectations, thus generating frustrations that radical organizations can exploit. For this purpose, relative deprivation is more significant than absolute deprivation. Unlike poorer, less educated elements of their societies—or equally educated, well-off members of our society—many educated, middle-class Muslims increasingly experience frustration with life as their potential opportunities are less attractive than their prior expectations. Frustrated with their future, the appeal of routine national life declines and suicide terrorism gives some perceived purpose to act altruistically, in the potential terrorist's mind, for the welfare of a future generation.

Revolutionary terror imprints itself into history when corrupt and corroded societies choke rising aspirations into explosive frustration.

4. Organization and the Banality of Evil

This frustrating confluence of circumstances helps to account for terrorism's popular support and endurance but not the original spark that ignites people's passions and minds. Most people in the world who suffer stifling, even murderous, oppression do not become terrorists. As with nearly all creators and leaders of history's terrorist movements, those who conceive of using suicide terrorism in the first place belong mostly to an intellectual elite possessing sufficient material means for personal advancement but who choose a life of struggle and sacrifice for themselves and who often require even greater commitment from their followers. Their motivations are not personal comfort or immediate material gain. Instead, their motivation is religious or ideological conviction and zeal, whose founding assumptions, like those of *any* religion, we cannot rationally scrutinize, and for which they inspire others to believe in and die. But arational motivations don't preclude rational actions.

Sponsors of martyrdom are not irrational. Using religious sentiments for political or economic purposes can be eminently rational, as when martyrdom or missionary actions gain recognition, recruits, and power in order to increase political "market share"[46] (to gain in the competition for political influence in a regional context, within the larger Muslim community, or with the rest of the world). Dwindling returns on individuals' future prospects in life translate into higher levels of recruitment and prompt returns for terrorist groups and leaders. But this degree of manipulation usually works only if the manipulators themselves make costly, hard-to-fake commitments. Through indoctrination of recruits into relatively small and closeted cells—emotionally tight knit brotherhoods—terror organizations create a family of cellmates who are just as willing to sacrifice for one another as a parent for a child. These culturally contrived cell loyalties mimic and (temporarily) override genetically based fidelities to kin and secure belief in sacrifice to a larger group cause. The mechanism of manipulation resembles that of the United States army (probably most armies), which trains soldiers in small groups of committed buddies who then grow willing to sacrifice for one another, only derivatively for glory or country.

Key to intercepting that commitment before it solidifies is grasping how, like the best commercial advertisers but to ghastlier effect, charismatic leaders of terrorist groups turn ordinary desires for kinship and religion into cravings for the mission they are pitching, to the benefit of the manipulating organization instead of the manipulated individual. Understanding and parrying suicide terrorism requires concentrating more on the organizational structure, indoctrination methods, and ideological appeal of recruiting organizations than on personality attributes of the individuals recruited. No doubt, individual predispositions render some more susceptible to social factors that leaders use to persuade recruits to die for their cause. But months—sometimes years—of intense indoctrination can lead to blind obedience no matter who the individual—as indicated in studies of people who become torturers for their governments.[47]

Part of the answer to what leads a normal person to suicide terror may lie in philosopher Hannah Arendt's notion of the "banality of evil," which she used to describe the recruitment of mostly ordinary Germans, not sadistic lunatics, to man Nazi extermination camps.[48] In the early 1960s, psychologist Stanley Milgram tested Arendt's thesis. He recruited Yale students and other American adults to supposedly help others learn better. When the learner, hidden by a screen, failed to memorize arbitrary word pairs fast enough, the helper was instructed to administer an electric shock, and to increase voltage with each erroneous answer (which the learner, actually an actor, deliberately got wrong). Most helpers complied with instructions to give potentially lethal shocks (labeled, 450 volts, but in fact, 0 volts) despite victims' screams and pleas. This experiment showed how situations can be staged to elicit blind obedience to authority, and more generally that manipulation of context can trump individual personality and psychology to generate apparently extreme behaviors in ordinary people.[49]

Social psychologists have long documented what they call "the fundamental attribution error," the tendency for people to explain human behavior in terms of individual personality traits, even when significant situational factors in the larger society are at work. This attribution error leads many in the West to focus on the individual suicide terrorists instead of the organizational environment which produces them. If told that someone has been ordered to give a speech supporting a particular political candidate, for example, most people in Western society will still think that the speaker believes what he is saying. This interpretation bias seems to be especially prevalent in individualistic cultures, such as those of the United States and Western Europe, as opposed to collectivist cultures, such as Africa and Asia. Portrayals by the United States government and media of suicide bombers as deranged cutthroats may also suffer from a fundamental attribution error: no instance has yet occurred of religious or political suicide terrorism resulting from the lone action of a mentally unstable bomber (a suicidal Unabomber) or someone acting entirely under his own authority and responsibility (for example, a suicidal Timothy McVeigh). The key is the organization, not the individual.

For organizations that sponsor suicide attacks to thrive—or even survive—against much stronger military foes, they need strong community support. Yet the reasons for that communal support can differ among people. Among Palestinians, perceptions of historical injustice combine with personal loss and humiliation at the hands of their Israeli occupiers to nurture individual martyrs and general popular support for martyr actions. Palestinian economist Basel Saleh observes that a majority of Palestinian suicide bombers had prior histories of arrest or injury by Israel's army, and many of the youngest suicide shooters had family members or close friends with such a history.[50] Shikaki has preliminary survey data suggesting that popular support for suicide actions may be positively correlated with the number of Israeli checkpoints through which Palestinians must regularly pass to go about their daily business and the time needed to pass through them (this can involve spending hours at each of several checkpoints, any of which can be arbitrarily closed down any time to prevent through passage). Humiliation and revenge are the most consistent sentiments expressed by not just recruits but also their supporters, though expressed more as community grievances than as personal ones.[51]

Although grievances generate support for terrorists and motivate some people to become recruits, debriefings with captured al-Qaeda operatives at Guantánamo Bay, Cuba, and with Jemaah Islamiyah prisoners in Singapore, suggest that recruitment to these organizations is more ideologically driven than grievance driven. Detainees evince little history of personal hardship but frequently cite relatives or respected community members who participated in earlier jihads, or close peers presently engaged, as influencing decisions to join the fight.[52] Ideology and grievance are not mutually exclusive. Jessica Stern's interviews with jihadists and their supporters in Kashmir reveal that both abound.[53]

Despite numerous studies of individual behavior that show situation to be a much better predictor than personality in group contexts, Americans overwhelmingly believe that personal decision, success, and failure depend on individual choice, responsibility, and personality. This perception is plausibly one reason many Americans tend to think of terrorists as homicidal maniacs. "If we have to, we just mow the whole place down," said Senator Trent Lott, exasperated with the situation in Iraq. "You're dealing with insane suicide bombers who are killing our people, and we need to be very aggressive in taking them out."[54] As Timothy Spangler, chairman of Republicans Abroad (a group of Americans living overseas that helps the Republican Party develop policy) recently put it, "We know what the causes of terrorism are—terrorists. . . . It's ultimately about individuals taking individual decisions to kill people."[55] According to last year's Pew Survey, most of the world disagrees.[56] Although we cannot do much about personality traits, whether biologically influenced or not, we presumably can think of nonmilitary ways to make terrorist groups less attractive to the community that supports them and undermine their effectiveness with recruits. That holds the key to defeating terrorism.

None of this necessitates negotiating with terrorist groups that sponsor martyrs in the pursuit of goals such as al-Qaeda's quest to replace the Western-inspired system of nation-states with a global caliphate. Osama bin Laden and others affiliated with the mission of the World Islamic Front for the Jihad against the Jews and Crusaders seek no compromise, and will probably fight with hard power to the death. For these groups and already committed individuals, using hard power is necessary. The tens of millions of people who sympathize with bin Laden, though, are likely open to the promise of soft-power alternatives that most Muslims appear to favor—participatory government, freedom of expression, educational opportunity, economic choice.[57] The historical precondition for such opening of society, and for the popular legitimacy of any form of governance to be effective, is to ensure that potential recruits in the Arab and Muslim world feel secure about their personal safety and cultural heritage. Such soft-power efforts may demand more patience than governments under attack or pressure to reform politically may tolerate in times of crisis. Forbearance is necessary to avoid increasingly catastrophic devastation to the Western democracies and to the future hopes of peoples who aspire to soft empowerment from a free world.

5. Conclusion: Can Humanity Renounce Planetary Rights of Interference and Control?

In the competition for moral allegiance, secular ideologies are at a disadvantage in the long run (no avowedly atheistic society has ever endured more than a few generations). For, if people learn that all apparent commitment is self-interested convenience or worse, manipulation for the self-interest of others, then their commitment is debased and withers. Especially in times of vulnerability and stress, social deception and defection in the pursuit of self-preservation is more likely to occur, as the Muslim historian Ibn Khaldûn[58] recognized centuries ago. Religion passionately rouses hearts and minds to break out of this viciously rational cycle of self-interest, to adopt group interests that may benefit individuals in the long run. Commitment to the supernatural underpins what French sociologist Emile Durkheim called the "organic solidarity" that makes social life more than simply a contract among calculating individuals.[59]

In breaking one vicious cycle, religions almost invariably set in motion another. The more strongly individuals hold to group interests, the more they risk excluding or fighting the interests of other groups. The absolute moral value that religions attach to in-group interests practically guarantees that the ensuing conflict and competition between groups will be costly and interminable, and only resolved in specific cases by banishment, annihilation, or assimilation of out-groups and their ideas. Principles of evolution do not discourage, and may in fact encourage, this sort of creatively destructive spiral.

Within this spiral, the secular democracies of North America and Europe have arguably lessened the compulsion of religious exclusion. They have done this not so much by dampening religious passion (more true anyway of Europe than America), as by channeling religious conviction into more or less *voluntary* association and action. The political and economic ideology of the nation-state system and globalization has taken on transcendental value that leaves little room for opposing or different conceptions of human social order.

Human minds—essentially unchanged in evolutionary structure since the Stone Age—have developed spiraling Space-Age arsenals for their ambitions. Jihadist suicide terrorism is not a psychological aberration, an exercise in social nihilism, or even a retrograde expression of traditionalism or fundamentalism, any more than Nazism was, despite the significance of some atavistic cultural elements. Jihadist martyrdom is a thoroughly modern, institutionalized counter-movement to recent dominant trends towards a New World Order. Defend against Jihadism we must, and help it to burn itself out. But let us not add life to its forlorn mission by unrelentingly muscling others with our mission.

Notes

1. Andrew Greeley, *The Sociology of the Paranormal* (London: Sage, 1975).

2. Scott Atran, *In Gods We Trust*, Evolution and Cognition Series (New York: Oxford University Press, 2002); and Scott Atran and Ara Norenzayan, "Religion's Evolutionary Landscape: Counterintuition, Commitment, Compassion Communion," *Behavioral and Brain Sciences*, 27 (2004), pp. 713–730.

3. Roy Rappaport, *Ritual and Religion in the Making of Humanity* (Cambridge, UK: Cambridge University Press, 1999).

4. Raymond Firth, "Offering and Sacrifice," *Journal of the Royal Anthropological Institute*, 93 (1963), pp. 12–24.

5. Garrison Keillor, "Faith at the Speed of Light," *Time Magazine* (3 May 1999).

6. Sören Kierkegaard, *Fear and Trembling and the Sickness unto Death* (New York: Doubleday, 1955 [1843]).

7. Max Weber, "The Protestant Sects and the Spirit of Capitalism," *From Max Weber: Essays in Sociology* (Oxford: Oxford University Press, 1946).

8. Emory Elliot, "Religion, Identity, and Expression in American Culture," *Social Science Information*, 24 (1985), pp. 779–797.

9. Adam Kuper, *The Chosen Primate* (Cambridge, Mass.: Harvard University Press, 1996).

10. David Sloan Wilson, *Darwin's Cathedral: Evolution, Religion and the Nature of Society* (Chicago, Ill.: University of Chicago Press, 2002).

11. Scott Atran, "Combating al Qaeda's Splinters: Mishandling Suicide Terrorism," *The Washington Quarterly*, 27 (2004), pp. 27–90.

12. David Rhode and C. J. Chivers, "Qaeda's Grocery Lists and Manuals of Killing," *New York Times*, 17 March 2002.

13. Michael Persinger, *Neurophysiological Bases of God Beliefs* (New York: Praeger, 1978).

14. Eugene d'Aquili and Andrew Newberg, *The Mystical Mind: Probing the Biology of Religious Experience* (Minneapolis, Minn.: Fortress Press, 1999).

15. Adolf Tobeña, "Benumbing and Moral Exaltation in Deadly Martyrs: A View from Neuroscience," Paper presented to the International Colloquium, "The Social Brain: Biology of Conflict and Cooperation," Barcelona, Spain, June 2004, see this volume chap. 7; and Scott Atran, "The Neuropsychology of Religion," *Neurotheology: Brain, Science, Spirituality, Religious Experience* (San Jose: University Press of California 2002), pp. 163–182.

16. Charles Darwin, *The Descent of Man and Selection in Relation to Sex* (Princeton: Princeton University Press, 1981 [1871]).

17. Cited in Louis Frazza, "Bush Committed to Iraq Handover in June," *USA Today*, 4 April 2004.

18. United States Department of State, *National Strategy for Combating Terrorism* (Washington, D.C., February 2003), p. 13.

19. "Address to a Joint Session of Congress and to the American People," White House news release, 20 September 2001; "Bush: 'al Qaeda Types' Committing Terror in Iraq," posted on FoxNews.com, 22 August 2003. http: www.foxnews.com/ story/0,2933,95481,00.html (accessed 15 October 2006); and quotes attributed to George W. Bush in "Iraqi City Can't Be Island of Resistance," op-ed posted online by tandd.com, 6 April 2004, http://theandd.com/articles/2004/04/ 06/opinion/opinion1.txt (accessed 15 October 2006).

20. "Views of a Changing World 2003: War with Iraq Further Divides Global Publics," Survey Report, Pew Research Center, 3 June 2003, http://people-press.org/reports/ display.php3?ReportID=185 (accessed 26 July 2006).

21. Mark Tessler, "Do Islamic Orientations Influence Attitudes toward Democracy in the Arab World: Evidence from Egypt, Jordan, Morocco, and Algeria." *International Journal of Comparative Sociology*, 2 (2002), pp. 229–249; and Mark Tessler and Dan Corstange, "How Should Americans Understand Arab and Muslim Political Attitudes," *Journal of Social Affairs*, 19 (2002), pp. 13–34.

22. Khalil Shikaki, "Palestinians Divided," *Foreign Affairs*, January/February 2002; and Public Survey Research Unit, Public Opinion Poll No. 9, Palestinian Center for Policy and Survey Research, 7–14 October 2003. http//www.pcpsr.org/survey/polls/ 2003/ p9a.html (accessed 26 July 2006).

23. "DoD Responses to Transnational Threats, vol. 2: DSB Force Protection Panel Report to DSB," (Washington, D.C.: United States Department of Defense, December 1997), p. 8, http://www.acq.osd.mil/dsb/reports/trans2.pdf (accessed 15 October 2006).

24. Colum Lynch, "Volunteers Swell a Reviving Qaeda, UN Warns," *International Herald Tribune (online)*, 19 December 2002.

25. Gary Becker, "Crime and Punishment: An Economic Approach," *Political Economy*, 76 (1968), pp. 169–217.

26. Alan Krueger and Jitka Malecková, "Seeking the Roots of Terror," *Chronicle of Higher Education, The Chronicle Review* (6 June 2003) http://chronicle.com/ free/v49/i39/39b01001.htm (accessed 26 July 2006).

27. Alan Krueger, "Poverty Doesn't Create Terrorists," *New York Times*, 29 May 2003.

28. National Research Council, *Discouraging Terrorism* (Washington, D.C.: National Academies Press, 2002), p. 2.

29. Michelle Ciarrocca and William Hartung, "Increases in Military Spending and Security Assistance Since 9/11," An Arms Trade Resource Center Fact Sheet, *Arms Trade Resource Center*, 4 October 2002, http://www.worldpolicy.org/projects/ arms/ news/ SpendingDOD911.html (accessed 26 July 2006).

30. Scott Atran, Response to "Individual Factors in Suicide Terrorism," *Science*, 304:5667 (2 April 2004), pp. 47–49.

31. Global Terrorism Index 2003/2004 (World Markets Research Centre, 18 August 2003).

32. United States Department of State, "Hope is an Answer to Terror," *September 11 One Year Later* (September 2002) p. 14. http://usinfo.state.gov/journals/itgic/0902/ijg e/gj03.htm (accessed 15 Oct 2006).

33. White House press release, 22 March 2002; and J. Jai, "Getting at the Roots of Terrorism," *Christian Science Monitor*, 10 December 2001.

34. Scott Atran, "Genesis of Suicide Terrorism," *Science*, 299 (7 March 2003), pp. 1534–1539.

35. Wesley Clark, Address to Veterans of Foreign Wars, Nashua, N.H., C-Span television, 20 December 2003.

36. David Von Drehle, "Debate over Iraq Focuses on Outcome," *Washington Post*, 7 October 2002.

37. Richard Bruce "Dick" Cheney, interviewed on Fox News with Brit Hume, 17 March 2004.

38. Rex A. Hudson, "The Sociology and Psychology of Terrorism: Who Becomes a Terrorist and Why," ed. Marilyn Majeska (Washington, D.C.: Federal Research Division of the Library of Congress, September 1999), p. 40 http://www.loc.gov/rr/frd/pdf-files/Soc_Psych_of_Terrorism.pdf (accessed 26 July 2006).

39. Scott Atran, "Who Wants to Be a Martyr," *New York Times*, 5 May 2003; and Scott Atran, cited in Corine Hegland, "Global Jihad," *National Journal*, 8 May 8, 2004, p. 1402.

40. "White Paper—The Jemaah Islamiyah Arrests," Ministry of Home Affairs, Singapore, 9 January 2003 http://www2.mha.gov.sg/mha/detailed.jsp?artid=667&type=4&root=0&parent=0&cat=0&mode=arc (accessed 26 July 2006).

41. Raphael Ezekiel, *The Racist Mind: Portraits of American Neo-Nazis and Klansmen* (New York: Viking, 1995).

42. *Al-Ahram Al-Arabi*, Cairo (3 February 2001).

43. Richard Nisbett, *The Geography of Thought: How Asians and Westerners Think Differently and Why* (New York: Free Press, 2003).

44. Jeremy Weinstein, "Resources and the Information Problem in Rebel Recruitment," Center for Global Development, Working Paper, November 2003.

45. Brian Barber, *Heart and Stones: Palestinian Youth from the Intifada* (New York: St. Martin's Press, 2003).

46. Mia Bloom, "Devising a Theory of Suicide Terror," *Dying to Kill: The Allure of Suicide Terror* (New York: Columbia University Press, in press); cf. Hamas Communiqué (Qassem Brigades), 9 August 2001. http://www.intellnet.org/resources/hamas_communiques/hamas/comm._text/2001/9_ aug_01.htm (accessed 15 October 2006).

47. See Mika Haritos-Fatouros, "The Official Torturer: A Learning Model for Obedience to the Authority of Violence," *Journal of Applied Social Psychology*, 18 (1988), pp. 1107–1120; and Peter Slevin, "Red Cross Describes Systematic Abuse in Iraq," *Washington Post*, 10 May 2004.

48. Hannah Arendt, *Eichmann in Jerusalem: A Report on the Banality of Evil* (New York: Viking, 1970).

49. Stanley Milgram, *Obedience to Authority* (New York: Harper & Row, 1974).

50. Basel, Saleh, "Economic Conditions and Resistance to Occupation in the West Bank and Gaza Strip: There Is a Causal Connection." Paper presented to the Graduate Student forum, Kansas State University, 4 April 2003.

51. Ariel Merari, "Social, Organization, and Psychological Factors in Suicide Terrorism," *Root Ccauses of Suicide Terrorism* (London: Routledge, in press).

52. Scott Atran, "Who Wants to Be a Martyr."

53. Jessica Stern, *Terror in the Name of God* (New York: Harper Collins, 2003).

54. Trent Lott, cited in *The Hill*, 29 October 2003.

55. Timothy Spangler, interviewed on *BBC News*, 21 January 2003.

56. "Views of a Changing World 2003."

57. Joseph Nye and Soft Power, *The Means to Success in World Politics* (New York: Public Affairs, 2004).

58. Ibn Khaldûn, *The Muqaddimah: An Introduction to History*, vol. 2, bk. 3 (London: Routledge & Kegan Paul, 1958 [1318]), p. 41.

59. Emile Durkheim, *The Elementary Forms of Religious Life* (New York: Free Press, 1995 [1912]).

Nine

ON THE PSYCHOLOGICAL DIVERSITY OF MORAL INSENSITIVITY

Shaun Nichols

When we learn of atrocities committed by psychopaths and by suicide terrorists, we are shocked by the evident lack of normal feeling for their fellow human beings. (By suicide terrorists, I mean to include not just the people who
have carried out suicide missions, but also the people who plan and organize
such attacks.) How could anyone be so callous to the suffering of others? We
recognize two significantly different psychological pathways to such insensitivity. I will maintain that psychopaths and suicide terrorists arrive at numbness through different routes. To see the two different paths to numbness, we
must speak more broadly about different psychological processing models that
can explain the appearance of deviant responses. In the first section, I will
distinguish between *midstream* and *upstream* effects on psychological processing. Once that issue is settled, I will turn to the task of placing psychopaths
into the framework. Psychopaths exhibit both insensitivity to suffering and a
deviance in moral judgment. This plausibly derives from *midstream* deviance
in the emotional processing system. We have no reason to think that the insensitiveness of suicide terrorists is similar at the psychological level. Psychopaths and suicide terrorists appear to have quite different moral psychologies.
I will then characterize the ways in which suicide terrorists plausibly are insensitive to suffering in others. Suicide terrorists, I will suggest, exhibit
numbness because of *upstream* psychological processes.

1. Two Paths to Deviance

To characterize the relations between suicide terrorists and psychopaths, we
must distinguish between two radically different psychological routes to
numbness. When a psychological system produces a deviant response to a
given stimulus, we might explain this deviance in terms of upstream, midstream, or downstream effects. Let me begin with an abstract characterization; examples follow.

Suppose that we know that presenting a stimulus S produces a characteristic response R in most people, and we know that psychological mechanism
M mediates the process. When we present S to a person who does not exhibit
R, several explanations are possible. An *upstream* explanation is that something happened in the overall psychological system prior to M's processing;
this upstream process either distorted or circumvented M's processing. A

downstream explanation is that something happened in the psychological system after M's processing; this downstream process prevented or distorted the normal response that follows M's processing. A *midstream* explanation of the atypical response is that M, the psychological mechanism itself, operated in a way that deviates from the norm. For our purposes, the key distinction will be between midstream and upstream paths to numbness. So I will elaborate a bit on the nature of midstream and upstream effects.

A. Midstream Effects

Midstream effects include, most obviously, effects that result from defects to the processing mechanism itself. People with Broca's aphasia often exhibit a peculiar deficit in syntactic recognition. For example, some such aphasics can evaluate active voice sentences, but not passive voice sentences. And a natural explanation of this is that brain damage has impaired the mechanism that does the job of syntax recognition. This would count as a midstream explanation of the atypical responses of Broca's aphasics. A related sort of midstream explanation appeals not to brain damage but to congenital defects. For instance, people with Specific Language Impairment make systematic syntactic errors in speaking their native tongue. One kind of explanation for this atypical linguistic behavior is that a congenital defect in their syntax production system is present. Such midstream defects might also be induced by environmental deprivation, as in feral children who never develop normal syntactic abilities. The key commonality to these midstream explanations is just that the atypical response is supposed to result from deviance in the psychological mechanism itself.

Another way that midstream effects might occur is by fatiguing a system not itself deviant. A phenomenon known as "semantic satiation" provides a good illustration. When we present a word to a subject repeatedly (either visually or auditorily), the subject appears to gradually lose the meaning of the word. This is a familiar phenomenon you can try yourself. Take a word like "architecture" and say it 100 times. Gradually, the word starts to appear weirdly disconnected from its semantics. These phenomenological ruminations are corroborated by work in psychology.

Linguists have studied semantic satiation for nearly a century, but one nice demonstration comes from a recent study by David A. Balota and Sheila Black.[1] They had subjects judge whether two visually presented words were semantically related (for example, royalty–king vs. royalty–box). Prior to this exercise, they presented subjects visual representations of one of the words (for example, royalty), either two, twelve, or twenty-two times. Results showed that for the younger subjects, exposure to more repetitions of the word resulted in worse performance in judging semantic relatedness. A natural explanation of these results is that the lexical access system is "satiated" with respect to this stimulus. Regardless whether semantic satiation is the right explanation, the suggestion provides an obvious sort of model for a different kind of midstream effect. The idea is just that a mechanism can become habituated to a kind of input, so that the mechanism will no longer produce the characteristic output given that input.

When we turn to the emotions, midstream effects might occur in either of these two ways. The emotion system might be deviant in some way, so that emotion system E in subject S does not produce the normal response for a given set of stimuli. For instance, a person might just fail to have a normal disgust system, and as a result he does not have the characteristic disgust response when encountering bodily fluids. Again, presumably such a defect could come about from a genetic defect, brain damage, or environmental deprivation. Significantly, the emotional mechanism itself is deviant.

Emotion systems might also exhibit the second kind of midstream effect. The emotion system in the subject might be perfectly normal, but the system gets habituated to an input so that it no longer produces the characteristic output. For instance, if persons are exposed to images of phlegm repeatedly over a thirty-minute period, their disgust system might gradually produce weaker and weaker responses to the input. Although the system is not damaged, it has become habituated to the visual presentation of phlegm and does not produce its characteristic output.

B. Upstream Effects

Sometimes a person fails to exhibit the modal response to a stimulus because of psychological processes that occur before input reaches the targeted mechanism. These kinds of upstream effects need not be the product of conscious intention, but they provide the best illustrations of upstream effects. Consider the Stroop Task. Subjects are presented with color terms (for example red, blue, yellow), which are printed in different colors (for example, the term "red" might be printed in blue ink). Subjects are told to report the color in which the word is printed. Subjects are much faster at the task when the color of the print matches the color word than when it does not. A clever subject might use upstream processes to beat the Stroop Task (or diminish the effect). If subjects intentionally blur their eyes, so that they cannot read the words, then the characteristic difference between matches and mismatches diminishes. In this case, the upstream cognitions have found a way to circumvent the typical processing that accompanies the Stroop Task. What subjects have done in such a case is prevent the input from getting to the lexical access system. So the lexical access system is perfectly normal, but it does not produce the characteristic output because it does not get the characteristic input. See Figure 1 for a tree that reviews the range of possible processing models we have considered. These kinds of upstream effects on psychological mechanisms can also occur for emotion systems.

Perhaps the best developed account of such upstream effects on emotion processing comes from Richard Lazarus' work on *coping*. On being presented with cues that typically lead to affective response, we can use strategies to avoid or diminish the characteristic response. Lazarus defines coping strategies as "cognitive and behavioral efforts to manage specific external or internal demands . . . that are appraised as taxing or exceeding the resources of the person." On his view, coping is crucial because it allows us to change or even prevent an emotional reaction. This can occur in several different ways.

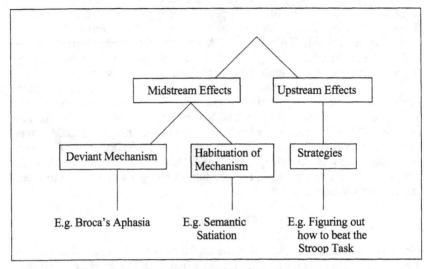

Figure 1. Processing models for deviant response patterns.

One way to cope is "by changing the way the relationship is appraised, and hence the relational meaning, and the resulting emotion"—if we change the way we conceive of the situation, this can alter the kind of emotional response we have. Coping can also occur "by affecting attention deployment, as in psychological avoidance, which takes a person's mind off the trouble." So, one obvious way in which we cope is by redirecting our attention away from thoughts about the troubling event or stimulus. Coping can provide a way to obviate the emotional process, and this is an upstream effect since this kind of coping occurs before emotion processing. The emotional mechanism itself, though, need not be deviant or habituated in any way. Instead, just as you can beat the Stroop Task by trying to prevent the input from getting to the lexical access mechanism, you can sometimes beat the emotional pain by preventing the input from getting to the emotion system.

2. Psychopaths: Moral Deviance and Midstream Numbness

Now that we have the general theoretical landscape laid out, we can try to see how psychopaths fit into it. We want to understand psychopaths' moral callousness. This callousness appears in two ways, as we will see in more detail below. First, psychopaths are insensitive to others' suffering; second, they have a shallow understanding of the character of moral prohibitions.

In James Blair's influential work on psychopathy, he finds that psychopaths show a general deficit in their sensitivity to suffering in others. Blair and colleagues showed images of people suffering to both psychopathic and nonpsychopathic criminals. While the subjects viewed these images, investigators measured subjects' physiological reactions over the next five seconds. Psychopaths exhibited significantly less physiological response than the nonpsychopaths did, suggesting that psychopaths have generally diminished basic responses to cues of suffering in others.[4]

In another series of experiments, Blair found that psychopaths show deviant performance on a standard measure of moral judgment, the moral/conventional task.[5] Previous work on moral judgment shows that subjects distinguish canonical examples of moral violations (for example, unprovoked hitting) from canonical examples of conventional violations (for example, standing up during story time). From a young age, children distinguish the moral violations from the conventional violations on several dimensions. For instance, children tend to think that moral transgressions are generally less permissible and more serious than conventional transgressions. Children are also more likely to maintain that the moral violations are "generalizably" wrong, for example, that pulling hair is wrong in other countries too. The children explained why moral transgressions are wrong in terms of fairness and harm to victims. For example, children will say that pulling hair is wrong because it hurts the person. By contrast, the children gave the explanation for why conventional transgressions are wrong in terms of social acceptability—talking out of turn is wrong because to do so is rude or impolite, or because "you're not supposed to." Further, they view conventional rules, unlike moral rules, as dependent on authority. For instance, if at another school the teacher has no rule prohibiting standing during story time, children will judge that standing during story time at that school is not wrong; but even if the teacher at another school has no rule against hitting, children claim that hitting is wrong.[6]

Blair found that people with psychopathic tendencies perform abnormally on the moral/conventional task. Children with psychopathic tendencies are more likely than other children to say that moral violations (for example, unprovoked hitting) are acceptable if no rule against them has been established.[7] While most people claim that moral violations like unprovoked hitting are wrong because they hurt the person, psychopaths tend to give social/conventional explanations for why the moral violations are wrong ("it's not the done thing").[8]

Psychopaths exhibit both emotional deviance and a deviance in moral judgment. Blair exploits this pair of deficits in psychopathy to develop an account of moral judgment. His theory splits into two parts. First, he maintains that normal humans have a "Violence Inhibition Mechanism" (VIM) triggered by distress cues, and this mechanism, he maintains, generates a sense of aversion when we witness cues of suffering. Second, he maintains that subjects treat events experienced as aversive in this way as nonconventional transgressions in the moral/conventional task.[9] This VIM mechanism is damaged in psychopathy, according to Blair, and this explains the psychopath's failure on the moral/conventional task. In normal subjects, the VIM produces negative affect, which generates moral judgment. Since psychopaths have a defective VIM, their moral judgment is correspondingly defective.

Blair's VIM account of moral judgment and psychopathy has several problems.[10] To see the deepest problem with the account, consider the crucial distinction between judging something *bad* and judging something *wrong*. Many occurrences regarded as bad are not regarded as wrong. Toothaches, for instance, are bad, but they are not wrong. The moral/conventional task is interesting primarily because it gives us a glimpse into judgments of *wrong*. For items in the moral/conventional task are explicitly *transgressions*, and the first criterion category is *permissibility*. The problem with Blair's account is that, while the proposal might provide a psychological model of judging something bad (in one sense), it does not provide a model of judging something wrong.

If the first part of Blair's theory is correct, VIM produces a distinctive aversive response. As with toothaches, we might regard the stimuli that prompt this aversive response as "bad." What class of stimuli is bad in this sense? Anything that reliably produces VIM activation. Distress cues will be at the core of this stimulus class.[11] The class of stimuli that will be accordingly aversive will include distress cues from victims of natural disasters and accidents. The class of stimuli that VIM will lead us to regard as bad includes natural disaster victims and accident victims. That these things are *wrong* is also quite plausible. Natural disasters are bad. But, barring theological digressions, we do not regard natural disasters as *wrong*. Similarly, if a child falls down, skins its knee, and begins to cry, this will produce aversive response in witnesses through VIM. Yet the child's falling down does not count as a moral transgression.

On the model that I prefer, the capability to draw the moral/conventional distinction depends on two quite different mechanisms. First, a body of information exists, a normative "theory" that specifies a set of harm-based normative violations. Second, Blair's data indicate that an emotional mechanism also plays a key role in mediating performance on the moral/conventional task—affective response appears to infuse norms with a special status. Since psychopaths have a deficiency in their affective response to harm in others, this plausibly explains why they fail to treat harm norms as distinctive.[12]

On this model, the normative theory and affective mechanism are plausibly dissociable. Children are sensitive to distress cues well before the second birthday.[13] But one-year-old children presumably do not make moral judgments because they have not yet developed an understanding of the normative theory that will guide their moral judgments in the coming years. Psychopaths, on the other hand, appear to have a dissociation in the other direction. They show a deficit in affective response to suffering and this appears to compromise their ability to respond normally on the moral/conventional task.

But psychopaths apparently have a largely intact knowledge of the rules prohibiting harming others.

Psychopaths exhibit a kind of deviance in moral cognition plausibly tied to a deviance in their sensitivity to suffering in others. But what is the nature of this affective deviance in psychopaths, this numbness to others' suffering? The most obvious explanation is a midstream explanation—in psychopaths, the emotional system that responds to distress cues is defective. This fits with Blair's own recent proposal about the psychopath's affective deviance—he maintains that the amygdala is centrally involved in responding to suffering in others and he finds that psychopaths exhibit amygdala dysfunction.[14] So, the insensitivity in psychopaths plausibly derives from midstream effects of the first variety—their emotional system is deviant.

If psychopaths instantiate the first type of midstream effect, what about the second type? Can a person with a normal emotional system come to have their emotional system habituated to the cues of distress? Presumably. A couple of years ago, as I was about to undergo a root canal, I casually asked the endodontist, "So, have you become inured to seeing people in pain?" To my dismay, she casually replied, "yeah." The endodontist was probably not a psychopath, but one explanation of her self-avowed numbness is that her emotional system has habituated to the signs of distress associated with root canals. Either her emotional system itself has habituated through long years of exposure, or perhaps in each particular surgery, the distress cues are initially upsetting, but the repeated exposure to a patient's distress cues leads to numbness. Even if the endodontist's numbness does not derive from habituation, the idea of habituation happening to people with normal emotional equipment is plausible. Just as our semantic system becomes less responsive in semantic satiation, our emotional systems will likely become less responsive in conditions of distress-cue satiation.

3. Suicide Terrorists and Psychopaths

In his contribution to this volume, Adolf Tobeña rightly notes that to compare psychopaths and suicide terrorists is instructive. But the differences, not the similarities, are what I view as especially significant.

We do not know whether suicide terrorists, like psychopaths, have generally diminished basic responses to the cues of another's suffering. In particular, we do not know how they would respond to the images that Blair shows his psychopaths. But we have no reason to think that most suicide terrorists would have generally diminished responses to suffering. Because suicide terrorists support suicide missions does not demonstrate an absence of responsiveness to suffering in others. A person can be emotionally bothered by witnessing a soldier kill his enemy and still think that the action was morally permissible. A soldier might be emotionally bothered by witnessing the suffering he inflicts on his enemy and still think that his action was right. George Orwell illustrates this possibility especially well in *Homage to Cata-*

lonia, writing, "When I joined the militia I had promised myself to kill one Fascist—after all, if each of us killed one they would soon be extinct." Orwell does not waver from this view, but when he reports his participation in a skirmish, we get a revealing glimpse into his emotional reaction. Orwell and his fellow soldiers are attacking the Nationalists' line and Orwell tries to throw a bomb at the point where an enemy rifle fired:

> By one of those strokes of luck that happen about once a year I had managed to drop the bomb almost exactly where the rifle had flashed. There was the roar of the explosion and then, instantly, a diabolical outcry of screams and groans. We had got one of them anyway; I don't know whether he was killed, but certainly he was badly hurt. Poor wretch, poor wretch! I felt a vague sorrow as I heard him screaming.

Although Orwell had wanted to kill a fascist, he cannot suppress his normal response to the salient cues of suffering coming from his enemy. But Orwell does not wallow in the feeling. He continues:

> But at the same instant, in the dim light of the rifle-flashes, I saw or thought I saw a figure standing near the place where the rifle had flashed. I threw up my rifle and let fly.[16]

Similarly, because suicide terrorists kill civilians does not exclude the possibility that the suicide terrorists would have a negative emotional response to the distress cues of their civilian victims.

When we turn to the moral/conventional task, we know that psychopaths exhibit deviant performance, but again, we have no reason to think that suicide terrorists would perform abnormally on the moral/conventional task. On the contrary, Islamic fundamentalist terrorists, for example, appear to treat their moral commitments with the utmost weight. To test the emotional sensitivity and moral judgment of suicide terrorists would be enlightening. Currently, the most plausible bet is that suicide terrorists typically have the same emotional equipment and the same basic capability to make moral judgment as the rest of us.

While we have no reason to think that suicide terrorists have a deviant emotional mechanism akin to that found in psychopathy, a difference between suicide terrorists and the rest of us is obvious. Suicide terrorists have different *norms* than we have. Many suicide terrorists think that killing United States civilians is permissible. On this dimension, they deviate from the average Western European and North American. This distinction also distinguishes suicide terrorists from typical psychopaths imprisoned in Western Europe and North America. So the comparison between suicide terrorists and psychopaths reveals salient differences instead of similarities. For a review of the contrasts between suicide terrorists and psychopaths, see Table 1.

Why do suicide terrorists have such different norms from us if, as I have suggested, we share basically the same intact emotional systems? The obvious answer is Culture. Cultural forces play a vital role in determining which norms a person embraces. So, even though suicide terrorists likely have the same low-level responses to suffering in others that we do, they have been enculturated in ways that lead them to have different norms.

If the foregoing suggestions about suicide terrorists are right, they provide a further illustration of the dissociation between norms and emotions. We

	Have normal basic responses to suffering in others	Perform normally on moral/conventional task	Maintain that killing U.S. civilians is wrong
Psychopaths	No	No	Yes
Suicide terrorists	Yes?	Yes?	No

Table 1. Psychopaths and suicide terrorists

share much the same emotional equipment as suicide terrorists, and yet we have quite different norms. So our basic emotional equipment does not immediately dictate our norms. Instead, the norms we accept are partly dictated by our culture, and cultural forces can promote norms that do not fit well with our emotional endowment.

4 Suicide Terrorists: Upstream Numbness

So far, I have been maintaining that suicide terrorists do not diverge from us at the level of basic emotional equipment. Instead, they differ from us in their normative commitments. But this difference in norms can generate crucial differences in their sensitivity to suffering in others. We might explain the callousness of suicide terrorists because of upstream processing, coping. If they have the basic emotional equipment that the rest of us do, then to avoid the unpleasant emotional consequences of contemplating and witnessing the suffering of civilians, the suicide terrorists must find ways to deal with their emotions. They engage in what we might call *norm-driven* coping. Their different norms, different values, lead them to believe that to kill and injure civilians is morally acceptable, in some cases morally commendable. Given these norms, they learn to manage the emotional consequences of the actions of their group. One way they do this, presumably, is by redirecting their attention from the distress cues of the victims to the perceived wrongs perpetrated on their group.

Two observations about norm-driven numbness are in order. First, while the kind of numbness on which we are focusing is numbness to another's pain, norm-driven numbness is not restricted to emotions in the moral domain. Plausibly, we have a norm that says you should tend your flu-stricken child, even though doing so is often quite disgusting. Children with the flu have trouble keeping bodily fluids confined to appropriate locations. But a parent who does not clean his child's vomit from the bathroom floor is a bad parent. So, as a parent, you know you ought to clean up the vomit, and you are bound to do so. The best you can do is cope with your disgust reaction. Presumably, we do. We try not to think about or smell the vomit while we are on the floor with the rags. Here then we have norm-driven numbness that does not stop up any emotions in the moral domain. You ought to clean up your child's vomit, and as a result, you use coping strategies for circumventing your disgust response.

The second point is that norm-driven numbness to suffering is not restricted to those against whom we moralize. Again, the parent-child relationship provides a good example. If your child has a bad laceration, then you should take the child to the doctor for sutures. But while you are there, you will likely try to cope with your emotions by not looking as the doctor pushes a needle through your child's skin. Doctors even tell parents not to look. When a parent copes with his emotional reactions in this way, we do not think the parent is morally corrupt (I hope!). We even think it morally admirable, or at minimum, appropriate and optimal, to be emotionally numb in some cases. If you need to suppress your distress response to best help an accident victim, obviously doing so is a good thing to do. The otherwise sensitive bystander who circumvents his emotional response to help a victim is praiseworthy.

Norm-driven coping is not restricted to emotions in the moral domain. Further, even for emotions in the moral domain, norm-driven coping is not intrinsically objectionable. In many cases to try to manage and restrain your emotions instead of letting them flourish makes sense. The kind of norm-driven insensitivity exhibited in suicide terrorists is not different in psychological kind from the kind of norm-driven insensitivity that characterizes most of us. Suicide terrorists, like the rest of us, exploit strategies for coping with the emotionally difficult situations in which they find themselves. Figure 2 provides an overview of the psychological routes to insensitivity.

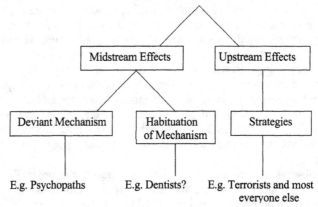

Figure 2. Processing models of insensitivity to others' suffering.

Although the callousness of suicide terrorists shocks us, what is centrally objectionable about suicide terrorists is not the numbness that they exhibit towards others' suffering. For if we shared their norms, to cultivate insensitivity by exploiting coping strategies would be sensible. No, what is objectionable about suicide terrorists is not the numbness but the root cause of their numbness—their norms. If the moral numbness of suicide terrorists is norm-driven, what does this tell us about policy? Depressingly little. The way to change suicide terrorists is to change the norms that they hold. We have no recipe for that.

5. Conclusion

One of the most significant developments in recent moral psychology has been the demonstration that emotions and emotional sensitivity play a crucial role in normal moral judgment. This advance has encouraged the oversimplification of identifying particular moral judgments with particular emotional responses. This oversimplification is plain in Blair's work, because he is admirably explicit about the emotional responses implicated in moral judgment. I have argued that, while emotions do play a crucial role in moral judgment, the culturally taught norms also play a vital role, and the contribution of the norms is partly independent of the contribution of the emotions. The moral insensitivity of psychopaths is not that they learned different norms from the ones we learned—psychopaths recognize which things their culture sanctions and which it prohibits. Instead, the moral insensitivity of psychopaths apparently comes from deviance within their emotional systems themselves. The moral insensitivity of suicide terrorists, on the other hand, does not seem to stem from deviance within their emotional systems. For all we can tell, they have normal emotional mechanisms. Instead, the moral insensitivity of suicide terrorists results from the norms they embrace.

Notes

1. D. A. Balota and S. Black, "Semantic Satiation in Healthy Young and Older Adults," *Memory & Cognition*, 25 (1997), pp. 190–202.

2. Richard S. Lazarus, *Emotion and Adaptation* (New York: Oxford University Press, 1991), p. 112.

3. Richard S. Lazarus, "Universal Antecedents of the Emotions," *The Nature of Emotion: Fundamental Questions*, eds. Paul Ekman and Richard J. Davidson (New York: Oxford University Press, 1994), pp. 163–171, quote, p. 166.

4. R. L. Blair, F. Jones, M. Clark, and L. Smith, "The Psychopathic Individual: A Lack of Responsiveness to Distress Cues?" *Psychophysiology*, 34 (1997), pp. 192–198.

5. R. L. Blair, "A Cognitive Developmental Approach to Morality: Investigating the Psychopath," *Cognition*, 57 (1995), pp. 1–29.

6. Elliot Turiel, M. Killen, and C. Helwig, "Morality: Its Structure, Functions, and Vagaries," *The Emergence of Morality in Young Children*, eds. J. Kagan and S. Lamb (Chicago, Ill.: University of Chicago Press, 1987), pp. 155–244; and J. Smetana, "Understanding of Social Rules," *The Child as Psychologist: An Introduction to the Development of Social Cognition*, ed. Mark Bennett (New York: Guilford Press, 1993), pp. 111–141.

7. R. L. Blair, "Moral Reasoning and the Child with Psychopathic Tendencies," *Personality and Individual Differences*, 26 (1997), pp. 731–739.

8. Blair, "A Cognitive Developmental Approach to Morality."

9. Blair, "Moral Reasoning and the Child with Psychopathic Tendencies."

10. Shaun Nichols, "Norms with Feeling," *Cognition*, 84 (2002), pp. 221–236.

11. Blair, "A Cognitive Developmental Approach to Morality"; and Blair, Jones, Clark, and Smith, "The Psychopathic Individual."

12. Shaun Nichols, *Sentimental Rules: On the Natural Foundations of Moral Judgment* (New York: Oxford University Press, 2004).

13. M. Simner, "Newborn's Response to the Cry of Another Infant," *Developmental Psychology*, 5 (1971), pp. 136–150; and C. Zahn-Waxler, M. Radke-Yarrow, E. Wagner, and M. Chapman, "Development of Concern for Others," *Developmental Psychology*, 28 (1992), pp. 126–136.

14. R. L. Blair, "The Neurobiological Basis of Psychopathy," *The British Journal of Psychiatry*, 182 (2003), pp. 5–7.

15. George Orwell, *Homage to Catalonia* (New York, Harcourt, Brace 1952), p. 70.

16. Ibid., pp. 96–97.

Ten

THE BENUMBING MORAL INDIFFERENCE OF THE WEALTHY: WHAT DOES IT TAKE TO MOTIVATE THE FULFILLMENT OF A MINIMAL NORM OF ECONOMIC JUSTICE?

William A. Rottschaefer

1. Introduction

In his provocative *One World: The Ethics of Globalization*, moral philosopher Peter Singer asks us to consider Bob and his prize collector's auto, a Bugatti.[1] Bob's Bugatti not only means a lot to him as a connoisseur of fine autos, but also is destined to serve as a source of retirement income. One day, Bob takes his Buggati for a drive. Deciding to do a little walking, he parks near a railroad track and starts to walk along the tracks. After proceeding for a couple of miles, he hears a train coming. At the same time, he notices a child trapped on the tracks of the approaching train. What to do? As it turns out, Bob has only two choices. He can turn a nearby rail switch allowing the train to proceed down a sidetrack, something that will lead to the inevitable destruction of his beloved Bugatti, but save the child. Or, he can do nothing, preserve his Bugatti, but lose the child. What should Bob do?

Singer contends that that most people have no doubt about what Bob ought to do. Bob should pull the switch, sacrifice his Bugatti, and save the child. If he does not, his failure is morally reprehensible.

Next, Singer asks us to consider a morally identical real-world situation. By giving $200 dollars to UNICEF, you can save the life of a destitute child in the third or fourth world. Your sacrifice is much less than Bob's. What ought you do? Our correct moral intuition about Bob and our ability to categorize the real case properly as morally identical with the imaginary case, should lead you, by means of our ability to appreciate consistency, to judge that you—and anyone else similarly advantaged—ought to give $200 dollars to UNICEF.

The duty of the relatively wealthy is apparent, but practice does not come near to meeting the moral norm. Why are relatively wealthy people morally indifferent—"benumbed," to use Adolf Tobeña's provocative word— to the sufferings of the vast majority? Tobeña considers the benumbed few, highly motivated to sacrifice their lives to an immoral cause that results in the death and injury of sometimes thousands of innocent people. To further his considerations, I propose to examine those many, some 900 million on Singer's account, who have little or no motivation to perform trivially self-sacrificial actions that together would save the lives of tens of millions. I will omit from consideration the equally pressing question of why these same people are motivated to participate in social and economic structures that enable this harm and destruction to continue. By considering this motivational indifference, I will address the issue of this dialogue, "the neurobiology of moral thought," conceived broadly to include the sciences of biology, psychology, and neuroscience. Examining some things that these sciences tell us about the sources and limits of moral motivation, I conclude that, though informative, we have much more to find out about moral indifference and concern.

Singer lays down a moral challenge to developed nations and their citizens, especially the United States of America. He challenges us to abide by an ethics suitable for a global community. If we pursue that ethics, we would seek to form a universal community in which the moral ideals of human rights, social justice, and environmental stability are manifest. His normative ethics springs from a fundamental normative principle that the highest ethical value is the greatest good, for the greatest number, impartially considered. He employs this standard to measure the morality of individual actions and social practices. Using a wealth of facts about climate change, world trade, and international relations, he details both the current crises and ethical demands facing humanity. Though not written for that purpose, his work embodies a bold attempt to address a focal concern of the Universal Forum of Cultures, Barcelona, 2004.

Besides questions about the defining and distinguishing characteristics of Singer's consequentialist moral ideal (and others, for instance, the Kantian ideal of respect for persons), we can raise questions about their attainability, adequacy, acquisition, and activation. Questions about attainability ask whether a moral ideal is within the evolutionary and learned capacities of human beings to acquire. Those concerning adequacy query whether adequate moral justification exists for an ideal. Questions about acquisition concern how achievable ideals are acquired, maintained and fostered and those about activation concern how, once acquired, these capacities might be exercised.

To focus our task, consider Singer's discussion of the moral ideal of human equality. The moral equality of all human beings is widely proclaimed, but not widely practiced. Singer suggests that our practice appears to follow more closely another moral ideal, one enunciated by the nineteenth-century British moral philosopher Henry Sedgwick: ideal of partiality of concern. This principle requires that we be most concerned morally about those closest to us, children, kin, lovers, friends, and those with whom we interact on a regular basis. We should be attentive, but in a lesser degree, to those who share our ethnic ties or who are fellow citizens, and to a still lesser degree with those of other races, cultures, and nations. Singer finds the moral ideal of partiality inadequate because it fails what he considers the crucial test of an adequate moral judgment, universalizability. The person making the moral judgment must be ready to prescribe that it be implemented in all circumstances, both actual and imaginary, and regardless of the affinity of the parties involved.

Universalizability implies impartiality. For the sake of discussion, I will assume the moral superiority of Singer's Consequentialist Ideal with respect to moral irrelevance of nationality in the impartial distribution of material goods.

Singer shows how practice, especially the practice of the government of the United States of America and its non-governmental agencies, fails to meet even the minimal standards set by the United Nations for eliminating poverty among the destitute peoples of the world. Some of this failure, he argues, is due to failure of political leadership. Another portion of the failure may be due to public ignorance and the consequent failure of citizens to demand more of their government. He discusses fascinating studies, the results of which indicate that the American public vastly overestimates the amount of foreign aid given by their government. These studies also indicate that those surveyed, when asked about what might be an appropriate level of giving for the United States, set the level far above the minimum United Nations standard. Apparently, on the national level, ignorance, and not the lack of ideal or motivation, is the problem. But, Singer notes that these studies may be misleading; they may only indicate the desire to appear morally upright. They do not tell us whether individual Americans hold Singer's moral ideal or, if they do, whether they would be motivated to follow it.

The World Bank estimates that $40–60 billion per year in additional aid for the next fifteen years would be necessary to achieve the United Nation's Millennium Summit goal to significantly reduce world poverty. What sort of fairly distributed burden would this put on the estimated 900 million people in high-income countries? A donation of about $100 per annum could achieve this goal, using the high end of the estimated need. The average per annum salary in the developed world is $27,500. A $100 per annum contribution is less than 0.4% of annual income, or less than one cent of every two dollars that a person earns. Singer rightly concludes that accomplishing this goal requires no "moral heroics." It demands only giving up a few trivialities and frivolities.

Achieving the bare minimum norm requires being motivated to do so. Singer thinks that we can be so motivated. As a moral philosopher in the rationalist tradition, he contends that reason provides both justification and motivation for moral ideals and actions. In his thought experiments about Bob and UNICEF, he appeals to three moral capacities: (1) a capability to form reliably correct ethical intuitions about imaginary cases; (2) an ability to discern morally relevant similar real world cases, when presented with them; and (3) a capability to consistently extend our reliable ethical judgments from the imaginary cases to the relevantly similar real world cases.

Do our best theories in evolutionary biology, neuroscience, and psychology support Singer's rationalist theory of moral motivation? If not, what do they tell us about the attainability, acquisition, and activation of the motivation to put the minimal norm into practice? A study of the history of modern scientific moral psychology finds three major contending approaches; behaviorist and social learning, Freudian, and the cognitive developmental theories of Jean Piaget and Lawrence Kohlberg.[2] By the 1960s, reason-emphasizing cognitive developmental theories of moral agency had achieved ascendancy. Developments since then have shown the limitations of the cognitive developmental approaches.[3] Besides most people appearing to achieve only the fourth stage of moral development, the stage in which what is moral is considered to be that which one's society says is moral, more serious problems appeared. That distinct irreversible stages of moral development exist is doubtful. Even more problematic, and especially key to our discussion, is the problem of moral motivation. At best, Kohlbergian theories of moral development account for moral reasoning. To the extent that Singer's moral psychology rests on similar rational methods to motivate moral practice, we have some empirically based reasons for thinking they are ineffective.

Around the same time, moral cognitive psychologists began to probe morality of infants and young children, populations not studied by Kohlbergians. Data examining emotional development and the efficacy of some sorts of parental discipline techniques indicate that emotions, especially those of empathy and sympathy, play key roles in moral development, especially moral motivation.[4] Studies of psychopaths appear to indicate that although their scores on standard measures of intelligence are not significantly different from normal individuals' scores, they are woefully lacking in terms of proper moral motivation.

Shaun Nichols has argued persuasively that psychopaths lack empathic capacities.[5] Finally, neurobiologists Antonio R. and Hanna Damasio and their colleagues have shown that lesions in the frontal orbital region of the brain, that have projections to the limbic area, cause profound deficiencies in decision making, including decisions concerning matters traditionally associated with morality.[6] Though patients suffering from such lesions appear to have normally functioning perception, memory, and intelligence, they are unable to make decisions involving planning and the assessment of long term consequences. The Damasios suggest that these patients are unable to narrow the range of possibilities generated in a given choice situation. They speculate that without properly working projections to the limbic area, patients are unable to use their emotional capacities to limit their decision space to a few evaluationally privileged choices. They have no "feel" for what is the right thing to do. They remain stymied in indecision or act on impulse for short-term immediate gratification.

These findings appear to point in one direction. Rationalist theories of moral agency must either be abandoned or supplemented by theories more akin to those of the British moral sentiment philosophers like David Hume's, that give pride of place to emotions in accounting for moral motivation.

Developments in evolutionary biology and their applications to animal behavior, including human behavior, sharply delineate the importance of emotions. The solution to the biological problem of altruism was central in this development. In organisms with sufficient neuronal gifts, these altruistic capacities become cognitive and motivational. Emotions are the prototype of such cognitive and motivational capacities. Charles Darwin understood our moral capacity to be founded on social instincts, especially empathic abilities. Studies in moral developmental psychology likewise emphasize the importance of the emotions in moral development.

Martin L. Hoffman pioneered psychological studies of moral internalization, what moral philosophers have traditionally called the development of conscience.[7] His work, and that of other researchers, has shown the superiority of inductive techniques in moral internalization. This technique appeals to developing children's empathic capability to appreciate the objective harm they cause. Moral internalization is superior to the technique of power assertion that makes use of fear of punishment and loss of privileges, and to the technique of love withdrawal that calls on anxiety concerning loss of parental affection and love. Finally, neurobiological findings, concerning patients with lesions in their orbital frontal cortex, also support the claim that for understanding agency, including moral agency, and for our ability to take on and act on moral ideals, we have to include a significant role for the emotions. Scientific findings also appear to indicate that emotions too have their limits. Evolutionary theory indicates not only the possibility of evolutionary altruism but also its limitations. The solution to the problem of biological altruism provides an evolutionary explanation of behavior directed toward non-kin and kin that are not direct descendants. But altruism toward direct descendants, indirect descendants, and the circle of reciprocators in a population does not extend the circle of altruism to the boundaries set by Singer's minimal norm, and, *a fortiori*, by his normative ideal. Since it appears to foster group competition and conflict, evolutionary altruism does not provide the motivation for the universality of ethical concern, implicitly or explicitly expressed in the ideal of any normative theory.

Hoffman has noted that empathy and sympathy are also subject to limitations.[8] We are prone to be empathetic primarily towards those with whom we have affinity and with whom we associate regularly. Empathy is subject to personal distress. Cues invoking empathy can overwhelm, leading us to feel distress and to withdraw from, or avoid, those cues. Empathy is also limited by being largely stimulus dependent. Because of these constraints on empathic motivation, Hoffman argues, it must be supplemented with the ethical principles of caring and justice. These enable a person to extend concern to those whom the person does not personally know and to provide for needs not immediately evident. He suggests that for these principles to be motivating, they have to become "hot": in some way associating themselves with the motivating power of emotions. The metaphorical character of this suggestion indicates that more empirical and theoretical work is required if we are to attain an adequate understanding of the motivating capacities that we need to fulfill Singer's minimal norm.

These studies on reason and emotion reflect the classical tension between Kantian moral norms that rely on reason for adequate moral motivation and Humean moral norms that rely on the passions. Reason can extend the circle with which we ought to be concerned to all human beings impartially considered, as Singer's minimal norm requires. But does it appear able to provide the motivational capability necessary to put the norm into practice?

On the other hand, emotions, especially empathy and sympathy, are motivationally potent. Still, their motivational power does not take us as far as Singer's minimal norm demands. These scientific theories and findings appear to indicate that neither reason nor emotion is adequate to do the job called upon them by something like Singer's minimal norm.

Another area of empirical research is salient in consideration of our question. Evolutionary considerations indicate that for living organisms to engage as agents in the struggle for survival and reproduction, we must distinguish self from non-self. They also suggest that when organisms acquire cognitive and motivational capacities, self-representation becomes a means to do that. Recent work in neuroscience indicates the significance of the role of representations of the self in basic motor actions.[9] I suggest that this work provides a neurological starting point and basis for understanding the importance of the conception of the self as moral agent.

Social cognitive psychologist, Albert Bandura, has developed a highly confirmed model of general human agency.[10] As applied to moral agency, the model indicates that any adequate account of moral motivation must include a conception of the self as a moral agent.[11] To be successful moral agents, persons must view themselves as having accepted moral standards as a measure of the adequacy of their actions in the moral realm, and reflectively taken on these standards as a source of motivation. They must also monitor, evaluate, and respond to their actions in the light of these standards. In addition, they must view themselves as capable of achieving the standards they set for themselves. On this account, agents will be motivated to achieve Singer's minimum norm, if they have internalized this norm, especially if they internalize it by taking it on themselves. In doing so, what makes them the moral agents they conceive themselves to be, is that they view themselves as the kind of people who value the sort of distribution of material goods that following the minimum norm entails. Such moral agents monitor and respond to their actions in light of this norm. In addition, they view themselves as capable of fulfilling this norm. That they view themselves as so capable is, itself, motivating.

If Bandura's account is correct, then persons acquire, maintain, and enhance this sort of self-referentially reflective agency in the same ways that they acquire the ability to perform other actions well. They do so by practice, observation of models, and by different sorts of symbolic learning. These findings suggest that conceptions of the self as moral agent may fill both the motivational gap left by rational considerations of impartiality and the restricted reach of motivationally effective emotional affiliation. But we need to exercise caution. Philosopher John M. Doris has recently argued that the classical studies of social psychologists Stanley Milgram and Philip Zimbardo, and more recent findings, make implausible different versions of moral agency based on moral character and virtue.[12] They show that moral action is highly sensitive to situational, as opposed to agent-centered factors. Do appeals to the role of the conception of the self as moral agent fall prey to these findings? Here we need to distinguish between accounts of moral character built on personality theories and those using social cognitive theories. The first sort appeals to such variables as temperament, disposition, trait, and attitude to account for behavior. The second appeal to specific cognitive and motivational capacities. In addition, while the first make personality central to their account of agency, the second maintain that not only internal "person variables" but also both the situation and the agent's behavior and its consequences are sources of behavior. Social cognitive theorists have been among the most prominent critics of personality theories of motivation and action. In addition, Bandura maintains that social and organizational contexts of action play a major role in shaping the moral actions of even those people who have developed the skills of moral agency.[13] Social and institutional practices bring about situations that enable agents to disengage themselves from moral responsibility. In this way, people are enabled to diminish or deny their moral responsibility by means of cognitive and motivational techniques.

On the other hand, some social practices enable individuals to extend the conception of themselves, so that it includes people from other groups. These practices foster ways in which the agent can implement an expanded sense of concern. They also model such activities and use symbolic modes to teach them. Social cognitive theories of moral agency, in contrast with personality theories, suggest that social structures also promote the situations in which people can understand not only how Singer's minimal norm applies to them but also adopt it and apply it to themselves. A problem remains, though, since the major means of acquiring moral motivation suggested by social cognitive theorists, those of practice, learning by modeling and by symbolic instruction, all appear to be morally neutral. They enable the acquisition of moral or immoral norms.

In conclusion, I have attempted to suggest some ways that the cognitive sciences, broadly construed, might shed light on both the sources for failure, and the possibilities for success, in achieving what appears to be a legitimate, but minimal moral challenge. I maintain that moral philosophers have much to learn from biology, psychology and neuroscience and that these sciences are only beginning to make a contribution to helping us to understand and remedy the moral evils perpetrated by the benumbed, whether they be sacrificial martyrs or the indifferently wealthy.

Notes

1. Peter Singer, *One World: The Ethics of Globalization* (New Haven, Conn.: Yale University Press, 2002).

2. William A. Rottschaefer, *The Biology and Psychology of Moral Agency* (New York: Cambridge University Press, 1998).

3. W. Kurtines and E. Grief, E., "The Development of Moral Thought: Review and Evaluation of Kohlberg's Approach," *Psychological Bulletin*, 81 (1974), pp. 453–470.

4. Nancy Eisenberg, *The Caring Child* (Cambridge, Mass.: Harvard University Press, 1992).

5. S. Nichols, "Mindreading and the Cognitive Architecture Underlying Altruistic Motivation," *Mind and Language*, 16 (2001), pp. 425–455.

6. R. Adolphs, A. Tranel, H. Bechara, H. Damasio, and A. Damasio, "Neuropsychological Approaches to Reasoning and Decision-Making," *Neurobiology of Decision-Making*, eds. A. R. Damasio, H. Damasio, and Y. Christen (Berlin: Springer Verlag, 1996), pp. 157–179).

7. Martin L. Hoffman, *Empathy and Moral Development: Implications for Caring and Justice* (New York: Cambridge University Press, 2000).

8. Ibid.

9. Patricia Smith Churchland, *Brain-Wise: Studies in Neuro-Philosophy* (Cambridge, Mass.: MIT Press, 2002).

10. Albert Bandura, *Social Foundations of Thought and Action: A Social Cognitive Theory* (Englewood Cliffs, N. J: Prentice Hall, 1986).

11. Rottschaefer, *The Biology and Psychology of Moral Agency*.

12. John M. Doris, *The Lack of Character: Personality and Moral Behavior* (New York: Cambridge University Press, 2002).

13. Bandura, *Social Foundations of Thought and Action*; and "Moral Disengagement in the Perpetration of Inhumanities," *Personality and Social Psychology Review*, 3:3 (1999), pp. 193–209.

Eleven

NATURALIST PERSPECTIVES ON MORALITY, LIMITS, AND POSSIBILITIES

Félix Ovejero

When we cannot solve a problem, one of the things we ask ourselves is whether our tools are adequate for understanding it. In the case of terrorism, it was only a matter of time before we looked toward neurosciences. Abundant reasons exist. In recent years, we have seen a progressive attempt to use a naturalist perspective to deal with many matters traditionally viewed as falling within the social sciences. This is especially the case of neuroscience research and, closely connected to it, evolutionary biology. Although "constructionist" theories persist, are even being revived—entrenched as they are in some university "Humanities" departments—this phenomenon is explained more by the logic of organizations and their inert need to justify their existence, than by the results obtained.

Such naturalist research has re-imposed a classical view of societies according to which human beings—emotionless, egoistic, highly rational creatures—agree to establish institutions, rules, which they will respect for as long as these are advantageous to maintain, in order to avoid confrontation. This view explains that human societies are maintained through spontaneous processes (the *invisible hand* or influence of the market) or reinforced through sanctions, such as state-mandated rules of the road or other state laws prescribed to discourage potentially conflictive behaviors. Yet this picture needs modifying in view of several naturalist-inspired results, which affect our ideas on society, our positive theories, and our rules.[1] Adolf Tobeña, among others, mentions two such results that have arisen in discussions that questioned theories thought to be fundamental in their respective spheres. In the normativist theory, the mental experiment presented by Philippa Foot, known as the trolley dilemma, has cropped up in many discussions on utilitarianism, the moral theory that holds correct actions are those that ensure maximization of aggregated wellbeing.[2] The second, the ultimatum game presented by Richard Thaler, has concerned many economists who view it as an objection to the *homo oeconomicus* (economic man) hypothesis, and by extension, to a significant part of economic theory that took it as a starting point.[3]

Recent research has reinstated a vision of society as a contract-agreement between calculating egoists with a series of results that appear reasonably consolidated:

(1) The anthropological theses of social theories—including their purest formulation, economic theory—do not correspond to the empirical results;[4]

(2) We participate from diverse, regular biases that distance us from rational behaviors in the sense of formal rationality theory;[5]

(3) Many of these biases distance us from "optimum" solutions, yet correspond to solutions to evolutionary problems (constrictions), for example, that we must make fast decisions under changing circumstances, using limited information and with a limited capability for analysis;[6]

(4) We are capable of recognizing such biases and recognizing our mistakes. In this reflective task, language is a powerful tool because it allows us to build theories and, with them, to escape from our perceived constrictions;[7]

(5) The presumption that human beings are purely egoistic is false, as false as claiming they are purely altruist;[8]

(6) Principles such as reciprocity or equity regulate many of our interactions in diverse human (and non-human) societies;[9]

(7) Human beings, and primates with an intense social life, are "natural psychologists": we make inferences regarding others' attitudes, reasoning and we second-guess their behavior, which forms a significant part of our communicative processes;[10]

(8) To rational egoists, the *homines oeconomici*, appear the closest to individuals suffering from affective blindness: they are incapable of making decisions, of valuing the emotional significance of events;[11]

(9) A society of *homines oeconomici*, with no emotional or regulatory bonds, sustained solely by its egoistic calculation, appears impossible: social interactions—including market exchanges—require trust, loyalty, and a sense of commitment;[12]

(10) Emotions operate in a coordinated manner (guilt with anger, revenge with fear) and, in this way, they resolve key social problems by avoiding conflicts from becoming destructive;[13]

(11) Emotions allow us to recognize the link between moral laws ("Thou shalt not kill.") and laws that are simple convention (pick up your fork with your left hand): people suffering from injuries affecting their emotional capability are incapable of distinguishing them;[14]

(12) Human beings present diverse emotional processes, repertoires of flexible commitments, and a variety of links between our rules and our emotions;[15]

(13) In each of us, different emotional and regulatory repertoires do not merely coexist, activated in diverse scenarios, but individuals widely differentiated in terms of motivation can coexist in the same scenario;[16]

(14) Our links to moral laws, except in pathological cases, are mediated by emotional links: injustice outrages us, arbitrariness humiliates us;[17] and

(15). Emotions have a biological substratum and are explained in evolutionary terms.[18]

All these results are significant and force us to review many of our preconceptions about human societies, institutions, and our manner of intervening in them. They also affect our idea of social sciences, like a "special" area, inaccessible using the theoretical or methodological strategies of naturalist sciences.[19] We must be prudent. Imagining what we might expect from naturalism in terms of explaining many problems that concern the social sciences would be difficult: inflation, World War II, urbanization processes, the crisis of feudalism, the break-up of the USSR. Yet they allow us to establish impossibility theorems, make affirmations on explanations that cannot be true, or those that do appear compatible with what we know of human cognitive dispositions.[20] For example, they would allow us to disqualify those social or economic theories that assume that individuals have a capability for analysis—or altruism—beyond human beings' scope. Meanwhile, they confirm for us that nothing astounding is inherent—they are compatible with our known biological substratum—in the solvent experimentation of social psychology. Results of studies in that field show that any of us, under some wholly unexceptional social pressures, can act like the Argentine military in Jorge Rafael Videla's time. Subject to exceptional circumstances (for example, a prison), we are capable of unleashing aggressive and cruel behavior.[21] Until now, we knew that a large part of that behavior is unleashed through changes in social roles. We can add that the form that that behavior adopts (aggressive, violent) depends on a repertoire established neurobiologically.

On the other hand, I do not see in what manner we could do away with the mentalist-intentional explanation strategies on which we build our social sciences—as has been suggested[22]—which include appeals to our emotions. For example, I am unsure how to explain the economic behavior of an agent without appealing to his or her beliefs (regarding the way things are; for example, how to increase profits) and his or her desires (obtaining profits). In any case, until we have come up with theories that explain processes without appealing to mental states such as beliefs or desires, I suspend my judgment on these suggestions. The best mode of showing that a strategy works is by showing results, solvent theories that resolve or dissolve the problems that concern social scientists. Currently, we generally find arguments concerning principle, based on historical comparisons, on analogies between the sterility of intentional strategies and the sterility of theories—such as the caloric, phlogiston or ether theories—that were unable to provide answers because the questions were senseless. I believe in this sense we must seriously practice what we preach. We need: more science.

1. Explaining Morality

Naturalist strategies can help solve the problems encountered, when attempting to explain laws, by social sciences' two customary theoretical approaches: the functionalist and the hyper-rationalist approach. (I prefer to talk of theoretical approaches as opposed to methodological strategies, because only rarely do the problems of theory compromise the "methods," in the explanatory strategies used in this case, respectively, the functional strategy and the intentional strategy.)[23] If my causal explanation (a blow to the head) for a headache is wrong, that just discounts my causal explanation, not causal explanations *per se*: another cause could explain my headache, for example, sunstroke. We should look at these social science problems to examine moral laws and see how naturalist theories can help us out of this impasse.

Both approaches begin by recognizing that moral laws are beneficial to some social system of reference. From that point on they diverge. Mostly sociologists develop the functional approach. Rules (for example, a prohibition on eating pork) are explained through their beneficial consequences for the social system (avoid squandering resources in societies with quite little water and not much vegetation).[24]

One branch of sociology has attempted a variant on this type of explanation, resorting to the economic theory of positive externalities: rules are subproducts of actions oriented towards distinct proposals for maintaining rules. They persist because they fulfill beneficial functions.[25] The fallacy of this explanation is immediate, like explaining away terrorist attacks by their beneficial effects on the pharmaceutical industry, as a consequence of the increase in tranquillizer sales. To recognize that functionalist sociologist explanations of rules do not help us, we still cannot afford to ignore that rules fulfill functions. Still, explanations taken from natural selection open the door to accepting those functions without falling victim to the functional fallacy—although problems and discussions are rife in this area.[26]

The hyper-rationalist approach, extremely popular with economists, consists of sketching out a scenario where some optimally rational egoistic agents behave morally or emotionally because it's "worth it" to them. Emotions or rules would have the same nature as the convention of driving on the right: an agreement we find convenient. The problem of this approach is not that the morality is not "worth it." Even a market economy, described by many people as a rational egoist's paradise, would be unworkable without a network of rules that force you to respect commitments, and to trust others.[27] We all want some moral sanction for those who respect our agreements. Also, occasionally, as the ultimatum game teaches us, not to be calculating, not just to consider benefits, is advantageous. If you know I am a rational egoist, you will offer me the minimum, knowing I will prefer something to nothing. If you know that I will get carried away by my indignation, or that I will behave vengefully, you will not make me manifestly unjust proposals. Unquestionably, emotions and rules are "worth it." The problem is that for emotions and rules to be "worth it" they must not be the result of a strategic calculation. We cannot make them "worth it." If everybody, in the end, behaved as calculating egoists, the rules would stop working.

On an individual level because, if I merely pretend to feel humiliated by your proposal when it violates an elemental rule of justice, and you know my moral indignation is "chosen," you will make me a miserable offer. You will be aware of my being a calculating agent and that, when push comes to shove, I will be content with what you are offering me, given that I do not have any other option. The only way the emotion serves my interests is that I cannot choose it. I cannot decide not to get emotional. We must be tied to our emotions. In the end, that bond points to biology, to selective pressures that favor that violating the rule unleashes the emotion. We can perceive the same in social interaction on the collective level: calculating behavior coerces others to respect the rules of trust while abstaining ourselves from doing so. In this manner, we benefit from the rules without paying the cost of maintaining them. Obviously, if we all acted like that, then nobody would respect the rules. We would not have any rules.

We also see that for the rules to fulfill their functions, we must be "tied" to them. This means they must have a biological substratum. There is no better link to moral norms than emotions. Emotions, coordinated, resolve the problem of rules and their sanctioning function. If you cannot avoid broadcasting a signal when you behave badly, do not respect agreements, or go your way, and the rest of us recognize that signal and cannot avoid penalizing you, then disloyal behavior will disappear. The emotions cemented into biological mechanisms are those signals: you cannot avoid feeling ashamed and blushing. I know what that color means and I cannot avoid becoming indignant. Briefly, with coarseness I hope you will forgive, the explanatory links—or explanatory constrictions—are: biology → emotions → rules → sociality.

2. Moral Evaluation

A naturalist perspective is helpful when we attempt to understand moral behavior. It can even help us to define operationally (or shed for good) significant concepts, such as utility or wellbeing, for empirical or normative theories. But moral behavior is not moral judgment. Explaining morality is one thing, valuing morality is another. Some behaviors in the distribution of goods are relatively generalized in human societies. You could even say that a set of extended

moral intuitions, or feelings of justice, exist. To formulate evolutionary explanations regarding these behaviors or intuitions is reasonable.[28] As Tobeña
highlights, moral behaviors and intuitions also occur in other species related
to us.[29] But we must adequately interpret this occurrence, and not confuse the
existence of such behaviors with the existence of moral and political evaluation. Distribution of food in different species follows regular, recognizable
patterns. To explore the criteria regulating these patterns is perfectly legitimate. We can analyze the distribution in any species, including insects. But to
engage in such analysis does not imply the assumption that we are facing
moral evaluations or moral theories carried into practice. To evaluate, we
must be able to govern our actions by alternative criteria; in this case, by alternative criteria for distribution, for example, effort, merit, need.

On the other hand, we do not have to believe that those moral practices,
even if fixed in our brain, are the final point in our moral judgments. We can
escape to our moral intuitions, evaluate, and correct them, regardless of
whether they have a biological base. A comparison helps clarify this circumstance. Human beings cannot perceive some colors or wavelengths. We see
the moon larger on the horizon than in the sky. Euclidian principles frame our
geometry and our "mental" physics are Aristotelian (so we say, "the sun
comes out," or "things fall"). In all those cases, those perceptions, fixed in our
neuronal wirework, are errors in several senses. We are able to evaluate them
as errors, to recognize that they are wrong. Those mental schemas have been
beneficial in evolutionary terms because they allow helpful adaptations—not
the best, but good—to ecological niches. For example, they let us access information quickly on average and draw inferences using fragmentary data.
Language—in this sense the same evolutionary process—lets us build theories
and artifacts that help us to escape those limitations. We can correct ourselves
and recognize our errors of perception: we can know the exact size of the
moon and that Aristotelian physics is false. Most of our best science presupposes systematic clashes with "intuitions" housed in our common sense with a
biological basis. If we were capable of escaping those limitations, firmly
seated in our biological basis, we are more able to escape much less determi-
nist dispositions, which we can naturally recognize and evaluate.

While I cannot perceive wavelengths beyond infrared or ultraviolet, I
can recognize that "I let myself get carried away" by an egoist or violent attitude, evaluate the attitude, and judge that I should not react in that manner.
The "trolley dilemma" is one of those cases for which we must correct our
moral biases, which tend to structure themselves as different situations identical in their relevant substance, under the spotlight of our analytical reflection
that shows, from a moral point of view, that no difference exists between
pushing a button and pushing a person.[30]

In this sense, our relationship to emotions would be no different from the
relationship to our inferential dispositions. Often we fall into these biases,
logical errors, many of which are systematic. We can even ponder the evolutionary reasons for such biases, conclude that in some sense, operating with

simplifying heuristics helps us make decisions.[31] But this does not stop us from recognizing those biases, their incorrect nature. This recognition is possible because we can evaluate our inferences from our logical theories. Concerning our moral behavior, we should also recognize some patterns, some heuristics, that run parallel to the heuristics of rationality, perhaps helping us to get many of our decisions right in some scenarios. Our having aggressive, jealous, or vengeful dispositions does not stop us from evaluating them. The closest comparison is to our gastronomic dispositions: millions of years of evolution, through hunger and scarcity, have contributed to us having a sweet tooth or being keen on greasy foods. We even like bodies that reflect—through their fatness—those tastes. Yet today, in our societies of abundance, such a disposition has pathological consequences like illnesses. Today we can recognize those circumstances and bridle our dispositions.

The existence of dispositions does not determine the moral principles that govern our collective life, although we cannot ignore them when designing our institutions. Let me describe an example. If human beings had egalitarian "instincts," it would be easy to split a cake into equal parts among a group. You would just have to let each person choose a piece. A simple institutional design based on a rule would be enough: "Everyone, please take the piece you want." Yet if we were the opposite, irremediable egoists, we could still have an egalitarian distribution.[32] In this case, instead of the above model, we should apply another one based on the rule: "Whoever divides the cake chooses their piece last." Propensities do not govern our moral principles—equality in this case—although they do govern how we carry them out, how we manage them. In this sense, knowledge of "human nature" imposes constrictions on our institutional proposals: for example, we cannot propose economic mechanisms that demand an impossible capability for computing information (some efficient market models) of individuals, or supererogatory generosity (some socialist models). In sum, we should recognize our ethical and emotional dispositions, yet these, which help us to explain, do not solve the problem of moral justification, of solving the problem of what we must decide or how we must organize our collective life.

In this reflective task, language fulfills a significant function. Not only does it help us evaluate our emotions, but also it can even enrich our emotional repertory. Some emotions—the emotions derived from feeling emotions, the second-degree emotions, for example, "shame at feeling fear"—require us to be able to recognize our first-degree emotion, the "fear," in this case, a task facilitated if we are able to designate it. We experience the first-degree emotion, whether we realize this, or whether we have a word to designate it. Yet the meta-emotion requires us to be aware that we are experiencing what we are feeling. For this reason, language is a crucial tool.

On the other hand, since emotions depend on judgment, they have a cognitive basis. Just like my fear disappears once I am told that there is no lion in the next room, my indignation at your behavior or my shame at my will depend on my judgments regarding what appears right to me.

3. On Terrorism

What can we say about suicide terrorism? I am not sure we can go far along naturalist lines. Above all, we are facing a serious characterization problem. I do not know how we could identify terrorist behavior in such a manner that our ponderings did not slip into vagueness or speculations on principle, transcendental arguments regarding the possibility that explanations exist, which we obviously cannot confuse with explanations. Terrorism does not appear to allow us the accuracy with which we can characterize language, processes of facial recognition, or dysfunctions like muscular dystrophy or dyslexia.

What are the behaviors we could recognize as unique to terrorist behavior? Obviously, after Hiroshima, the "willingness to sacrifice innocent people with the aim of achieving political objectives" does not count as terrorism for many people. I will focus on two Tobeña mentions, typical of standard analyses of terrorism, or more accurately, analyses of the relationship between emotions and morality: the terrorists' absence of empathic capability and the supposed disdain they have for their life in the name of an idea of good. Neither of these is satisfactory as a description of the terrorists' emotional behavior: academics in this area remind us of the difficulty, if not impossibility, of obtaining a reasonably satisfactory definition.[33]

Regarding the first, the supposed incapability of terrorists to place themselves in the other's role, to grant the other humanness, I believe that largely, the case is just the opposite. First, the negation of the human condition of the other is not unique to terrorists. As Tobeña reminds us, this negation forms part of most warlike strategies: without delving further, a large part of the antiterrorist fight begins by qualifying terrorists as "animals and vermin." Then, we should not forget that in the sophisticated theological discussions that accompanied the so-called discovery of America, many people defended the humane treatment of the natives, in the manner we treat children today, for paternal reasons—because they were not fully developed human beings, or so they thought. Today, we can also defend the rights of animals without appealing to empathies. Above all, terrorists do not lack empathy either. A large part of the terrorist strategy involves assuming that the other is so human they will accept the blackmail of violence. The potential victims, terrorized, will pressure politicians, transmitting the message that the terrorists are like inexorable mechanisms, that whatever happens, they will never cease. Terrorists never forget that their victims are human and that they are afraid to die.

The other aspect of many popular definitions is terrorists' supposed disdain for their lives in the interests of communal justice. This idea does not help us to characterize terrorist behavior, especially for anybody not a suicide terrorist. First, the subordination of life to justice is not a necessary condition for terrorism, since it is also brandished by a large number of those who refuse to yield to terrorist blackmail. The idea takes in that case the form of the following thesis: what is important is not life in any form, but dignified life. This is a sophisticated standard thesis that, with nuances, has arisen in discussions between moral philosophers concerned with abortion and euthanasia. In the case of those who resist terrorism, for example, in the Basque Country, its formulation is unequivocal. We know that if we accept the terrorist demands, the threat of death—terrorism—will disappear, but at the price of a life without freedom or dignity: a price that we are not prepared to pay, because we do not think life is the supreme value.[34] We can even reasonably sustain that politics is born at the moment we resignedly accept the threat of death as a final argument that forces us to comply with any arbitrariness. Yet this is not a sufficient condition either: whoever believes that conservation of their own life is a final undisputable principle, implicitly accepts that they are ready to kill—precisely to preserve their life.

We can naturally establish some ideas regarding aggressiveness, in a more or less precise sense. Yet terrorism, as Tobeña says, is more than this. Or less: the explanations that concern us in social sciences have a date. For example, we want to understand the 1929 Wall Street Crisis, the 11 September 2001 attacks in New York City and Washington, D.C., and Basque terrorism from the 1960s until now. We should not forget that any action we can seriously qualify as terrorism, of those in which we are interested, goes back less than a few centuries. This is a completely irrelevant period in terms of affecting our emotional and cognitive dispositions. To appeal to general dispositions confuses more than it clarifies. It would be like trying to explain nationalisms by appealing to the presence of territorial dispositions.

Notes

1. Félix Ovejero, *"Del Mercado al Instinto (o de los Intereses a las Pasiones),"* *Isegoría*, 18 (1998); and *La Libertad Inhóspita* (Paidós: Barcelona, 2003).

2. Philippa Foot, *Virtues and Vices and Other Essays in Moral Philosophy* (Oxford: Basil Blackwell: Oxford, 1978).

3. Richard Thaler, "Anomalies: The Ultimatum Game," *Journal of Economic Perspectives*, 2:4 (1988), pp: 195–206.

4. Kenneth Joseph Arrow, *The Rational Foundations of Economic Behaviour: Proceedings of the IEA Conference Held in Turin, Italy* (Basingstoke, UK: Macmillan, 1999 [1996]).

5. J. Bettman, J. Johnson, and J. Payne, "Consumer Decision Making," *The Handbook of Consumer Behavior*, eds. Thomas S. Robertson and Harold H. Kassarjian (Englewood Cliffs, N. J.: Prentice-Hall, 1991); and Isabelle Brocas and Juan d. Carrillo, eds., *The Psychology of Economic Decisions* (Oxford: Oxford University Press, 2003).

6. Jerome H. Barkow, Leda Cosmides, and John Tooby, eds., *The Adapted Mind: Evolutionary Psychology and the Generation of Culture* (New York: Oxford University Press, 1992); Gerd Gigerenzer and Todd M. Peter, *Simple Heuristics that Make Us Smart* (Oxford: Oxford University Press, 2000); Dan Sperber, David Premack, and Ann James Premack, eds., *Causal Cognition: A Multidisciplinary Debate* (New York: Oxford University Press 1995).

7. Daniel C. Dennett, "The Role of Language in Intelligence," *What Is Intelligence?* ed. J. Khalfa (Cambridge, UK: Cambridge University Press, 1994); and

Peter Carruthers and Andrew Chamberlain, eds., *Evolution and the Human Mind: Modularity, Language, and Meta-cognition* (Cambridge, UK: Cambridge University Press, 2000).

8. John H. Kagel and Alvin E. Roth, *The Handbook of Experimental Economics* (Princeton, N. J.: Princeton University Press, 1995); and S. Bowles and H. Gintis, "Homo Reciprocans," *Nature*, 405 (2002).

9. Peter Hammerstein, ed., *Genetic and Cultural Evolution of Cooperation* (Cambridge, Mass.: MIT Press, 2003).

10. Nicholas Humphrey, *The Inner Eye* (London: Faber in assoc. with Channel Four, 1986); and Dan Sperber and Deidre Wilson, *Relevance: Communication and Cognition* (Oxford: Blackwell, 1995).

11. Antonio R. Damasio, *Descartes' Error: Emotion, Reason, and the Human Brain* (New York: Putnam, 1994).

12. L.-A. Gérard-Varet, Serge-Christophe Kolm, and J. Mercier Ythier, eds., *The Economics of Reciprocity, Giving, and Altruism* (London: Macmillan, 2000); and Walter J. Schultz, *The Moral Conditions of Economic Efficiency* (Cambridge, Mass.: Cambridge University Press, 2001).

13. Alan Gibbard, *Wise Choices, Apt Feelings* (Oxford: Clarendon Press, 1990).

14. Sue Taylor Parker and Michael L. McKinney, eds., *Origins of Intelligence* (Baltimore: Md.: Johns Hopkins University Press, 1999).

15. Alexandra Maryanski and Jonathan H. Turner, *The Social Cage: Human Nature and the* Evolution of Society (Stanford, Calif.: Stanford University Press, 1992); and Y.-A. Hu and D.-Y. Liu, "Altruism versus Egoism in Human Behavior of Mixed Motives: An Experimental Studies," *American Journal of Economics and Sociology*, 62 (2003), p. 4.

16. Hans Werner Bierhoff, Ronald L. Cohen, and Jerald Greenberg, *Justice in Social Relations* (New York: Plenum Press, 1986); Alan Page Fiske, *Structures of Social Life: The Four Elementary Forms of Human Relations: Communal Sharing, Authority Ranking, Equality Matching, Market Pricing* (New York: Free Press, 1991); and J. Elster, "The Empirical Study of Justice," *Pluralism, Justice, and Equality*, eds. David Miller and Michael Walzer (Oxford: Oxford University Press, 1995).

17. S. Bowles and H. Gintis, "Prosocial Emotions," Santa Fe Institute Working Paper #02-07-028 (2003); and Michael Lewis and Jeannette M. Haviland-Jones, *Handbook of Emotions* (New York: Guilford Press, 2000), pp. 91–115.

18. W. G. Rundman, John Maynard Smith, and R. I. M. Dunbar, eds., *Evolution of Social Behaviour Patterns in Primates and Man: A Joint Discussion Meeting of the Royal Society and the British Academy* (Oxford: Oxford University Press, 1996); and William A. Rottschaefer, *The Biology and Psychology of Moral Agency* (Cambridge, Mass.: Cambridge University Press, 1998).

19. Barkow, Cosmides, and Tooby, *The Adapted Mind*; and H. Gintis, "Towards the Unity of the Behavioral Sciences," Santa Fe Working Paper #03-02-015 (2003).

20. Félix Ovejero, *La Quimera Fértil* (Barcelona, Spain: Icaria, 1992).

21. Arthur G. Miller, ed., *The Social Psychology of Good and Evil: Understanding Our Capacity for Kindness and Cruelty* (New York: Guilford, 2004).

22. Paul M. Churchland, "Folk Psychology and the Explanation of Human Behavior," *The Future of Folk Psychology*, ed. John D. Greenwoee (Cambridge, UK: Cambridge University Press, 1991).

23. Daniel C. Dennett, *The Intentional Stance* (Cambridge, Mass.: MIT Press, 1987).

24. Marvin Harris, *Cows, Pigs, Wars, & Witches: The Riddles of Culture* (New York: Vintage, 1974).

25. James Samuel Coleman, *Foundations of Social Theory* (Cambridge, Mass.: Harvard University Press, 1990).

26. André Ariew, Robert Cummins, and Mark Perlman, eds., *Functions: New Essays in Philosophy of Psychology and Biology* (Oxford: Oxford University Press, 2002).

27. Robert H. Frank, *What Price the Moral High Ground? Ethical Dilemmas in Competitive Environments* (Princeton, N.J.: Princeton University Press, 2004).

28. S. Bowles, "Strong Reciprocity and Human Sociality," *Journal of Theoretical Biology*, 206 (2000).

29. Christopher Boehm, *Hierarchy in the Forest: The Evolution of Egalitarian Behavior* (Cambridge, Mass.: Harvard University Press, 1999); F. B. M. de Waal, *Chimpanzee Politics: Power and Sex Among Apes* (Cambridge, Mass.: Harvard University Press, 1989); and *Good Nature* (Cambridge, Mass.: Harvard University Press, 1996).

30. C. Sunstein, "Moral Heuristics," University of Chicago Law & Economics, Olin Working Paper, No. 180 (2003).

31. Daniel Kahneman, Paul Slovic, and Amos Tversky, eds., *Judgment under Uncertainty: Heuristics and Biases* (Cambridge, UK: Cambridge University Press, 1982); and Gigerenzer and Peter, *Simple Heuristics that Make Us Smart*.

32. John Rawls, *A Theory of Justice* (Oxford: Oxford University Press, 1972).

33. I. Sánchez-Cuenca, *"Son todos los Terrorismos Iguales,"* ("Are All Terrorisms the Same?") *Claves de Razón Práctica*, 144 (2004).

34. A. Arteta, *"Arquíloco como Pretexto: Un Ética de la Deserción,"* (Archilochus used as a Pretext: An Ethics of Defection), *Claves de Razón Práctica*, 128 (2002).

Twelve

SUICIDE TERRORISTS, NEUROSCIENCE AND MORALITY: TAKING COMPLEXITIES INTO ACCOUNT

Antoni Gomila

In these comments, I will focus on a central question regarding the neurobiological basis of morality: whether trying to found moral competence in some sort of neuronal structures makes sense, and correlatively, whether viewing moral incompetence as some sort of psychopathology or brain malfunction makes sense. True, Adolf Tobeña's paper does not explicitly make this claim, but elements in the second part suggest or encourage such a view.[1] Be that as it may, I think that this is a relevant question in its own right, one to which previous authors have already answered in the affirmative.[2]

In a sense, the issue is analogous to that of whether an account of good health in exclusively biological terms is possible. As Georges Canguilhem showed, though, such a concept involves normative considerations that refer to social values.[3] As regards morality, these normative, and social dimensions are even more evident and explicit; more so, given that the foundation of morality is even more ambiguous than the foundation of good health, which in the end must appeal to some sort of functional aspects. In the case of morality, though, the nature of the good is not as patent, an individual can consider something good that a whole society deems repugnant (and vice versa).

Because of these considerations, we should be prudent when interpreting the research that Tobeña reviews, to avoid the risk of falling into the reductionist temptation of equating amorality with mental illness, and to avoid viewing immorality as psychopathological.

This last issue surrounding the nature of amorality, what morality comes to, rank among the most important propellers of ethical thinking. The acknowledgement of human diversity, in historical and geographical terms, which also involves moral values and behaviors, gave initially rise to judgments of non-humanity to those whom are different. At the same time, rejection of such a simplistic judgment threatens to call the spectrum of relativism, if every human behavior is to be equally acceptable. But relativism appears to be inconsistent with the very possibility of morality, of judging right and wrong, given their characteristic inconditionality. To think of those with different moral views, or with quirky behaviors, as "mentally ill" or "neurobiologically disordered," would amount to a similar mistake, and might generate a similar dialectics.

Apparently, such an approach seems to recommend itself in the case of psychopathy, the features of which Tobeña nicely describes as an extreme case of amorality. But as he acknowledges, no such biological basis of psychopathy has been found yet. Even so, we can reasonably expect some sort of correlation between psychopathy and brain functioning given that the "immunity" to moral considerations and lack of fear of consequences of these subjects are kinds of mental activity, which must have their neurobiological grounding. But it could consists in some kind of global functional disconnection of different motivational systems, instead of some kind of localized lack of neuronal activity.

In the case of the suicidal terrorists, though, we have good reasons—such as those for which Scott Atran argued in his contribution to this symposium—to reject their assimilation to some kind of psychopaths.[4] On the contrary, they appear to be people with a strong moral sense, understood as sense of duty towards their group, which they view as an innocent victim of a situation of injustice forced by a stronger enemy. In this regard, the usual concepts of endo- and exo-group are not enough to account of this phenomenon. the sense of belonging may contribute to increase consensus within the endo-group, and exaggerate communalities, while magnifying differences with the exo-group. But this is not enough to account for the bursting of violence between them. A history of violence was always present in the precedent of the phenomenon of suicidal attacks, and it appears to also have been a necessary condition.

From this point of view, the brain of a suicidal terrorist could turn out to be boring and uninteresting for Neuroscience. In effect, most experimental studies have used practical dilemmas designed to get subjects to feel a conflict. Suicidal terrorists might not feel any such conflict. Perhaps if scanning the brain of a terrorist were possible, we might find nothing of interest regarding this contentious issue.

The idea of using conflict to understand human decision making has been common currency in game theory since the prisoner's dilemma. I believe that Neuroscience has imported the approach wholesale. True, such an approach fitted naturally into neuroscientific experimental designs. Cognitive conflict (such as between semantics and syntax in language processing), has also been used in Neuroscience to highlight neural processes corresponding to mental systems differentially engaged in a task depending upon how the task is worded. In the current case, I think that Neuroscience has just assumed game theory background, and in so doing, has inherited the same problems that affect such a view of human decision in terms of weighing costs and benefits.

To focus on what is of interest here, let us remember that a dilemma for this approach appears when a subject faces the commensuration of two different sets of costs and benefits. The footbridge dilemma is illustrative of that: On the one hand, utilitarian considerations provide a reason in favor of the course of action that produces the best (or less bad) outcome. On the other hand, we have the "you shall not kill" sense of duty. We can also view the ultimatum game as a dilemma for offers between 30 and 10 percent less than the total, where a sense of conflict may arise, while at that point, rejection—altruistic punishment—becomes mandatory for the subject. On the contrary, the trolley "dilemma" is not properly a dilemma, because researchers ask the subject whether hitting the switch is "all right," not what the subject would do. Investigators elicit a judgment, not a decision. [5]

For a situation to be a dilemma, two courses of actions must be available, each of which has some *prima facie* reasons in its favor, such that the subject must deliberate to reach a decision. Moral dilemmas are comprised of situations wherein one or both of the horns of the dilemma must have its *prima facie* appeal out of moral considerations. Yet a person can deem something right, or proper, but not morally right or proper, and still prefer it. The moral reasons are not the only, much less the final, reasons for a person's options (despite our competence at rationalization or ideology). This is common practical knowledge among business "sharks," crooked politicians, military commanders, or even university professors: life is hard and keeping our hands clean is not possible if we are to succeed.

Genuine moral dilemmas are situations in which both options have moral reasons in their favor, so that the question faced by the deliberator is to weigh their moral principles or values in such a case. These are the kind of situations where, according to post-war French existentialism, a person may act by chance or without a reason (just as Buridan's ass, in the end, before dying of hunger, might choose one source of food over the other for no particular reason). More poignantly, these sorts of situations led Isiah Berlin to conclude that reducing all values to one is not possible, and expecting to be able to always reconcile all of them is not reasonable given their incommensurability. [6]

We should keep in mind these complexities of morality to avoid a too fast and ready interpretation of the experimental results. As I see them, they all turn on situations where the conflict exists between different combinations of costs and benefits. The issue is to ascertain to what extent human beings prefer the most rational—understood as the best trade-off—of interests. Game theory dilemmas are interesting because they appear to show that human beings are not rational in this sense. Their interest is limited because game theory does not take the complexities of human morality into account. [7] The reason is that game theory's descent is nineteenth century Utilitarianism. On this view, morality and rationality are equated, and rationality is understood as self-interest. Even on its own grounds, though, this approach fails, because it is inconsistent with an adequate theory of the moral subject (Derek Parfit showed this, but stuck to the self-interest view of rationality, and rejected the idea of a moral subject [8]).

One of the problems of Utilitarianism is that it gives the same weight in the deliberation to all the reasons and all the people concerned. This is an impersonality requirement, which appears to be psychologically implausible. One of the best examples of that debate, also of current renewed interest, is

that according to Utilitarians, we should give the same weight to future generations and their interests as we afford to currently living people. But considering the interests of people who may live in the next century is quite difficult.
That is why the appeal to future generations usually takes the form of taking
the interests of our children into account, a twist in the way of personal involvement. While being concerned with the future consequences of our decisions may be reasonable, Utilitarianism does not prove a good way to make
anyone so concerned because of this impersonality.

We can work out a better picture of human morality if we distinguish the
basic, natural level of human motivation, from a second, reflexive, level. The
first is the level of preferences, interests, spontaneous motivational states,
which mediates human relationships. In this sense, it involves a basic reference to "good" or "bad" The second is the level of explicit morality (norms,
values, reasons), where the subject becomes morally accountable, can deliberate, and inhibit level one inclinations. This distinction allows us to realize that
conflicts can already arise at level one: "I am thirsty and hungry at the same
time: what I do first, eat or drink? What should I do if I have to choose just
one action?" It can also appear at level two (as when a father thinks his duty is
to be protective but also respectful of the autonomy and freedom of his adolescent girl). It can also arise at the interaction of both levels (I feel inclined to
hate this rival that defeated me, while I have reasons not to do so because it
would be childish and shameful). To comply with duty is difficult.

This distinction helps explain why the same people that may judge, or
have reasons to believe, that it is right to kill one person to save five others,
may not be willing to do so themselves. Personal—not merely emotional—
involvement may mobilize level-one motivational states, the most powerful
(some, following David Hume, contend that personal involvement is the only
motivational force).

At this personal level, in addition to moral principles, "level one" inclinations, natural preferences, and motivations matter. The "moral sense"
Charles Darwin mentions, and understands in terms of spontaneous "sympathy" (following the lead of Hume and Adam Smith) and what could nowadays
be termed "humanitarian feelings," corresponds to this basic level of moral
life, below and previous to the moral concepts (goodness, duty, worth), and to
abstract moral reasoning. Emotions, especially moral, self-conscious ones,
such as remorse, pride, shame, or resentment, also belong with the basic level
of moral experience. Indignation, which appears in the ultimatum game, is
also relevant here: Persons believe that others have treated them unfairly, even
if they lack the (explicit) concept of justice (such as the chimps).

Tobeña, in the section "The Neuroimagery of Amorality" provides indirect, neuropsychological evidence of the psychological plausibility of these
different levels. There, he reviews neurobiological evidence of dissociation
between what I have called "level one" (motives, preferences, natural inclinations) and "level two" (reasons, norms): he mentions the finding of patients

who, after brain injury, retained their ability for moral reasoning while their behavior was no longer influenced by it.

I would recommend that Neuroscience should take this broader approach to morality, to understand how the brain reflects genuine moral conflicts such as the addict contemplating whether to quit, the obese person considering whether to stop compulsive eating, the compulsive liar considering whether to repent, or the fundamentalist's inability to even consider in imagination a "taboo-breaking" statement.

From this standpoint, we should plainly see that game theory dilemmas do not pose a problem for ethical theories in general, but just for utilitarian theories, which are the descent of game theory. How "human beings [can] tend to consider it acceptable to sacrifice deliberately the life of one person in exchange for five when all required is the flick of a switch, but not when it would involved pushing the actual person to be sacrificed," appears enigmatic if we merely assume a simplistic view of human action.[9] We can find a distinct parallel in the difference people normally find in killing as opposed to letting someone die, or between action and omission. The intention is the same, the outcome is the same, but the actions are not. Most people do judge these sorts of oppositions to be morally different. For example, many who countenance passive euthanasia (letting a person die) would be reluctant to engage in active euthanasia, such as administering a lethal injection. Even in the case of brain stem death where vegetative functions continue (breathing and pulse), most people still respect a moral difference between active and passive euthanasia, despite the person already being "dead" by some definitions.

In the trolley experiment, a different wording of the problem could suffice to obtain a different answer. If the wording called attention to the way the outcome must be accomplished and by whom, it would make subjects aware of their personal involvement.

Lacking that awareness, we can reasonably expect a different decision in the footbridge dilemma as that obtained in the trolley dilemma, because of the personal—not merely emotional—involvement. This does not show that we are morally inconsistent, but that when we reason in abstract moral terms, we do it differently from when we deliberate about what to do. The reader could reply that to be palatable, my reinterpretation heavily depends on the crucial effect of wording, as if whether explicit reference to morality could be decisive. We do find that available evidence points in this direction in the area of "judgment under uncertainty."[10] To ask "What would you do in such and such circumstances?" and, "Do you think doing X in such and such circumstances is morally right?" are not equivalent questions. Persons could be unable or unwilling, to do what they think is morally right, or they might be unable to reach a reasoned decision about which moral principles, of those that they respect, they should give priority. This amounts to the difference between a Kantian categorical understanding of duty without exceptions versus a utilitarian trade-off of costs and benefits.

With all this as background, we can now turn to the central issue I want to consider: why we should not conceive of a behavioral anomaly, such as suicide terrorism, in psychopathological terms. The complexities of human morality may help us understand why, in extreme circumstances, some people may feel obliged to do extreme things and why some people may suffer from adaptation problems because of how they value what they did, or what they failed to do. Again, we should not buy into the game theory assumption that rationality only amounts to weighting costs and benefits. Morality also involves appeal to values and norms the scope of which includes persons' self-evaluation. This caution comes from consideration of past abuses of psychiatry, which, in retrospect, we view as obvious mistakes (such as the Soviet psychiatric practice of diagnosing political dissidents as "fools" and institutionalizing them in psychiatric hospitals).

Maybe an example can help clarify and emphasize this point. The case of Claude Eatherly, pilot of a weather reconnaissance aircraft Straight Flush that flew over potential targets before the Enola Gay dropped the atomic bomb on Hiroshima, Japan, on 6 August 1945, is illustrative. Acclaimed as a hero, soon after the end of World War II, he began to experience terrorizing nightmares during which the faces of the victims of the bombing appeared to him. He became depressed and began to drink alcohol. In 1950, he made a suicide attempt. After that, he started voluntarily six-week psychiatric treatment at a military hospital. His life did not improve; by 1953, he began to commit small crimes such as breaking into banks and post offices without ever taking anything. His reported intention was to debunk his war hero status because of his overwhelming feelings of guilt. Condemned, he returned to the hospital instead of entering the prison. There he stayed for a few years. The clinical description of his state, described by Dr. McEtroy, head of the hospital, is interesting:

> His regret feelings and consciousness of guilt are considered pathological; his sensitivity, which distinguishes him from all their unconcerned fellows, is interpreted as "dull feelings" and his fixed ideas will be treated with shocks of insulin.[11]

On the contrary, Paul Tibbets, the pilot of the Enola Gay, felt no such remorse, and always considered that what they did was right and proper.[12] But should we consider Eatherly's case a psychiatric one? Were not his feelings understandable and morally justified? The pang of consciousness that Eatherly experienced after the realization of the damage and evil he had been instrumental in causing, may well have generated mental health problems for him. I contend that these problems stemmed from an extremely acute moral sense. It was because of his moral values that he could not stand what he had contributed to cause.

Karl Adolf Eichmann, the German SS chief who facilitated and managed the program of extermination camps during World War II, exemplifies the counterpoint to Eatherly. Israeli secret agents captured Eichmann, who had taken refuge in Argentina after the war. They brought him to trial in Israel. Eichmann's testimony inspired Hanna Arendt's expression "the banality of evil," meaning that we can cause the greatest of evils without acknowledging its moral significance, as if evil were something banal, void of significance for the agent.[13]

Something similar may happen with torturers, able to live a perfectly adapted life, apparently hearing the agonizing screams of their victims as noise associated with their work. We could be inclined to view examples such as these as the sick, pathological cases. Instead, what we have here is lack of a "moral sense," a lack of basic empathy for human suffering, and lack of a sense of responsibility: a lack of personal involvement in the production of evil—typically attributed to a higher authority.

I do not mean, though, to keep separate the study of psychopathology and the study of moral sensitivity. Instead, my conclusion is that we should better acknowledge their intricate and complex relationships. Morality depends upon the values and social norms that a person has internalized; sometimes, in extreme circumstances, a person may be unable to cope with his or her own standards and the outcome may be a psychopathology.

Claude Eatherly's inability to rationalize all the damage he had indirectly helped to cause led him to be socially maladapted. But his feelings evince something admirable, and most of his contemporaries probably shared his feelings. Eichmann's moral dumbness at the level of personal involvement helps us understand how totalitarian regimes are viable and suggests that we should expend more effort on the moral education of youngsters.

More than merely teaching abstract norms and reasons, moral education should be a sentimental education, a self-constitution of patterns of emotional interaction (nowadays, children learn more about these values from situational comedy programs on television than from educators or parents).

Another, different, example of how intricate the links between mental health and moral sensitivity can be is the case of Siegfried Sassoon, a British poet who took part at the Battle of Somme, during World War I. That battle best exemplifies the cruelty and stupidity of war (half a million British and German soldiers and two hundred thousand French troops died without any territorial gain by either party). Sassoon, after sustaining injuries twice, took a stand against war, threw his Military Cross into the river Mersey, and decided not to return to the front. Instead of the court-martial he expected, the military authorities decided that he was unfit for service and sent him to a psychiatric hospital, where he was officially treated for neurasthenia ("shell shock"; the modern diagnosis would be Post Traumatic Stress Disorder). Finally, though, he decided to return to the front, out of a feeling of guilt for having abandoned his colleagues.

In Sassoon's case, we find a conflict and then a resolution between the mental health effects of a life experience and the strength of some of the values—companionship, patriotism, enforced by military training—needed to block the natural compassionate reaction of the moral sense. Yet based on reports of post-traumatic effects caused by torture and cold-blood killings by American soldiers in Iraq, such training is not always enough to block these emotions. Moral principles may appear to be neat and unambiguous, but the application in real life, in personal involvement, is not so neat; it may affect our mental life. To come back to World War II, Primo Levi and Jean Améry committed suicide, while another vivid writer, Jorge Semprún, not Jewish but a communist, found a way to make sense of that episode in his life.

Further development of these considerations would probably require discussion of the notion of defense mechanisms and related views of the structure of human subjectivity. We would probably need to question the Freudian notion and suggest a more adequate understanding of the self as a moral subject. I dare not do that here. I will just mention that writings in Neuroscience have already begun to reintroduce such a notion.[14] I believe that this notion has much to contribute if such a discussion would manage to get the complexities right. In any case, neuroscientific research undoubtedly helped to clarify these complexities and the nature of personal involvement, and it may continue to advance knowledge in this respect.

Acknowledgments

I am deeply indebted to Josep E. Corbí for discussion of the thoughts contained in the final section of this chapter, and introducing me to the Eatherly case. I have received support for writing from the Spanish Ministry of Education, through project BFF2003-129. I also want to thank the organizer of The Social Brain Forum for allowing me to be part of this great event, and the English editor for her help.

Notes

1. Adolf Tobeña, "Benumbing and Moral Exaltation in Deadly Martyrs: A View from Neuroscience," paper presented to the International Colloquium, "The Social Brain: Biology of Conflict and Cooperation," Barcelona, Spain, June 2004 (see this volume chap. 7).

2. Cesare Lombroso, *Crime: Its Causes and Remedies* (Montclair, N.J.: Patterson Smith, 1968).

3. Georges Canguilhem, *The Normal and the Pathological* (New York: Zone Press, 1991).

4. Scott Atran, "Religion, Suicide, Terrorism, and the Moral Foundation of the World," paper presented to the International Colloquium, "The Social Brain: Biology of Conflict and Cooperation," Barcelona, Spain, June 2004 (see this volume chap. 8).

5. Tobeña, "Benumbing and Moral Exaltation in Deadly Martyrs," pp. 77–79.

6. Isiah Berlin, The Crooked Timber of Humanity (Princeton, N.J.: Princeton University Press, 1958).

7. F. Schick, *Making Choices: A Recasting of Decision Theory* (Cambridge University Press, 2003).

8. Derek Parfit, *Reasons and Persons* (Oxford: Oxford University Press, 1984).

9. Tobeña, "Benumbing and Moral Exaltation in Deadly Martyrs."

10. D. Kahnemann and A. Tversky, "The Framing of Decisions and the Psychology of Choice," *Science*, 211 (1982), pp. 453–458.

11. Gunther Anders and Claude Eatherly, *Burning Consciousness* (New York: Paragon Hause, 1961), p.47.

12. Paul W. Tibbets, *The Tibbets Story* (New York: Stein & Day, 1978).

13. Hannah Arendt, *Eichmann in Jerusalem: A Study on the Banality of Evil* (New York: Viking Press, 1963).

14. V. S. Ramachandran and Sandra Blakesly, *Phantoms in the Brain: Probing the Mysteries of the Human Mind* (New York: Quill, 1999).

Thirteen

FOUNDATIONS OF MORALITY IN THE INFANT

David Premack

As a rule, American schools do not teach morality. Educators believe morality is a private matter that parents should teach to their children. This is a mistake, I would suggest. The parents are too late; their children already know morality. Evolution taught them.

Human beings lived 95 percent of their existence as a species in small bands of twenty-five to forty individuals, women gathering plant food, men hunting. Most bands were egalitarian; they had no social hierarchy or permanent leaders and people shared food. Selective pressures arising from the lifestyle of the hunter-gatherers are likely to have led to the evolution of morality. Test evidence supports the evolutionary view. Children show moral knowledge from an early age.[1] Three principles summarize children's moral knowledge: (1) Do not harm the other one; (2) Deal fairly with other; and (3) Care for those who are in distress.

These simple principles owe their power to their fecundity. Each can take indeterminately many forms, for example, "harm" can be mental or physical, "fairness" is subject to enormous diversity, and "distress" takes many forms. More important than the fecundity of the principles is that people can recognize all of the forms that the principles take.

But if we are so nicely endowed as a species with moral knowledge, so well equipped with intuitions for recognizing the moral alternatives; if morality can be captured by three simple, though extraordinarily fecund principles, which take infinitely many conditions all of which humans can recognize—if we are, in sum, so beautifully endowed with moral competence, why is the world in such a mess?

Knowledge does not automatically produce performance. Regrettably, while evolution has prepared us nicely with moral competence, not surprisingly, it has "failed" us with regard to self-control. Although our lifestyle as hunter-gatherers—small bands of twenty-five to forty, living in close proximity, sharing food—led to selective pressures for the evolution of morality, it did not lead to selective pressures for self-control. People need self-control when they live alone, but they must independently control selfish desires. Hunter-gatherers were never alone. If a hunter-gatherer harmed his neighbor or dealt unfairly with him, others would quickly detect his doing so. This will not lead to self-control, though it may induce susceptibility to social control.

Our social intelligence is legendary. We have an elaborate theory of mind, attribute mental states to others, and do so recursively. Human beings worry not only about what John thinks of them, but also what John thinks, Mary thinks, Joe thinks, Delores thinks, Henry thinks, of them. Evolution may have "short-changed" us in self-control, but it did not deny us sensitivity to the minds of others.

Self-control comes not from evolution, but from training of the young by the mother. All mammalian infants form close attachments to their mothers, but only the human mother exploits this fact, using her powers of reward and punishment to train the infant. Her many injunctions include toilet training, chewing with the mouth closed, and not hitting your sister. The children feel the training at two levels. First, motivationally, for rewarded acts increase in frequency, while punished ones decrease. But the cognitive level is far more important. Children are not just a passive recipient of mothers' rewards and punishments—they induce a rule that will help them summarize their mother's training. The rule they induce is something like: do NOT do what comes naturally, inhibit your natural dispositions, try hard! This rule is critical because it enables the child's learning to transfer to adulthood. Though the challenges faced as adults are quite different from those faced as children, they make the same internal demands. To not to cheat on tests, not to steal, and not to engage in adultery, the adult (like the child) must: "inhibit natural impulses," "try hard!" and "not do what comes naturally."

How effective is self-control? Millions of Americans have quit smoking. How did they do it? Some of them quit by the method we call "cold turkey." After having smoked for twenty years or so, they make a decision not to smoke, and then never smoke again. Surveys suggest that 80 percent of American smokers who try to quit succeed. Approximately 30 percent (three of every eight successful "quitters") did it cold turkey, suggesting that they evinced self-control. What accounts for the remaining 50 percent? Apparently, they did not have the self-control required to quit by themselves, but were "forced" by social control to try it by other, assisted methods.[2] In America, jail is about the only public place where smoking is permissible. The federal government has banned smoking in most public places. In forcing people to smoke on the sidewalk like social outcasts, the government turned a sophisticated act into a socially disreputable one. This outcome of almost twice as much social control as self-control is reminiscent of the hunter-gatherer band.

Though many people think that shame and guilt play a large role in self-control, we have no evidence for this assumption. Studies have shown that fearful children are more inclined to restrain themselves. A fearful child, who, when placed in a novel environment clings to his mother instead of explore, shows more guilt if he is caught violating a rule. He looks down, his face changes color. Also, he is less likely to violate injunctions such as "Don't touch those toys" and the like. But suppose that fearful, guilt-prone children turn into fearful guilt-prone adults. Are we looking at morality or obedience? I smell the stale aroma of obedience, not morality.

Interestingly, morality is the only evolved ability—as compared with language, number, music, theory of mind, or social competence—where we violate our competence. We do not usually produce ungrammatical sentences, miscalculate, sing out of key, or attribute flagrantly false states of mind. Since misbehaving yields no profit, the transition in these cases from competence to performance is straightforward. But this is not the case in moral knowledge. Violating our moral competence can be considerably profitable. Moral action can be extremely costly, not only in terms of the profit that I lose by not cheating you, but in terms of the cost, I might have to pay to prevent others from not cheating you.

Let us look at the three principles, which summarize our moral knowledge. Consider briefly how these principles appear in the child. In the eighteen-month-old, we see strong evidence for the third principle, "Care for those in distress." Doris Bischof-Kohler showed fifty eighteen-month-old infants an individual familiar to them, holding a broken Teddy Bear, who was crying and moaning.[3] Forty-eight children came to the rescue of the victim. The infants patted the individual, consoled her, and even tried to mend the Teddy Bear. Two of them recognized the victim's distress and vulnerability, but instead of helping, they behaved sadistically, marching around like soldiers, shouting and stomping. Still, ninety-six percent of the children acting in favor of morality is pretty good for any species.

Now let us consider the second principle, which commands the child to treat the other one fairly. A simple way to demonstrate the young child's sense of fairness is to show the child two dolls, and then, in one case, give both dolls equal pieces of candy; in another case, give them unequal pieces. Do the children react differently? Do they smile when we give the dolls equal shares, frown when we give them unequal shares? Do they shout, "No! No!" in the one case, even try to hit the tester? Unfortunately, most developmental psychologists do not test children in this manner (as chimpanzees would force us to do). Instead, they interview the children and ask questions. Ample evidence exists to demonstrate the child's recognition of the propriety of fair division. We also find that, while young children are strict in equating fair with equal, older children sanction giving more to those who contribute more, or need more. The child's recognition of what is fair does not mean that he will always share his goods in a fair manner. Knowledge does not guarantee performance.

Do infants recognize the moral principles? We showed computer-generated animations of spontaneously moving balls to ten month-old infants, using looking time as a measure of interest.[4] Infants do not appear to prefer looking at one object caress another instead of hitting another, as you might think they would if they recognized the moral principle, "Do not harm others." They look at one case as long as at the other. Still, this is not a discerning test of their moral judgment and may indicate merely that they find hitting as interesting to look at as caressing. A better test would give the infant an opportunity to determine whether one object hit or caressed another, say, by turning its head in one direction of the other. But researchers have not conducted tests of this kind for any of the moral principles.

While we have not tested morality with infants, we found evidence for the foundations of morality in children as young as ten months old. To begin with, infants distinguish physical from psychological objects: this distinction is a precursor of morality, since psychological, not physical, objects are the locus of morality. Physical objects move only when acted upon by another object: psychological objects are self-propelled and move autonomously.

Infants interpret the movement of physical objects in terms of force and size. For example, if a big ball hits a little one and the second one hardly moves, infants show surprise; if a little ball hits a big one and the second moves a lot, they again look longer than usual.

Psychological objects, in addition to being self-propelled, move in a distinctive, goal-directed way, for instance, they maintain a fixed trajectory "aimed" at an object. When infants see objects that are both self-propelled and move in goal-directed ways, they attribute intention to them; they then no longer interpret the movement primarily in terms of force. Value (positive/negative) is the main parameter they now compute.

If one intentional object contacts another, the infant assign value to the interaction, either positive or negative depending on the force of the contact. A caress or soft contact is coded positive, a hit or hard contact, negative. Infants also recognize when one object helps or hinders another object to achieve a goal. For instance, if shown an object trying to escape through a hole in a wall, and a second object lifts the first one to reach the hole, they interpret this as help, and assign a positive value. If, on the other hand, the second object blocks the escape of the first, they interpret this as hinder and assign a negative value.

What is interesting here is that infants equate the two positives and they equate the two negatives. Caress and help, they equate, even though these acts are not physically similar. They equate hit and hinder, too, though they are not physically similar. A simple test shows they have equated both. When infants have lost interest in looking at caress (help), they do not regain interest when shown help (caress); similarly, when they have lost interest in looking at hit, they do not regain interest when shown hinder.

To restore the infants' interest, we must change the value of what we show them. An infant habituated on hit (or hinder), will regain interest if shown either caress or help. Similarly, an infant habituated on caress (or help), will regain interest if shown either hit or hinder. In the infant's book, value takes priority over physical similarity. That already shows a propensity toward morality.

We may say that infants interpret the world in a pro moral way. They recognize some things in the world as being intentional and goal-directed, and attribute value to their interaction. This is already a foundation of morality, an essential precursor of morality, present in the ten month-old and probably even younger infants.

Can we show similar precursors in animals? I see no reason why we should not. In a recent experiment, biologists tried to demonstrate a sense of fairness in capuchin monkeys.[5] When the experimenter gave one monkey a preferred object, and the other a non-preferred one, the animal given the non-preferred object objected. Still the animal did not object when researchers gave it the preferred object, and gave the non-preferred object to the other monkey. But this case is no less immoral than the first. So the monkey's objection to being given the non-preferred object is not a demonstration of morality but only of injured self-interest. You do not need a monkey to make this point. If you shift a bee from a sweet to a less sweet substance, it will buzz "angrily." You may object by saying that the bee is merely reacting to the difference in the two sweetnesses, whereas the monkey is objecting to its not being the preferred individual. Perhaps the monkey is chagrinned by its inferior social status; but to prove this will require a different experiment. Demonstrating injured self-interest does not require testing two animals at the same time. If you test a single monkey, and downgrade its food, the monkey will complain as angrily as the bee.

Classic evolutionary models, designed to explain altruism, do not contribute to an understanding of the three basic moral principles in human beings. William Donald Hamilton's kin selection explains quite elegantly the altruism in insects.[6] A bee that loses its life while saving two or more sisters will perpetuate its own genes (since it shares three quarters of its genes with them, and two times three-quarters makes one and a half.) But this has no bearing on human moral knowledge, which is not restricted to kin. In addition, religious and political convictions override kinship. In civil wars and revolutions brothers kill brothers, and fathers and sons kill one another. Human beings and insects are not good models of one another (contrary to sociobiology).

Robert L. Trivers' reciprocal altruism (if you scratch my back I will scratch yours, to oversimplify), presupposes both recognition of the identity of others and memory, both of which are well developed in children.[7] Yet Trivers' model does not explain human morality any more than does Hamilton's do. Children do not restrict empathy to those who have been empathic to them; nor do they deal fairly only with those who have dealt fairly with them; nor do they refrain from harming only those who have refrained from harming them. Tit for tat is not the basis of morality.

We cannot find the selective pressures that explain the evolution of human morality in either of the models designed to explain altruism. They arise instead from the lifestyle of the hunter-gatherer. On the other hand, the altruism models, especially that of Trivers, do help explain why human beings share food and are especially likely to do so when the food supply is unreliable.

We tend to ignore one kind of sharing, perhaps because men largely write anthropological literature. Women routinely collect more plant food than they need, and give it to other women, who also routinely collect more than they need, and so on. This mode of sharing does not fit any evolutionary model. On the contrary, it suggests that giving, is an intrinsic disposition in women. So is receiving, since in that situation, giving is not possible unless the other receives. Women have given to infants, and sometimes to strangers (for example, Rose O'Sharon in John Steinbeck's *Grapes of Wrath*[8]) for thousands of generations. The marvelous lines in James Joyce's *Ulysses*, where Molly Bloom whispered fiercely: "Yes...Yes...Yes!" well illustrates their intrinsic disposition to give and receive.

An intrinsic disposition to share may be present in men, too, though it may be weaker than in women. In any case, it is less likely to appear, because the meat men share is more costly to obtain than plants, and the extra cost may suppress a baseline of intrinsic giving.

The moral principles of all human groups, though modified by their distinctive environments, are the same except for this: Groups do not apply the principles to the same people. The Nazis did not apply moral principles to Jews, whites did not apply them to blacks, the rich do not apply them to the poor, and Muslims do not apply them, and so on. Group boundaries often override morality.

Infants, according to our model, have the concept of group, and recognize group under two conditions.[9] If shown two or more intentional objects that appear to be moving together willingly, they regard them as a group. If one object, instead of moving willingly with the other, forces the other to move, the infant sees, not a group, but sees the object as forced to move as the "possession" of the other.

Physical similarity is the second condition under which infants perceive group. When shown a set of black and white objects, infants expect the black objects to move together, and the white objects to do likewise. But if we show the infant is shown white and black objects willingly move together, it regards them as a group; free co-movement takes priority over physical similarity.

According to our model, infants expect group members to co-reciprocate. If a nonmember attacks one group member, infants expect other group members to reciprocate, to attack the assailant, or other members of his group. These are the presently unverified assumptions of our model. To test them, and other models, is essential to understand the disastrous effect of group boundaries on our observance of moral principles.

To sum up: thanks to our hunter-gatherer past, we are well endowed with moral knowledge, as summarized by the three moral principles: (1) Do not harm the other one. (2) Deal fairly with others. (3) Care for those who are in distress. But the same evolutionary history has left us ill endowed in self-control and subject to a disastrous group effect. Our conversion of moral knowledge into moral performance is shaky.

Notes

1. Elliot Turiel, *The Development of Social Knowledge: Morality and Convention* (Cambridge, UK: Cambridge University Press, 1983).

2. Center for Disease Control, "Cigarette Smoking among Adults—United States 2000 and 2004," *Morbidity and Mortality Weekly Report*, 54:44 (11 November 2005).

3. Doris Bischof-Kohler, "The Development of Empathy in Infants," *Infant Development: Perspectives from German-speaking Countries*, eds. Michael E. Lamb and Heidi Keller (Hillsdale, N.J.: Erlbaum, 1991), pp. 245–273.

4. David Premack and Ann J. Premack, "Infants Attribute Value +/- to the Goal-Directed Actions of Self-Propelled Objects," *Journal of Cognitive Neuroscience*, 9:6 (1997), pp. 848–856.

5. Sara F. Brosnan and Frans B. M. deWaal, "Monkeys Reject Unequal Pay," *Nature*, 425 (2003), pp. 297–299.

6. William Donald Hamilton, "Altruism and Related Phenomena, Mainly in Social Insects," *Annual Review of Ecological Systems*, 3 (1972), pp. 193–232.

7. Robert L.Trivers, "The Evolution of Reciprocal Altruism," *Quarterly Review of Biology*, 46 (1971), pp. 35–57.

8. John Steinbeck, *The Grapes of Wrath* (New York: Viking Press, 1939).

9. David Premack and Ann J. Premack, "Origins of Human Social Competence," *The Cognitive Neurosciences*, ed. Michael S. Gazzaniga (Cambridge, Mass.: MIT Press, 1995), pp. 205–218.

Part Three

EVOLUTIONARY ROOTS OF
SOCIAL BEHAVIOR

Fourteen

CONFLICT AND COOPERATION
IN HUMAN AFFAIRS

Arcadi Navarro

Who trusted God was love indeed
And love Creation's final law–
Tho' Nature, red in tooth and claw
With ravine, shriek'd against his creed–[1]

Although the idea of Nature being mercilessly violent and bloody, "red in tooth and claw," is still seen as following naturally from Charles Darwin's ideas, nowhere in the *Origin* did Darwin quote Alfred Lloyd Tennyson's verses or mention such an extreme notion. Instead, he wrote about competition for food and mates and about the ability to withstand unfavorable climates. Still, Darwin's powerful description of the "struggle for life," a concept contained in the title of his book, *The Origin of Species by Means of Natural Selection or the Preservation of Favoured Races in the Struggle for Life,* caused a lasting impression in the minds of biologists, economists, and sociologists alike.[2]

The idea of a struggle for life, from which the better adapted emerge victorious to engender the following generations, has been extremely fruitful. Derived concepts such as competition, predation, and parasitism are at the root of our understanding of nature. They have empowered us to act upon it in previously unconceivable ways. But, most importantly, Darwin's ideas and its derivations have allowed us to recognize ourselves as another animal species and to reevaluate our position in the universe. Our capacities as a species, as wonderful and complex as they are, strongly depend on our genes, just as the traits that characterize any other organism (this is not necessarily the case for our differential capacities as individuals; this is a key caveat). Human nature is the product of evolution. Over millions of years, natural selection has been able to shape it. This realization is in the basis of this chapter.

After a century and a half of successfully explaining the world, we now widely accept that a struggle for life is constant and that nature is fundamentally competitive. This conceptualization does not imply that the consensus among scientists is that nature is always "red in tooth and claw." Quite obviously, nature is not a continuous and ruthless fight between self-interested creatures. The natural world is bursting with counterexamples, full of well-documented cases of cooperation and altruism. Wolves do get their teeth and claws red when hunting and killing deer, but they do so in cooperative packs; pigeons and petrels regurgitate food for their offspring; worker bees sacrifice their lives by stinging attackers of their beehive. Human beings provide the best and most elaborate examples of cooperation and altruism in nature: they live in enormously complex societies whose norms, laws, and customs gravitate around mutual aid and how to ensure it. Human beings die for king and country, have hyper-specialized and sometimes quite boring jobs, pay taxes and join nongovernmental organizations. All around us we can see people contributing to the welfare of other people. Human beings are so used to this high level of co-operation that, traditionally, we have not cared much about what might be the explanation of such behavior or about its socio-cultural implications.

An overly simplistic view of evolution causes the apparent paradox of a competitive nature that presents so many instances of cooperation and the difficulties in explaining what we know about human societies in terms of sheer competition. In sharp contrast to the early misinterpretations of the struggle for life within a human context, which were presented as justifications for some of the most hideous policies in modern history, today we know that co-operation, just like conflict, is deeply ingrained in the evolutionary history of our species. In what follows, we will try to show how an evolutionary view of human nature and society can help us, not only to explain why we are the way we are, but also to push forward the limits of our political and social thought.

1. Teaming Up: The Hierarchical Nature of Life

With some brilliant exceptions, until the late 1960s, scientists tended to focus on the study of the conflictive interactions mentioned above: competition, parasitism, or predation. They paid far less attention to cooperation because they believed it to be of limited significance, only useful to explain some peculiar groups of organisms—such as ants or termites—but of little relevance for the rest of life forms on the planet. A deeper understanding of the organization of living organisms has changed this view. This improved knowledge comes from the realization that, since the appearance of life on Earth about three and one half billion years ago, teamwork has allowed the emergence of increasingly complex life forms.

The organization of the living world is hierarchical. Every form of life, from the simplest bacteria to complex eukaryotic, multi-cellular organisms, whose functions are coded by thousands of genes, and which may live in large social groups, is constituted by lower-level units that group together and co-operate to form higher-level units of organization (genes, chromosomes, bacteria, eukaryotic cells, multi-cellular organisms, and societies). The major landmarks in the diversification of life have involved cooperation-driven transitions between these hierarchical levels.[3] Every level in the hierarchy is formed by members that, in their individual state, might have fiercely competed but that, in their present form, display excruciatingly complex and self-less cooperative behaviors.

Consider individual cells in a multi-cellular organism. Instead of trying to out-compete and out-reproduce each other in a mad race for resources, like bacteria in a culture would, the cells in our bodies grow in a harmonious and cooperative manner. Coordination is so complete that most of our cells renounce the ultimate goal of all living things: contributing to the next generations. Cells in our skin, intestines, and brains delegate their reproductive functions to a few specialized sperms or ova. Still, conflict is possible. Some cells may act selfishly and go back to their old ways, reproducing without control and causing havoc in our bodies. We call that kind of conflict cancer. It illustrates how crucial cooperation is in our bodies to keep us alive. Let us now consider eusocial organisms, such as ants, termites, bees or the naked mole rat. In all these cases, cooperation is so extreme that workers have delegated reproduction to a few members of the colony: the queens. Again, selfish reproduction is possible in limited cases, but it is so harmful for the community that these species have evolved amazing repressive strategies to prevent it, sometimes resembling a police state.[4]

We could keep describing analogous situations in other levels of organization such as cooperation between genes to form genomes or cooperation between different genomes to form eukaryotic cells and so on, but the central idea should be patent by now. Cooperation has allowed all this complexity to exist. In the highly competitive struggle for life, cooperative strategies repeatedly have proven successful.

We can draw an obvious parallel between the examples above and human society. We can think of society as an organism comprised of many specialized units working in a coordinated way. Almost every aspect of social life can fit in this framework: school, religious institutions, hospitals, armies, laws. But is this a correct analogy? Can we be positive that we can apply the same biological mechanisms underlying cooperation in the natural world to human society? Are there any lessons to be learned from the study of these questions? To tackle all these issues, we first need to understand how cooperation can come about in general, and in human societies in particular.

2. Different Paths to Cooperation

Cooperation can be defined in terms of cost/benefit. Whenever an individual incurs a cost in order to provide a benefit for another individual or set of individuals, we say that the first individual is cooperating or acting altruistically.[5] The cost can be anything, ranging from food, money, or time, to the donation of an organ. Evolutionary studies provide five different models of how such behavior can be promoted by natural selection. We will discuss these models separately, but their common underlying principle is simple: cooperation can be a successful adaptive strategy if individuals that cooperate tend to help other cooperators.[6] Intuitively, we can say that if cooperators help selfish individuals equally or preferentially over other cooperators, selfishness will prevail. Selfish individuals will incur lower costs, yet reap the benefits of altruism: to be a cooperator will not be profitable. Natural selection has favored the evolution of mechanisms that allow cooperators to focus their benefits on individuals who are likely to be cooperators themselves.

Selfish genes: George C. Williams and William Donald Hamilton discovered the first way in which selection favors cooperation in the 1960s.[7] Their work triggered the "Sociobiological Revolution," popularized by Edward O. Wilson in *Sociobiology: The New Synthesis* and *On Human Nature*.[8] Most famously, the central concept of this revolution is embodied in the title of Richard Dawkins' bestseller, *The Selfish Gene*.[9] The underlying idea is simple: if a cooperator's behavior is genetically coded, a cooperator can safely help its relatives, since they share genes and they will also tend to be altruists. We can better understand this idea from the point of view of a gene-promoting cooperation. The gene will increase its frequency in the population not only if the individual carrying it reproduces, but also if the individual carrying it helps other individuals who share the same gene to have their offspring, even if, by doing so, the cooperator incurs in a large cost.

Imagine a gene that makes me help my brothers and sisters. Because, on average, I share 50 percent of my genes with any of my brothers (we have the same mother and father), if I die to save the lives of, say, four of them, I will still be helping two copies of my genes (50 percent of four) to be passed on to the next generation. From the genes' point of view, this is a great deal. By causing the cooperator to help its relatives, the gene is selfishly helping to copy itself. It follows that the closer the relatives, the more advantageous is cooperation with them.[10] This mechanism is known as *kin selection* and is based on a simple principle, Hamilton's rule, according to which, cooperation is evolutionarily advantageous if costs to the cooperator are lower than the total benefits bestowed upon the individuals it benefits, corrected by the degree of kinship of these individuals with the cooperator.[11]

Hamilton's rule proved to have enormous explanatory power. It accounted perfectly well for multi-cellular organisms (all the cells are genetically identical, so it makes sense for them to delegate reproduction) and eusocial organisms (we can show that for a worker bee to help its queen reproduce is more efficient than for the worker bee to reproduce herself). Kin selection has a privileged role in human affairs. It helps explain nepotism, for instance. But in both human beings and other animals, cooperation also extends to non-relatives. The selfish gene does not explain it all.

Reciprocity: Another way to guarantee that a cooperator helps other cooperators is to make sure that the individual that profits from a cooperative act will, sooner or later, repay.[12] Getting an intuitive idea of this mechanism is easy, since it is based on common sense and we all became familiar with it in nursery school: "if you scratch my back, I'll scratch yours." By applying reciprocity, individuals can interact preferentially with other cooperators. It plays a role in our day-to-day life, whenever we go shopping, for example. Even so, detailed mathematical models show that reciprocity is far less powerful in promoting cooperation than kin selection. We find little evidence of reciprocity in nonhuman beings.[13] Also, human beings and other organisms cooperate far beyond reciprocity. In our large and complex societies, we do sometimes scratch the back of individuals who we are unlikely to meet again.

Indirect reciprocity: Mathematical and simulation studies show that some of the problems posed by reciprocity are solved if individuals can keep tract of each other's helping records.[14] If a cooperator helps someone who has previously been shown to be a helper (someone who has a *good reputation*), then cooperators will tend to interact with other altruists and the possibility for cooperation will evolve. We can readily see examples of how this operates in our society but, again, obviously we cooperate with people we have never met. What compels us to do so?

Social norms and punishment. Human societies are regulated by law or by some kind of norms and traditions only loosely dependent on rational choices of the individuals that implement and obey them. We can define norms as several shared prescriptions about how to behave in interactions with both known and unknown individuals. They present interesting features that fall under the common name of *strong reciprocity*.[15] Experiments show that third parties will reward law-abiding individuals, even at a cost for the re-warders. This behavior has been termed *altruistic rewarding*.[16] On the other hand, when individuals do not adhere to norms, third parties may undertake punitive actions. Experimental work shows that these punitive actions are a form of altruism: individuals that punish lawbreakers do it at a cost for themselves. Both the lawbreaker and the punisher pay a cost and the punisher enjoys no direct profits from that action. The benefits are indirect; punishment induces the correct behavior in potential lawbreakers. Known as *altruistic punishment*, researchers have recently proven its crucial importance in securing high-level cooperation.[17]

Altruistic rewarding and punishment constitute powerful incentives for cooperation even when direct or indirect reciprocity are not possible and information about reputation is not available, because cooperators will reward those whom they view as cooperative and punish those whom defect.

Human societies evince many examples of such norms and their enforcement: from dress codes and table manners to rules for community living, marketplace regulations, and religious beliefs. Mathematical models, simulations, and experiments based on these ideas show how these mechanisms can help fix maladaptive attitudes in a society.[18] Once a reward and punishment system is installed, a society can establish almost any norm, independently of whether the norm is beneficial to anyone or even if it is indisputably detrimental (clitoridectomy, for example). This kind of mechanism fails to explain why are there so many cooperative social norms instead of senseless sets of arbitrarily determined rules.

Group selection: We can understand that cooperative norms that make adaptive sense are more frequent than fanciful laws by considering a further level in the hierarchy of nature: groups of individuals within a species. The idea behind models of *group selection* is that groups can compete among themselves just as individuals or species do. Social groups with more cooperative norms that improve their access to resources increase their reproductive rates or make their warfare techniques more efficient may dominate or conquer other groups, either by the force of arms and demography or by prestige-biased transmission, which induces individuals to preferentially imitate successful groups. Investigators have shown that the norms of a successful group can preferentially spread from group to group relatively rapidly.[19] Because cooperation fosters success, these processes can lead to the preferential proliferation of cooperative norms. The ethnographic, archaeological, and historical record evinces many such examples.[20]

The above list includes mechanisms of increasing complexity which are not mutually exclusive. The most complex mechanisms (group selection, rewarding and punishment), which require extremely advanced mathematical or simulation tools to describe and study them, are intuitively more lucid to us than the simpler, gene-based, kin-selection ideas. This just goes to show how accustomed we are to acting according to such complex mechanisms.

3. Identity and Cheating

Besides the commonality that all of these mechanisms promote interactions between cooperators, another feature they have in common is that they all rely on distinguishing cooperators from selfish individuals. For multi-cellular organisms, this is no big problem. Being attached to the same body guarantees that, if one individual (a cell) is a cooperator, the individuals it will interact with will be cooperators as well. If we consider social groups the situation becomes more intricate. How can a cooperator be sure to be helping other cooperators? Unambiguous identity markers are needed.

A straightforward possibility is a "green beard gene."[21] If individuals with green beards (or, for that matter, any patently distinguishable feature) cooperate, but do so exclusively with other green-bearded individuals, cooperation will quickly spread and the world will become a peaceful paradise of green-bearded cooperators. But this fairytale world is fragile. It can easily be invaded by mutant cheaters who, despite boasting luxuriant green beards that induce others to help them, would never cooperate with their fellow beings. Cooperators would soon vanish, as their world was quickly overtaken by such selfish individuals. Ensuring that an apparent cooperator is an authentic a cooperator is the key issue.

Inextricably tied to higher levels of cooperation, new opportunities for cheating and conflict arise. The increasingly complex cooperation-promoting mechanisms outlined above depend on increasingly complex identity markers. These have been studied in detail and the overall picture is that, parallel to the addition of hierarchical levels in nature, continuous arms races are being waged between cheaters, who try to cunningly disguise themselves as cooperators, and cooperators who try crafty strategies to uncover them.[22] Because of the everlasting conflict between cheaters and cooperators, these identity markers are a fundamental part of cooperation mechanisms.

Consider, for example, kin selection. Kinship creates many possibilities to distinguish relatives, with whom one cooperates, from other individuals. Close kin, besides sharing the tendency to cooperate, may share a similar appearance or smell that natural selection may use as cues to build an instinct like "help those who look like you." In other cases, when family groups tend to remain in the same territories, simple proximity can be used as a cue: "help those who are around your parents."[23] Kin selection is crucial for human beings and, because we have elaborate cognitive capabilities, our kin-recognition systems are sophisticated. The available evidence suggests that human beings use a variety of cues to assess kinship, including physical similarity to oneself and other family members, scent, proximity during youth and social learning of relationships.[24] Interestingly, researchers have shown that men are more kindly disposed towards babies that resemble themselves.[25]

In the case of higher primates, especially human beings, multilevel recognition systems operate because cooperation is also multileveled. More intricate cooperation mechanisms depend on correspondingly complex identity-recognition systems. At the highest level, the importance of group-recognition mechanisms is a consequence of the enormous importance of group structures in primate evolution. Our species has only recently (over the last few thousand years) started organizing itself in large societies formed by several million individuals. Until then, hominids lived in loosely organized small groups; so evolution has shaped us to exist under this social condition. This fact is central to any adaptive explanations of human behavior.[26] (Incidentally, some traits adaptive in one environment may not be adaptive or may even be detrimental under our present conditions). By getting together in small bands, hominids not only protected themselves from predators but also created boundaries between groups and generated the conditions for selection among hominid groups.

According to research conducted in recent decades, inter-group conflict among hominid groups has been a crucial force in the evolution of human beings.[27] It not only allowed the extension of the cooperation-inducing norms that made some groups more successful than others, but also posed a difficult challenge to our ancestors: to quickly distinguish in-group members from out-group individuals, so that each could be treated accordingly. Conflict between groups may have selected individuals with higher cognitive abilities and generated not only strong in-group cooperative bonds and recognition methods, but also other typically human features, for example intra-group status hierarchies, to facilitate the coordination of group work toward a common goal.

Because group identity recognition is so complex, social learning of the appropriate identity markers is far more important than in the case of kin-recognition systems, for example. These markers are complex and, like a Russian doll, include markers of lower level. Appearance-related markers, such as pigmentation, stature or facial resemblance, and proximity markers, such as close territory sharing since childhood, which are key as kin-recognition systems, can be used, since an individual's blood relatives tend to belong to the same group. Other markers are mostly social, such as clothing or tattoos. Interestingly, the social conventions and norms that these cooperation mechanisms have been crucial to establishing are themselves identity markers. Religion, rituals and language are among the most important. Language, in particular, has been studied in detail as a group marker, and surprising results have been obtained. In a series of famous (and polemical) experiments performed in the United Kingdom, black youth stigmatized a recording of speakers of Black vernacular English as low class, but simultaneously picked the speakers as a likely source of support in a fight, compared to voice speaking Standard English.[28]

Identity recognition systems are coded in our genomes in an extremely complex way whose details researchers still ignore. Current evidence suggests that no genetic determination of these markers exists, which is not as paradoxical as it may appear. The tendency and capability to become skilled in the detection of some markers is what is coded in our genes, but not the form they take in any given culture.[29] Our brain is ready to become tuned to some classes of signals, but we learn the signals themselves after we are born. This is also the case in chimpanzees. Experiments performed with chimpanzees raised in human families show that the chimps can distinguish and classify images of other chimpanzees and of human beings in different groups. They usually make one mistake: they classify their image with those of their human families, because they have learned to recognize them as their group.

4. What Have We Learned?
A Short List of Questions and Proposals

I hope that this brief overview has shown how our knowledge about human altruism has advanced over the last two decades. Some of the newest results may defy long-cherished yet naive prejudices. They raise interesting questions and suggest avenues of research that we must explore. A short list of examples follows:

(1) Experimental evidence indicates that reputation formation, rewards and, crucially, punishment, have been, and are, powerful determinants of human behavior.[30] Altruist punishment allows for the success of cooperation because it dissuades people from breaking laws and generally reduces deception and conflict. For instance, we altruistically keep criminals in jail not only because we want to reeducate them, but as an example to potential noncooperators. Should this second and, from an evolutionary point of view, more important social role of punishment receive more attention? Should "punishment as an example" be limited to primary school, or perhaps completely ruled out of our societies? What would be the social consequences of a reevaluation of the roles of reward and punishment in our educational system?

(2) Different human groups are characterized by different social norms. Some of these are cooperative, some not. Some norms may have been produced by rational or adaptive choices from the groups that practice them, but a good number of them were not. Some norms are indisputably maladaptive—the by-product of innate and extremely efficient norm-formation systems.

Some of these undesirable norms, on the other hand, have been transformed into robust group identity markers. To what extent are they dependent situation (environment)? How should we act upon these norms? What could be the consequences of these actions for the identity of the affected groups?

(3) Campaigns to suppress identities that exclude and create an increasing feeling of "comprehensive human identity," are usually based on the promotion of overly abstract concepts, such as "solidarity." Because such abstractions do not reflect any identity markers, they do not make use of innate predispositions to distinguish members of our group, but they actually fight these predispositions. Early formation of multicultural and multiethnic social groups, together with the early promotion of common human physical and cultural traits and universal values (such as those proposed by the Forum) as group markers, should be an efficient way to promote the feeling of belonging to a single "human group."

I am aware that these ideas are too schematic. The systematic study of sociological problems from an evolutionary perspective and the use of both theoretical and empirical techniques have produced amazing results. But this is a relatively young field. Lots of interesting research is currently being conducted which might add surprisingly significant pieces of information or help reinterpret available evidence. Yet, on these scientific grounds, we can try to push our understanding of identity and society. Perhaps we can contribute to one of the major goals of humanity in our times: making our cultural differences our main asset, instead of our main problem.

Notes

1. Alfred Lord Tennyson, *In Memoriam (A.H.H.)[i.e. Arthur H. Hallam]* (London: n.p., 1850).

2. Charles Dawin, *The Origin of Species by Means of Natural Selection or the Preservation of Favoured Races in the Struggle for Life* (Cambridge, Mass.: Harvard University Press, 1989 [1859]).

3. J. Maynard Smith and E. Szathmáry, *The Major Transitions in Evolution* (Oxford, Oxford University Press, 1995); Richard E. Michod, "Cooperation and Conflict in the Evolution of Individuality, 1. Multi-level Selection of the Organism," *American Naturalist*, 149 (1997), pp. 607–645; and Richard E. Michod, *Darwinian Dynamics, Evolutionary Transitions in Fitness, and Individuality* (Princeton, N.J.: Princeton University Press, 1999).

4. F. L. W. Ratnieks and P. K. Visscher, "Worker Policing in the Honeybee," *Nature*, 342 (1989), pp. 796–797.

5. Axelrod, *The Evolution of Cooperation* (New York: Basic Books, 1984).

6. Steven A. Frank, *Foundations of Social Evolution* (Princeton, N. J.: Princeton University Press, 1998).

7. George C. Williams, *Adaptation and Natural Selection* (Princeton, N. J.: Princeton University Press, 1966); and W. D. Hamilton, "The Genetical Evolution of Social Behaviour," *Journal of Theoretical Biology*, 7 (1964), pp. 1–52.

8. Edward O. Wilson, *Sociobiology: The New Synthesis* (Cambridge, Mass.: Harvard Univ. Press, 1975); and *On Human Nature* (Cambridge, Mass.: Harvard Univ. Press, 1978).

9. Richard Dawkins, *The Selfish Gene* (Oxford: Oxford University Press, 1976).

10. S. A. West, I. Pen, and A. S. Griffin, "Cooperation and Competition between Relatives," *Science*, 296 (2002), pp. 72–75.

11. Hamilton, "The Genetical Evolution of Social Behaviour."

12. Robert M. Axelrod, *The Complexity of Cooperation* (Princeton, N. J.: Princeton University Press, 1997).

13. P. Hammerstein, "Why is Reciprocity so Rare in Social Animals?" *Genetic and Cultural Evolution of Cooperation* (Cambridge, Mass.: MIT Press, 2003).

14. Axelrod, *The Complexity of Cooperation.*

15. E. Fehr, U. Fischbacher, and S. Gaechter, "Strong Reciprocity, Human Co-operation and the Enforcement of Social Norms," *Human Nature*, 13 (2002), pp. 1–25; and E. Ferh and U. Fischbacher, "The Nature of Human Altruism," *Nature*, 425 (2003), pp. 785–791.

16. Ferh and Fischbacher, "The Nature of Human Altruism."

17. E. Fehr and S. Gachter, "Altruistic Punishment in Human Beings," *Nature*, 415 (2002), pp. 137–140; and Ferh and Fischbacher, "The Nature of Human Altruism."

18. R. Boyd and P. J. Richerson, "Punishment Allows the Evolution of Coopera-tion (or Anything Else) in Sizable Groups." *Ethology and Sociobiology*, 13 (1992), pp. 171–195.

19. R. Boyd and P. J. Richerson, "Group Beneficial Norms Can Spread Rapidly in a Structured Population," *Journal of Theoretical Biology*, 215 (2002), pp. 287–296.

20. Robert Boyd and Joan B. Silk, *How Human Beings Evolved* (New York: Norton, 2000); and Boyd and Richerson, "Group Beneficial Norms Can Spread Rapidly in a Structured Population."

21. Dawkins, *The Selfish Gene.*

22. Axelrod, *The Complexity of Cooperation.*

23. West, Pen, and Griffin, "Cooperation and Competition between Relatives."

24. Arthur P. Wolf, *Sexual Attraction and Childhood Association: A Chinese Brief for Edward Westermarck* (Stanford, Calif.: Stanford University Press, 1995).

25. S. M. Platek, R. L. Burch, I. S. Panyavin, B. H. Wasserman, and G. G. Gallup, "Reactions to Children's Faces: Resemblance Affects Males More than Females," *Evolution and Human Behavior*, 23 (2002), pp. 159–166; and S. M. Platek, S. R. Critton, R. L. Burch, D. A. Frederick, T. E. Myers, and G. G. Gallup, "How Much Paternal Resemblance is Enough? Sex Differences in Hypothetical Investment Decisions but not in the Detection of Resemblance," *Evolution and Human Behavior*, 24 (2003), pp. 81–87.

26. Boyd and Silk, *How Human Beings Evolved.*

27. Richard D. Alexander, "Evolution of the Human Psyche," *The Human Revolution*, eds. Paul Mellars and Chris Stringer (Edinburgh, UK, Edinburgh University Press, 1989).

28. William Labov, *Sociolinguistic Patterns* (Philadelphia: University of Pennsylvania Press, 1972).

29. Boyd and Silk, *How Human Beings Evolved.*

30. Ferh and Fischbacher, "The Nature of Human Altruism."

Fifteen

A COMMENT ON "CONFLICT AND COOP-ERATION IN HUMAN AFFAIRS" BY ARCADI NAVARRO

Sandro Nannini

1. Conflict and Cooperation in Human Nature

Arcadi Navarro's paper confirms how wrong all interpretations of Charles Darwin's natural selection theory are when trying to base on biological evolution right-winged political ideologies such as "social Darwinism" in the nineteenth century or some forced applications of sociobiology nowadays. The belief that aiming at enhancing equality and justice in human societies is doomed to failure is false. Human nature includes a tendency both to conflict and cooperation.

Still more interesting for a philosopher in Arcadi Navarro's paper is that he shows that the forms of cooperation available in animal life are hierarchically ordered. Human forms of cooperation, such as "social norms and punishment" or "group selection," typically develop through biological evolution from natural forms of cooperation such as "selfish genes" and direct or indirect "reciprocity." This means that norms, values, and all other cultural traits can promote cooperation and make human societies possible only insofar as they are based on a kind of interaction between human beings that has a biological basis. If norms do not respect the limits imposed by human nature, they cannot promote any cooperation.

To my way of thinking, neglecting this fact was one of the fundamental reasons why the "experiment," implemented in the USSR and other socialist countries for about seventy years, to found a society based on equality and social justice failed. For the same reason, we must base programs of international cooperation (for example to reduce poverty or air pollution) or more generally attempts to promote "virtuous behavior" inspired by principles of "public ethics" on a realistic account of the ability of human beings to understand such programs and accept such moral values. For these programs to be successful, we must take into account persons' human nature and their cultural background. Promoters need to ensure that the people understand the programs and that the programs are consistent with their moral values. The risk for human beings to be followers of the Latin motto, *Video meliora proboque deteriora sequor*—I see the better way and approve it, but I follow the worse way—is always around the corner!

Utopian programs of social policy that do not take account of the constraints imposed by biological human nature fail. People continue to act in
selfish ways; they are willing to cooperate only with other human beings who are
members of the same restricted group to which they belong. But such failures do
not warrant the conclusion that racism and mistrust of foreigners is inevitable
because these traits appear to be in agreement with the biological basis of human
behavior. On the contrary,—and this emerges also from the final proposal of
Navarro's paper—we can shrewdly exploit the natural tendency to cooperate
only with those that we recognize through "identity markers" as belonging to our
own group to create international solidarity and cooperation instead of conflict
and war. We can do this by introducing into human cultures "identity markers"
that make all human beings members of a single "group," humankind.

2. Facts and Norms

So far, I agree on the whole with Navarro's considerations. I believe that we
need to more deeply investigate the relationship of cultures and societies to
human minds and indirectly to their biological basis if we want to avoid two
opposite but symmetrical misunderstandings. On the one hand, we must avoid
succumbing to the naive view of "ethical naturalism" maintained by many
philosophers in the nineteenth century such as John Stuart Mill.[1] On the other
hand, the mere validity of a norm cannot explain why an individual executes
an action.

Regarding the first point, according to ethical naturalism, ethics can be
directly derived from empirical knowledge. But ethical naturalism is wrong
since no socio-biological theory can directly imply what is just or unjust from
a moral or political point of view, or what is right or wrong from a prudential
point of view. Thinking otherwise would bring us to forget what we have
learned from David Hume and logical empiricists: No "ought-sentence" is
entailed by premises that are all "is-sentences." Knowing how things are
never implies what we have to do. Ethics and politics have a *normative* dimension necessarily missing in a scientific *description* and *explanation* of
reality. The reason is simple: Even if we endorse a statement of the kind,
"People have the natural tendency to behave so and so" we may always *without contradiction* affirm "Nevertheless, behaving so and so is morally unjust
(or prudentially wrong, or irrational)." Therefore, a biological theory that *explains* why people behave so and so cannot *justify* the moral or legal principle
that people ought to behave so and so.

As for the second point, the mere validity of a norm can *justify* a designated action but cannot *explain* why an individual executed it. For example, if
the traffic light I have in front of me is red, my stopping the car is justified but
not explained by that fact. I could have crossed the intersection had I not *seen*
that the light was red, or if I had not *known* the Highway Code, or if I had
decided not to respect the code. My action is not explainable by an objective

state of affairs and a norm but by psychological, subjective facts: my knowledge of that state of affairs and my desire to respect that norm.

A norm is a cultural trait that exists only insofar as members of a culture usually accept and respect it. A norm can causally determine behavior only if it forms the content of individual intentional mental states of the people who recognize it. For us to more fully comprehend biologically based forms of cooperation, we must further investigate the relationship between social or cultural facts and individual human minds.

3. The Mind-Body Problem

With regard to the relationship of social and cultural facts to individual human minds I will show that from one point of view, such a relationship is formally analogous to the mind-body relationship. From another point of view, the relationship is different and autonomous from the mind-body relationship. As for the first problem, common sense suggests that a cultural trait exists insofar as it is implemented by individual mental acts or mental dispositions. For example, a language like Spanish or English exists insofar as it is spoken and understood through mental acts and actions of single human beings. Philosophical views like Georg Wilhelm Friedrich Hegel's idealism, according to which the *Weltgeist* (World Spirit) is the true reality and individual human beings in the flesh are only its "manifestations," appear to be implausible nowadays, even among philosophers.

On the contrary, the traditional Cartesian view that the mind is a substance different from the body and could exist in principle without it, is still widespread. But just as cultures cannot exist without their human individual bearers, I cannot see any good reason to think that mental states could exist without being implemented by physical and neurophysiological processes. According to the naturalistic view I endorse, mental states are *virtual* states that need a neurophysiological implementation (unless they are mere illusions, idealizations, or *façons de parler* (ways of speaking)). Mental states are a re-description of physiological processes by means of psychological concepts. For example, in the language of folk psychology, the firing of C-fibers is termed "pain."

The mind-brain relationship is not a cause-effect relationship similar for example to the relationship between fire and smoke. If the emerging of mental states was the effect of brain processes, then mental states would be ontologically independent of brain processes: fire and smoke are two distinct things. Therefore, the brain and the mind would also be two distinct things if the brain were to be the cause of the mind. The mind-brain relationship is similar instead to the relationship between woods and the trees that comprise it. From an ontological point of view, the woods exist only as a re-description of the trees that comprise it, although the wood has properties (for example, a form, an extension), which are not properties of the single trees that make it up. Similarly, mental states are ontologically reducible to brain processes, but their explanation may require psychological concepts that belong to a *level of analysis* different from the level of analysis of neurophysiological concepts. Psychology is not reducible to neurosciences. But this does not mean that psychology may be completely independent of neurosciences. The neurophysiological implementation of mental states imposes *constraints* on their psychological explanation.

Not only might mental states be implemented by different brain processes, but also they are sometimes not completely reducible to neurophysiological processes without a residue, especially if they are not described through concepts of scientific psychology but through concepts of folk psychology. Let us distinguish in mental phenomena a *virtual* part implemented by neurophysiological processes and a *fictitious* part not implemented at all, that is an illusion (or an idealization, or a mere *façon de parler*) whose introduction in our language sometimes may be quite useful but that strictly speaking does not exist.

This distinction between virtual states and fictitious states among mental states has an important consequence from an epistemological point of view. Even if, for example, we apparently have sufficient *prima facie* evidence to think that the mental state C is the cause of the mental state E, we may accept this hypothesis in scientific psychology only if C being implemented by a (may be unknown in detail) neurophysiological process C^* is plausible, E is implemented by a (may be unknown in detail) neurophysiological process E^*, and C^* is the cause of E^*. If this causal relation is possible according to known biological theories, then we may plausibly say that the virtual mental state C *virtually* causes the virtual mental state E. If C is a fictitious state, and E has, on the contrary, a neurophysiological implementation, then to think that C (even virtually) causes E, is absurd, since a fiction does not exist and therefore cannot cause any effect whatsoever in the real world. We must, in this case, re-interpret our evidence and find out a different explanation of the observed facts.

For example, let us assume that I am going to the station to catch a train. My action may be explained by saying that I am going to the station (action A) because I want to catch a train (mental state W) and believe that I can catch my train only if I will go to the station (mental state B): "A because W and B." This explanation follows the fundamental schema S of folk psychology to explain voluntary actions:

$$(S) \text{ Want} + \text{Belief} \rightarrow \text{Action}.$$

Is S transferable to scientific psychology independently of its neurophysiological implementation? Theorists have offered four major responses to this question:

(1) Yes, S is transferable because mental states are not reducible to brain processes; therefore, psychology is independent of neurosciences. The

explanation of an action by bringing out the reasons it was executed is independent of any neurophysiological explanation of the bodily movement that implemented that action (many kinds of dualism).

(2) Yes, *S* is transferable because brain processes and mental states have the same formal *symbolic* structure. Folk psychology can offer to scientific psychology models of explanations that do not care about the neurophysiological implementation of mental states even if mental states are virtual states that exist only insofar as they are implemented (somehow, in a way that we ignore) by neurophysiological processes. If "*A* because *W* and *B*," is true, then *somehow* "*A** because *W** and *B**" is also true (Jerry Fodor's "language of thought hypothesis");

(3) Yes, *S* is transferable because by *attributing* to me *W* and *B* you can bring out some psychological features and regularities of my behavior that are not visible at the level of a neurophysiological description of my body although mental states are virtual states that exist only so far they are implemented by neurophysiological processes. The difference of this theory as compared with (2) is that the psychological ("personal") description and the neurophysiological ("subpersonal") description of the same events are not necessarily isomorphic: minds with the structure of a serial Turing Machine might be implemented by brains that have the structure of a parallel "neural network" (Daniel C. Dennett's view of consciousness and his "intentional stance")

(4) No, *S* is not transferable because folk psychology is fundamentally wrong. Wants and beliefs do not exist *under the description given to them by folk psychology*. Therefore, *S* is fundamentally wrong and must be substituted by more adequate psycho-neurophysiological theories (eliminativism).

All strong naturalists reject dualism (response 1) as contrary to all empirical findings and to the "closure" of the physical world. Whereas the language of thought hypothesis (response 2) appears to be implausible from a biological point of view: The brain is no serial hardware and for it to directly work as a Turing Machine is impossible. Dennett's view (response 3) appears instead to be more in agreement with empirical findings and with the use of psychological concepts in everyday life. In addition, eliminativism (if correctly understood) opens a useful cooperation of philosophy and psychology with neurosciences. Overall, to maintain a view of the mind that tries to keep the best parts both of (3) and (4) appears to be plausible.

We must analyze the introspective and behavioral data in such a way that the mental states, the topic of folk psychology, are re-defined from a scientific point of view and divided into two groups: virtual and fictitious states. (1) *Virtual* states are real insofar as they are implemented by neurophysiological processes (although brain processes and mental processes under their respective neurophysiological and psychological descriptions are likely not isomorphic); and (2) Strictly speaking, *fictitious* states do not exist (although their preservation in our language might be quite useful, even necessary sometimes).

If we come back to the evaluation of the appropriateness of S, we will see that if a voluntary action is explained through mental states that are virtual states, our explanation is sound and might be true. In the case that our explanation mentions instead fictitious states, it might still be useful if such "fictions" are idealizations or *façons de parler* that have a minimum of biological basis. But if they are mere illusions, then our explanation is false.

4. The Society (and Culture)-Mind Problem

We can apply the conclusion discussed above to causal explanations of social facts and cultural traits through other social facts and cultural traits since a strong analogy exists between the relationship of the mind to the body and the relationship of the culture (or society) to the mind. Even social facts and cultural traits are virtual realities that exist only insofar as they are implemented by human beings who act in a some way because they have particular wants and beliefs. Even among social facts and cultural traits, we must distinguish virtual states that really exist because they have a psychological implementation from other social facts or cultural traits that, strictly speaking, do not exist because they are idealizations, *façons de parler*, or illusions.

In this case, too, some of these fictions may be very useful in everyday life or even in science. For example, the concept of a perfectly rational agent of which economists speak is essential in classical economics. But if I want to explain the economic fact *A* by saying that *A* is caused by the economic fact *B*, my explanation is false if *A* and *B* are not implemented by any individual actions or if, according to our psychological knowledge, the actions that implement A cannot be the cause of the actions that implement *B*. For example, economists generally admit that increase in demand often causes inflation. Such an explanation would be false if it was not psychologically plausible that if an article is in great demand, shopkeepers who sell it will be induced to increase its price.

Nowadays, economists interested in the so-called cognitive economics censure classical economics exactly because they think that we should not use many idealizations of classical economics such as the concept of "perfectly rational agent" or of "perfect market," since such concepts are devoid of any plausible psychological implementation.[2] Real markets are *systematically* different from the perfect market, and real people are systematically different from the perfectly rational agent. I do not discuss here whether such new economists are right. What is interesting here is how we can reconstruct the dispute between them and classical economists as a discussion about the nature of economic concepts like the perfectly rational agent or the perfect market. Do these concepts refer to virtual states or to idealizations provided with a sufficient psychological implementation? If they do, then classical economics is empirically grounded. Are concepts such as perfectly rational agent or perfect market, on the contrary, ideological constructions without any empirical basis and devoid of any power of prediction? In this case, classical economics completely misses its mark.

To sum up, analogies between the mind-body problem and the "culture (or society)-mind problem" are striking. We may conclude that on the one hand, social sciences are *epistemologically* independent of psychology in the same (limited) measure as psychology is independent of neurosciences. On the other hand, social facts and cultural traits are *ontologically* dependent on mental states as mental states are ontologically dependent on neurophysiological processes. The epistemological independence is, in both cases, limited by the ontological dependence. Only virtual states (or virtual things), can have causal efficacy on the real world; fictitious states cannot.

In spite of this analogy, a big difference exists between "the mind-body problem" and "the culture (or society)-mind problem." A social fact or a cultural trait, if real, is a *second order* virtual reality since its psychological implementation needs a neurophysiological implementation in its turn. Social sciences are limited not only by the constraints imposed by psychology but also indirectly by the constraints imposed to the very psychology by neurosciences and biology. The social sciences also inherit the neurophysiological constraints of psychology.

5. Biological Evolution and Cultural Evolution

Now let us return to Navarro's paper and analyze the two forms of cooperation, "social norms and punishment" and "group selection" in the light of the above mentioned remarks on the relationship of social facts and cultural traits to their psychological (and indirectly biological) basis. On the one hand, in social sciences, thinking of social facts and cultural traits as states that can have a causal efficacy on human behavior only if they have a psychological and biological implementation perfectly meets a socio-biological and evolutionistic approach. But we may not forget that the ontological dependence of social facts and cultural traits from a psychological and biological basis does not prevent a limited autonomy of social sciences from psychology and biology. In addition, socio-biologists such as Dawkins and philosophers such as Dennett have spoken of cultural traits as "memes" that settle in human minds and proliferate from a mind to another like viruses in cells.[3] The concept of meme is quite controversial and I do not want to discuss it here. But the above mentioned remarks on the nature of cultural traits are sufficient to understand that a cultural trait, if it is psychologically and biologically implemented, can keep its identity passing from a mind to another and can be the object of a kind of "cultural selection". Such a selection is based on the psychological and biological mechanism of the transmission and proliferation of cultural traits.

Therefore, a cultural evolution exists that, although dependent on biological evolution, enjoys a certain degree of autonomy at its own level of analysis.

This nature of cultural traits gives both opportunities and risks to humankind. On the one hand—as Navarro emphasizes—the psychological mechanisms that implement the proliferation of cultural traits allow maladaptive traits to have success sometimes. On the other hand, the (although limited) autonomy of cultural traits from their psychological and biological implementation allows also "virtuous" forms of cooperation to develop beyond the simplest ones which human beings have in common with many other animals. For example, virtuous traits can improve the efficacy of group selection beyond the effects of the demographic success. To sum up, cultural evolution cannot act against biological evolution but it can act beyond it.

Notes

1. John Stuart Mill, *Utilitarianism* (London: Parker, 1863).
2. Paul Bourgine and Jean-Pierre Nadal, *Cognitive Economics: An Interdisciplinary Approach* (New York: Springer, 2004).
3. Richard Dawkins, *The Selfish Gene* (Oxford: Oxford University Press, 1976); and Daniel Clement Dennett, *Consciousness Explained* (Boston, Mass.: Little, Brown, 1995).

Sixteen

CULTURAL NICHE CONSTRUCTION
AND HUMAN EVOLUTION

F. John Odling-Smee

1. Introduction

Anyone who attended the Dialogue on "The Social Brain," at the Universal Forum of Cultures, Barcelona, 2004, is likely to have come away from it convinced that contemporary human societies are facing unprecedented problems and unprecedented opportunities. Most of our problems and many of our opportunities appear to be caused by conjunctions of "old" human behaviors, often generated by our "social brains," and "new" human technologies generated by contemporary cultural processes. For once, the word "unprecedented" is fully justified. In this context, unprecedented does not just relate to recent human history, but refers to the entire history of human evolution and even to the entire history of life on Earth. Nothing like what is happening now, to us and because of us, has happened before in evolution, even though different events of comparable significance and magnitude have happened. We appear to be taking part in what John Maynard Smith and Eörs Szathmary have called one of the major transitions in evolution; it continues today.[1]

So how can we understand ourselves if doing so requires understanding the unprecedented? It cannot be easy, but if we wish to avoid our problems, or take advantage of our opportunities, we need to try. Given the scale of these events, the obvious place to start is with evolution.

A preliminary obstacle is that contemporary evolutionary theory, hereafter called standard theory, does not provide a sufficient basis for understanding human evolution. Standard evolutionary theory has the potential to tell us lots about human nature and human behavior, including human social behavior. But the standard theory is weak in dealing with human cultural processes, partly because potent cultural processes are unique to human beings. Cultural processes do not even exist in most other species. Standard theory also fails to deal satisfactorily with the role of human technology in human evolution. Richard C. Lewontin points out that for standard evolutionary theory, "The environment 'poses the problem'; the organisms posit 'solutions.'"[2] Human technology, obviously poses problems and posits solutions, if only because it keeps changing the environments that pose the problems. Does that put human technology outside the pale of evolution? I think not. But it probably does put it beyond the reach of standard evolutionary theory.

In this article, I will place human evolution in the context of a more comprehensive approach that my colleagues and I have been working on for some time. We call it "extended evolutionary theory," and claim it offers a more accurate and empirically useful theoretical framework for making sense of prior human evolution and our contemporary lives.[3]

2. Niche Construction

Extended evolutionary theory differs from standard evolutionary theory primarily by adding a new process, called "niche construction," to the concept. First, I will describe how niche construction affects evolution in general. Then I will apply it to human evolution. Finally, I will discuss how the resulting altered view of human evolution may help us understand ourselves better. Figure 1a summarizes the standard theory. Natural selection pressures in environments (E) act on populations of diverse organisms (or phenotypes) and influence which individuals survive, reproduce, and pass on their genes to the next generation via genetic inheritance. The adaptations of organisms are assumed to be products of natural selection molding organisms to fit pre-established environmental templates. The templates are dynamic because processes independent of organisms frequently change the worlds to which organisms have to adapt. The changes that organisms bring about in their worlds are seldom thought to have evolutionary significance.

Fig. 1a   Standard evolutionary theory

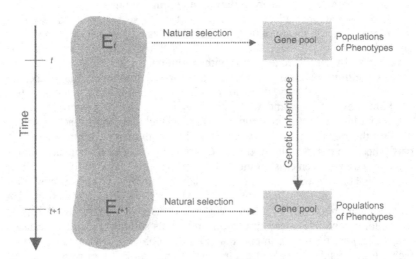

One difficulty with this traditional view is that it largely ignores the feedback in evolution caused by the modification of natural selection pressures by the activities of organisms. Organisms, through their metabolisms, behaviors, and choices, partly define, create, and destroy their environments.[4] In doing so, they inevitably transform some of the natural selection pressures that act on themselves and on others. Subsequently, these transformed selection pressures feedback to select for different genotypes in populations.[5] Adaptation cannot be just a matter of organisms responding to autonomous natural selection pressures in environments. Sometimes it must also involve organisms responding to natural selection pressures previously transformed by organisms. We call the transformation of natural selection by the actions of organisms "niche-construction."

Elsewhere, we have given many examples of niche construction from all the kingdoms of life.[6] Space is limited here, so I will only give a single non-human example. I will choose earthworms, which adds piquancy because Charles Darwin originally described them.[7]

By burrowing, dragging organic material into the soil, and mixing it up with inorganic material, and by their casting, earthworms dramatically change the structure and chemistry of soils. Soils that contain earthworms demonstrate enhanced plant yield, less surface litter, more topsoil, more organic carbon, nitrogen, and polysaccharides, and better porosity, aeration, and drainage. It follows that earthworms must live in partly self-constructed worlds. Some of the selection pressures that act on earthworms must have been transformed by the prior activities of earthworms.

Turner examined the consequence of the soil-changing activities of earthworms. He compared the physiological characteristics of earthworms, in particular the characteristics of their kidneys, to those of other animals, and discovered a surprising fact. Earthworms are equipped with the "wrong" kidneys. Different kinds of kidneys are typically found in different animals, depending on where they live. Animals living in freshwater are in danger of being flooded by excess water; freshwater kidneys excrete surplus water. Animals living in the sea are in danger of being killed by excess salts; marine kidneys get rid of salts. Animals living on land are in danger of drying up, so terrestrial kidneys prevent desiccation by retaining as much water as possible. The crucial point is that terrestrial earthworms are equipped with nearly typical freshwater kidneys. What appears to have happened is that earthworms have retained the freshwater physiology of their aquatic ancestors and are poorly equipped physiologically for living on land. They do live on land, but only because they niche construct. Turner devotes an entire chapter to explaining exactly how they do it. I will give his conclusion:

Earthworms when they came onto land, seem to have . . . pursued a strategy of using ATP energy to work against soil weathering. Along the way, they essentially co-opted the soil as an accessory organ of water balance. The advantage of adopting this strategy is clear: it is accomplished much more rapidly than a retooling of internal physiology.[8]

What earthworms tell us is that adaptation is a two-way process. Adaptation is not just a matter of natural selection selecting for adaptive traits in organisms. It is also a matter of organisms transforming some of the natural selection pressures in their environments to suit themselves, by niche construction.

3. Extended Evolutionary Theory

For this reason, we proposed an extended theory of evolution that explicitly incorporates niche construction.[9] The basic idea is summarized in Figure 1b, which illustrates a scheme in which the evolution of organisms depends on natural selection and niche construction. Ancestral organisms transmit genes to their descendents under the direction of natural selection pressures in their environments, exactly as shown in Figure 1a. These same organisms pass on selected habitats, modified habitats, and modified sources of natural selection in those habitats to descendents via an "ecological inheritance," under the direction of niche construction. The net result is that the selective environments encountered by organisms are partly determined by independent sources of natural selection, for example, by climate, weather, or physical and chemical events. They are also partly determined by what organisms do, or previously did, to their and to each others' environments, by niche construction.

Fig. 1b   Extended evolutionary theory

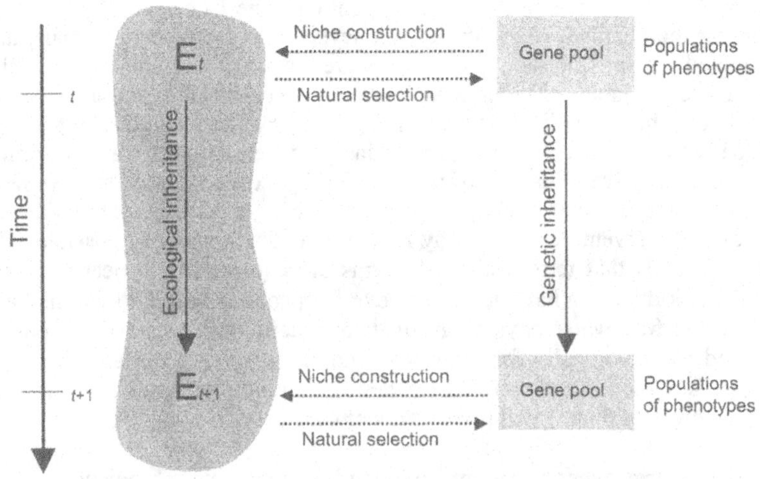

Ecological inheritance (Figure 1b) is also a proposed new process in evolution. It refers to the inheritance, via an external environment, of one or more natural selection pressures previously modified by niche construction. It is a second general inheritance system in evolution, but it works quite differently from genetic inheritance.[10]

4. Implications for the Human Sciences

What are the implications of extended evolutionary theory for our own species? Given that most human niche construction depends on cultural processes, I will begin with a well known example of human cultural niche construction.

When our pastoralist ancestors first domesticated cattle and drank milk, they set up self-induced natural selection pressures in favor of genes that increase lactose absorption in human adults, by synthesizing an enzyme, lactase, which breaks down the lactose in milk. Consequently, between 70 and 100 percent of human adults who come from parts of the world with a long history of dairy farming can continue to drink milk long after their childhood is over. Others cannot.[11] This example shows that, through cultural niche construction, human phenotypes can sometimes influence human genetic evolution. Yet according to standard evolutionary theory, phenotypes are not supposed to be able to influence their genetic evolution. The idea sounds suspiciously like Lamarckism even though it is not. Niche construction is Darwinian because it only modifies orthodox Darwinian natural selection pressures. This lactose tolerance example and others like it, pose problems for the standard theory. I will show this by considering two ways in which biologists have previously tried to relate human cultural processes to evolution.

The first, sociobiology, is firmly based on standard evolutionary theory and suffers the consequences.[12] The standard theory only models a single inheritance system in evolution, genetic inheritance (Figure 1a). The only way in which any organisms can possibly contribute to evolutionary descent must be by passing on their genes to their descendents. Since human sociobiology is based on the standard theory, it has to assume this limitation also applies to human beings beings. Scientists assign human phenotypes the same status as the phenotypes of every other species. We are just "survival machines" or "vehicles" for our genes. Our only evolutionary function is differential survival and reproduction relative to natural selection and chance.[13] This leads to the version of human evolution summarized in Figure. 2a. Sociobiology recognizes the existence of human cultural processes and it can recognize cultural inheritance within cultures. But, the most that it permits any of these cultural processes to do for human evolution is to influence which individuals are the fittest and which the least fit, and thereby, who contributes their genes to genetic inheritance in each generation.

Fig. 2a   Human sociobiology: single inheritance

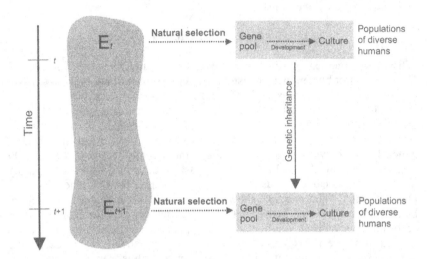

The drawback of this approach is that it fails to explain how our human ancestors, by inventing agriculture, contributed to human evolution in a second way, by transforming natural selection pressures in their environments by "agricultural" niche construction. For this to have happened, human beings must be more than survival machines in evolution. To an extent, we must also be active "co-directors" in our evolution.

The second approach is gene culture co-evolutionary theory, which fares better. Like the sociobiologists, the gene-culture co-evolutionary theorists recognize that human culture exists. Unlike the sociobiologists, they also realize that human cultural inheritance sometimes promotes the transformation of natural selection pressures in human environments in ways that do have consequences for human evolution.[14] The dotted feedback arrows in Figure 2b symbolize this point.

Gene-culture co-evolutionary theory is an advance on sociobiology because it can explain more data, but it still faces two problems. First, it regards the transformation of natural selection pressures in environments as an exclusively human affair, something only human beings can do, and only because of culture. Earthworms demonstrate this assumption is false. Niche construction

Fig. 2b   Gene culture co-evolution: dual inheritance

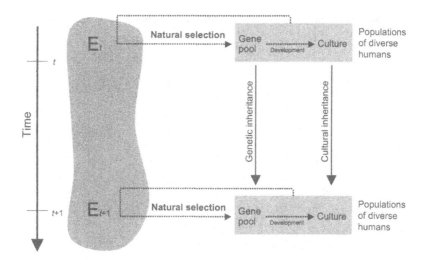

is a general phenomenon. All organisms do it, and it does not depend on culture.[15] Second, gene-culture co-evolutionary theory did not initially incorporate either niche construction or ecological inheritance. Yet without these intermediate processes, this so-called dual inheritance approach is poorly equipped to explain exactly how human cultural processes can influence human genetics.

To meet these criticisms we proposed that, instead of basing gene-culture co-evolution on standard evolutionary theory, we should base it on extended evolutionary theory.[16] Figure 2c illustrates what happens when we do this. Extended evolutionary theory converts gene-culture co-evolution from a dual inheritance to a triple inheritance theory. It now incorporates: (1) genetic inheritance directed by natural selection, (2) ecological inheritance directed by niche construction, and (3) cultural inheritance directed by cultural processes. Cultural inheritance is different from genetic and ecological inheritance in that it is not a general inheritance system in evolution, but almost exclusively human. It works by influencing both of the other two general inheritance systems in human evolution.

It influences human genetic inheritance by contributing to differential survival and reproduction in human populations in the manner that sociobiology and the earlier versions of gene-culture co-evolutionary theory say it does. But cultural inheritance also influences human ecological inheritance by contributing to the transformation of natural selection pressures in human environments by cultural niche construction. Subsequently, natural selection pressures previously modified by human cultural niche construction may select for different human genotypes.

Fig. 2c   Gene-culture co-evolution: triple inheritance + niche construction

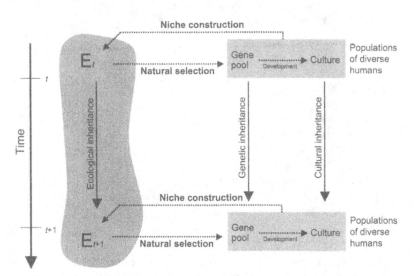

5. An Evolutionary Framework for the Human Sciences

We suggest this triple inheritance version of gene culture co-evolution (Figure 2c) is a step closer to the comprehensive theory we are going to need to understand ourselves. More complicated than earlier theories (Figures 2a, 2b), it is still incomplete. For instance, it completely omits human developmental processes and is too general to be immediately useful.

So how can we make the theory work? Answering this question would require a detailed explanation of all the ways human genetic and cultural processes can interact with each other and is beyond the scope of this chapter. The most we can do is to consider one component of this theory in greater detail. I will focus on the different ways in which human cultural niche construction can affect human lives. Figure 3 summarizes three routes via which human cultural niche construction can potentially influence either human history, or human genetics.

Fig. 3   Alternative responses to feedback from cultural niche construction

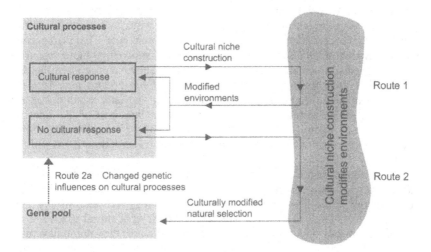

Route 1, the feedback loop at the top, depicts a scenario in which cultural niche construction modifies a human environment in some way that feeds back to a human population and subsequently causes a further cultural change in that population. Suppose human cultural niche construction changes a human environment by polluting it. The pollution may subsequently feed back to cultural selection and transmission processes in the human population, to favor the invention and spread of a new technology, to counteract the pollution. Route 1 refers to all cases in which cultural niche construction only affects cultural processes. It changes human history, but it does not affect human genetics.

Route 2 (Figure 3) does affect human genetics. Here cultural niche construction changes an environment as before, but this time, either because no cultural response to the change occurs, or because the cultural response is insufficient, the feedback from the changed environment eventually acts as a modified natural selection pressure that subsequently selects for different human genes.

The evolution of human lactose tolerance is one example. Another comes from Kwa-speaking cultivators in West Africa.[17] A genetic change occurred in these people as a consequence of their cutting clearings in tropical rainforests to enable them to grow their crops. The clearings increased the amount of standing water which provided better breeding grounds for malaria-carrying mosquitoes. That increased the prevalence of malaria, which apparently modified natural selection in favor of an increase in the frequency of the hemoglobin S allele because, in heterozygotes, the S allele confers a degree of protection against malaria.

Route 2a (Figure 3) is the same as Route 2 except that the genotypes selected by culturally modified natural selection underpin the evolution of culture itself. A candidate example is the evolution of the human brain. Leslie C. Aiello and P. Wheeler proposed that our ancestors may have used their increasingly large brains to improve their diets in ways that caused modified natural selection pressures to select for smaller human guts. That then permitted the evolution of still larger brains, because apparently more resources were diverted from smaller guts to larger brains. They also proposed that this happened in two episodes, initially when our *Homo erectus* ancestors improved their diets through more efficient hunting and later when our *Homo sapiens* ancestors started to cook. Cooking externalizes part of the digestive process, which again permits the digestion of food by smaller guts. Since cooking is an obvious example of cultural niche construction, it exemplifies Route 2a.[18]

Interactions can also occur among all three of these routes depending on exactly how human populations respond to the consequences of their niche-construction. If the Kwa speakers had realized they were intensifying their selection by malaria, they might have altered their agricultural practices. Alternatively, if they had had access to modern medicines, they might have used drugs to counteract the malaria. Either of these responses could have converted Route 2 to Route 1, because the additional counteractive cultural niche construction could have cancelled out the need for any genetic response. Conversely, today we do not always realize the harmful consequences of our contemporary cultural niche-construction, or if we do, we are not always prepared to pay for remedies. For example, global warming probably is a consequence of our contemporary, technologically amplified niche-construction. If we are unwilling to invest in corrective technology, it might eventually cause Route 1 to revert to Route 2 by exposing human populations to natural selection pressures that could affect human genetics.

6. Conclusion

The main innovation introduced by extended evolutionary theory is the replacement of the idea that human phenotypes are just "vehicles for genes," dedicated to the single evolutionary task of differential survival and reproduction, by the realization that human phenotypes, like phenotypes in every other species, also modify natural selection by niche construction.

In human beings, this second task in evolution is immediately enhanced by two species-specific traits: (1) cultural processes, which because of human technology, are now uniquely potent; and (2) human consciousness, inclusive of our knowledge about evolution. The second carries the astonishing implication that, in our species, the processes of evolution might eventually become self conscious, but is nowhere near doing so yet. As David L. Hull points out, "the vast majority of human beings have never heard of Darwinian evolution."[19] Yet no matter how distant that prospect, it remains implicit in the "major transition in evolution" we represent.

These unique human traits are also largely responsible for the unprecedented problems and opportunities stemming from current human cultural niche construction. Derek Bickerton describes one of these problems as "runaway niche construction."[20] Because niche construction poses problems and posits solutions, the extreme potency and pace of modern cultural niche construction risks posing new problems so rapidly, and on such a large scale, that we will not be able to respond to them adaptively by either cultural or genetic processes (Figure 4). That could happen if, for example, our previously evolved social brains inhibit adaptive cultural responses capable of countering the threatening consequences of our own cultural niche construction. A second problem has already been demonstrated by history. The premature illusion that we already understand evolution led to Social Darwinism in the nineteenth century. This was a false theory of evolution due primarily to non-biologists (Lewis Henry Morgan and Herbert Spencer). It eventually promoted catastrophic forms of social engineering in the twentieth century that nearly destroyed civilization. We have got to get the theory right.

A central theme at the Barcelona meeting was the resolution of human conflicts. Here we have an opportunity to make progress by gaining insights into the fundamental functions of conflict and cooperation in evolution. Conflicts will always be with us. The logic of evolution ensures that. A better understanding of the mechanisms of conflict mediation and cooperation in evolution could make a major contribution to the peaceful resolution of future human conflicts.[21]

There may also be philosophical opportunities. For many people, Darwinism, as described by standard evolutionary theory, raises doubts about the meaning of human life. The prospect of being no more than a variant trial-and-error vehicle for whatever genes you happen to carry is not flattering. The Darwinism expressed by extended evolutionary theory tells a different story. Human beings are also conscious, potent, cultural niche constructors. As such, we are co-directors in an evolutionary process that we will never control, but might consciously influence. That conceptualization could re-introduce meaning into many individual human lives, on the basis of science, not myths.

Notes

1. John Maynard Smith and Eörs Szathmary, *The Major Transitions in Evolution* (New York: W. H. Freeman Spektrum, 1995).

2. Richard C. Lewontin, "Gene, Organism, and Environment," *Evolution from Molecules to Men*, ed. D. S. Bendall (New York: Cambridge University Press, 1983), p. 276.

3. F. John Odling-Smee, Kevin N. Laland, and Marcus W. Feldman, *Niche Construction: The Neglected Process in Evolution*, Monographs in Population Biology, 37 (Princeton, N.J.: Princeton University Press, 2003).

4. Lewontin, "Gene, Organism, and Environment."

5. Odling-Smee et al., *Niche Construction*.

6. Ibid.

7. Charles Darwin, *The Formation of Vegetable Mold through the Action of Worms, with Observations on their Habits* (London, Murray, 1881).

8. J. Scott Turner, 2000. *The Extended Organism: The Physiology of Animal-Built Structures* (Cambridge, Mass.: Harvard University Press, 2000), p. 119.

9. Odling-Smee et al., *Niche Construction*.

10. Ibid.

11. W. F. Bodmer and L.L. Cavalli-Sforza, *Genetics, Evolution and Man* (San Francisco, Calif.: W. F. Freeman, 1976); William H. Durham, *Coevolution: Genes, Culture, and Human Diversity* (Stanford, Calif.: Stanford University Press, 1991); and E. J. Hollox, M. Poulter, M. Zvarik, V. Ferak, A. Krause, T. Jenkins, N. Saha, A. I. Kozolov, and D. M. Swallow, "Lactose Haplotype Diversity in the Old World," *American Journal of Human Genetics*, 68 (2001), pp. 160–172.

12. Edward O. Wilson, *Sociobiology: The New Synthesis* (Cambridge, Mass.: Harvard University Press, 1975).

13. Richard Dawkins, *The Selfish Gene*, 2nd ed. (New York: Oxford University Press, 1989).

14. L.L. Cavalli-Sforza and Marcus W. Feldman, *Cultural Transmission and Evolution: A Quantitative Approach* (Princeton, N.J.: Princeton University Press, 1981); Robert Boyd and Peter J. Richerson, *Culture and the Evolutionary Process* (Chicago, Ill.: University of Chicago Press, 1985); and Durham, *Coevolution*.

15. Odling-Smee et al., *Niche Construction*.

16. Ibid.; and K. N. Laland, J. Odling-Smee, and M. W. Feldman, "Niche Construction, Biological Evolution, and Cultural Change" *Behavioral and Brain Sciences*, 23 (2000), pp. 131–175.

17. Durham, *Coevolution*.

18. Leslie C. Aiello and P. Wheeler, "The Expensive-Tissue Hypothesis," *Current Anthropology*, 36 (1995), pp. 199–221.

19. David L. Hull, "Taking Memetics Seriously: Memetics Will Be What We Make It," *Darwinizing Culture: The Status of Memetics as a Science*, ed. Robert Aunger (Oxford: Oxford University Press, 2000), p. 55.

20. Derek Bickerton, personal communication, 2004.

21. Peter Hammerstein, ed., *Genetic and Cultural Evolution of Cooperation* (Cambridge, Mass.: MIT Press, 2002).

Seventeen

WHAT DO WE KNOW OF
THE SOCIAL BRAIN?

Camilo José Cela Conde, Miguel Ángel Capó,
Marcos Nadal and Carlos Ramos

The objective of this study is to analyze scientific findings capable of describing the mechanisms underlying the human behaviors of cooperation and conflict on a biological and cognitive level. The underlying question we aim to answer is whether we can understand these behaviors in a more profound way than through mere folk psychology models. Such an understanding, based on the certainty that conflict and cooperation involve mechanisms fixed by natural selection, would necessitate explanation of the appearance of cognitive processes related to these behaviors and identifying the causal biological mechanisms. To do so we review three types of approach to this question: the sociobiological, neurobiological, and genetic approaches.

1. The Sociobiological Approach to Social Behavior

Modern study of the biological roots of social behavior goes back to the flourishing of a new approach toward animal behavior constructed from ethology in the sixties and consolidated in the mid-seventies of last century as a field called sociobiology. Edward O. Wilson described sociobiology as the systematic study of the social bases of any social, animal, or human behavior.[1] The factors differentiating sociobiology from ethology is the adoption of the so-called gene's point of view, and development of a conceptual apparatus based on that perspective. Before the consolidation of sociobiology, many ethologists assumed that natural selection would have favored the appearance of behavior that was costly for the individual yet favorable toward the group. Accordingly, we could explain many aspects of animal social behavior as a sacrifice by the individual for the collective good. Vero Copner Wynne-Edwards was one of the researchers who contributed most in this field.[2] He argued that groups of individuals or species that limited their growth according to their environmental resources had greater survival rates than those that overexploited their habitats because the behavior of some individuals altruistically foregoing reproduction.

George C. Williams' criticism of group selection models, and his convincing arguments in favor of more parsimonious explanations, prepared the way for the work of Edward Wilson and Richard Dawkins, who popularized adoption of the genetic perspective to adequately understand social behavior.[3]

From that perspective, they considered animal behavior, including social behavior, as a medium developed by the genes to ensure their transmission to descendents. As Kevin N. Laland and Gillian R. Brown stated, scientists came to think of the body and its functions as mere vehicles to transport and transmit genes.[4] But this stance interferes with explanation of altruist behavior. If the objective of genes, and the social behavior related to them, is to maximize their chance of being transmitted to future generations, how can we explain the behavior of an individual who reduces their chances of survival and reproduction to increase those of another individual?

William Donald Hamilton based his answer, known as kin selection, on our knowledge that closely related individuals share copies of many genes.[5] Accordingly, animals can increase the presence of those common genes in the next generation by favoring reproduction in close relatives. Although the altruist act of sacrificing yourself to help someone else might reduce your chance to transmit your genes, the probability of transmitting other copies of your genes increases whenever the beneficiary is a close relative. Hamilton predicted that this behavior would be selected whenever the cost to the altruist individual was less than the benefit for the receiver or receivers, multiplied by the probability that the relative possessed an identical gene. The closer our kin, the greater the sacrifice we are prepared to make through an altruist act.

After reviewing Hamilton's work, Robert Trivers introduced the idea of reciprocal altruism to answer the question of altruistic behavior between unrelated organisms.[6] He suggested that altruist behavior, which was initially costly for the agent yet beneficial for the recipient, could appear among unrelated individuals who interacted during a long period, whenever there was a high probability that the other individual would reciprocate the altruist act in the future. Under these conditions, over time, both individuals would have gained more through their altruistic interaction than if they had not cooperated. In cases such as these, reciprocal altruism runs against certain individuals' tendency not to reciprocate—or to deceive. To avoid deceivers appearing or those deceivers re-offending, human beings have developed procedures such as altruistic punishment.[7]

Currently, we approach the biological bases for social behavior from perspectives inherited from sociobiology, such as evolutionary psychology, human behavioral ecology, the theory of dual inheritance or memetics. Although these perspectives differ in their objectives, methods and spheres of application, they all assume that a special characteristic of the human brain enables human social behavior, tied to cooperation or conflict. Even though no wide consensus exists regarding the human brain's special characteristics, which allow our cognitive and behavioral sophistication in the sphere of social relationships, a good chance exists that we need to review them. In the next section, we do this from an evolutionist approach.

2. Evolution of the Human Brain

Ralph L. Holloway indicates four serious difficulties surrounding study of human brain evolution.[8] First, the only organisms available for study are live organisms. From an empirical perspective, no direct evidence exists of the brain's evolution or of the forces of natural selection that influenced this evolution. Clues to the relationship between morphological aspects of the brain and behavior are contained in fossil records, but they are fragmentary and require much interpretive effort. Second, we do not fully understand the relationships between the neuronal variables (such as brain size, or neocortex size), and behavior. Third, the only available evidence on the brain's evolution involves the brain's superficial characteristics, which can provide information about only one part of the behavioral range. Fourth, knowledge is sorely lacking about how the variations between species are related in terms of cerebral organization and behavior. For these reasons, researchers into human brain evolution support their findings mainly on two types of evidence: evidence from fossil specimens and evidence from comparative neuroanatomy. Traditionally, researchers have focused attention on two aspects of the brain from this phylogenetic perspective: size and organization.

The comparison of different vertebrate species' brains, including those of human beings, reveals that brains vary not only in size but also in structure. Still, brains are all constructed on the same basic plan, comprising three principle embryonic divisions: prosencephalon (telencephalon and diencephalon), mesencephalon, and rhombencephalon (metencephalon and myelencephalon). Apart from size, all vertebrate brains have the same principle subdivisions. The main differences among vertebrates have to do with the relative and absolute size of different brain regions. The difference in absolute sizes has a strong positive correlation with the organism's body size: the larger the animal, the larger the brain needed and the diverse structures that comprise it. Yet the relative size differences of encephalic components are more revealing. Evolutionary biologists tend to relate them with diverse behavioral adaptations. Different animals, with differing evolutionary histories, show contrasting solutions to the dilemmas of adaptation. As a rule, the relative size of a region serves as a guide for the functional significance of that region in the specie's adaptation.

According to the traditional view, more "primitive" vertebrate groups would have developed relatively simple neuronal circuits that would constitute the basis of elementary behaviors and relationships to surroundings. More "advanced" groups would have additional, more refined, and complex neuronal circuits that would allow more sophisticated behavioral adjustments and cognitive capabilities. Researchers use the term encephalization to refer to this progressive increase in the size of the more rostral regions of the nervous system in relation to body size. The most caudal structures of the nervous system, for example, the medulla and the brain stem, would have changed little during evolutionary progress, containing circuits common to all vertebrate groups.

Yet the more rostral regions, such as the telencephalon, would be more highly developed in the more advanced vertebrate groups, incorporating new, more complex mechanisms and neuronal systems. According to this view, the highest creation level would have culminated with the appearance of the neocortex in mammals, above all in primates and in human beings, which enables and explains their superior behavioral and cognitive capabilities.

A. When Did Hominids' Brains Grow?

Human lineage separated from that of chimpanzees around seven or eight million years ago. Initially, brain size did not grow significantly, as evinced by estimations of the cranial capacity of the early australopithecines (400 to 500 cm^3), such as *Australopithecus afarensis*, that reveal figures which are very similar to those of living chimpanzees. In ratio to body size, cranial capacity within the robust lineage has not significantly varied. But with the appearance of the first of our genus, *Homo habilis*, the brain grew extra-allometrically. This means that although no solid evidence exists suggesting that the body size of the *Homo habilis* was different from that of the australopithecines, the cranial capacity of *Homo habilis* is estimated to be approximately 700-750 cm^3. This increase in cranial capacity, of approximately 250 to 300 cm^3, compared with the australopithecines, is a significant figure. From *Homo habilis* to *Homo erectus*, absolute brain size increased again up to 900 to 1000 cm^3, although, in view of the significant increase in stature of these hominids, authors such as Holloway consider that this was an allometric increase, an increase due to general body size growth.[9] After *Homo erectus*, most brain growth was extra-allometric, because no significant variations in body size compared to brain size occurred. The final stage in evolution of the hominid's brain involved an extra-allometric increase of approximately 400 to 500 cm^3, with the appearance of *Homo sapiens*, whose brain is approximately 1350 cm^3. In addition to mere validation of brain size increase, theorists have proposed explanations regarding possible factors that have contributed to this tendency throughout our evolution. Let us review the most significant parts.

B. Why Did Large Brains Appear?

Brain tissue is, to quote Leslie C. Aiello, "very expensive."[10] The large brains favored by selective pressures in *Homo* require a great amount of biological and energetic resources. What cognitive capacity was worth such a costly investment associated with increasing brain size and complexity? Its benefits should necessarily overcome the consequent costs.

Nicholas Humphrey suggested one possible answer to this question: brains became larger and more complex in order to understand the highly complex rules of social interaction.[11] Interestingly, the cognitive mechanisms that enabled us to introduce and understand social rules must have appeared prior to the divergence of the human and chimpanzee lineages. Plenty of evidence shows that chimpanzees, and other primates for that matter, lead far from simple social lives.

Following Daniel C. Dennett's model, the strategies that any individual belonging to a community maintains when they encounter their fellows—or generally, any individual *A* who interacts with individual *B*—depend on how *A* considers its behavior will influence *B*.[12] In the ebb and flow of expectations, these calculations can become as complicated as those of a chess player considering future moves. The capability of certain primates to evaluate the world and their role in it in such a manner requires a considerable amount of "intelligence." With the concept of *Machiavellian intelligence*, Dennett wanted to express the range of cognitive processes needed for any species to reach the third order intentional system, which he was describing. This system allows an individual *A*, who is interacting with another individual *B*, to attribute *B* with a mind complex enough to harbor desires and beliefs regarding *A*. Accordingly, we suppose that *A* will act as well as possible to ensure *B* interprets *A*'s behavior in the way *A* wants. Dennett's assumption is that we are social actors, and we wish to manipulate others. Yet, who are "we"? Does this description apply just to human beings, or both to human beings and chimpanzees?

A sibling group to the *Pan+Homo* group, the biological group most closely related to us and to chimpanzees is the genus *Gorilla*. Gorillas construct social groupings of a dominant male, several females, and their corresponding young; so they need a similar level of Machiavellian intelligence. In contrast, Orangutans, *Pongo*, are solitary animals with respect to males, so they cannot establish the higher intelligence barrier among the them. Sarah F. Brosnan and Frans B. M. de Waal have shown through a clever experiment how capuchin monkeys, *Cebus apella*, have a highly developed sense of justice. They learn to exchange cards for food with their human keepers yet refuse to do so if the treatment offered is worse than that shown to another monkey whose exchange they have watched and evaluated.[13]

Behavior like this reveals several significant keys regarding the emotional component of intelligence and its influence on our decisions and actions. For example, it forces us to ask whether we should change the mathematical models that describe human behavior in terms of calculation and decision to introduce the emotional variable. Yet we still do not know how to do this because we do not know enough about the way our brains relate feelings and judgments. Increase in brain size, whether absolute or relative, obviously is not enough to account for the social cognition capabilities of human beings. We need to focus on the structural reorganization processes occurring during the brain's evolution in the primate line, especially within our family.

C. The Hypothesis of Frontal Expansion

Holloway was one of the first researchers to realize that the visual areas of the human brain occupied a surprisingly small region of the cerebral cortex.[14] Although this region is not small in absolute terms, in comparison with other primates, our visual cortex is smaller than what we might expect in the brain of a primate as large as modern human being. Along with other observations, Holloway argued that evolution of the human brain does not just imply an increase in size but significant modification in its organization.

In a more thorough study into human brain reorganization throughout evolution, taking into account knowledge on the mechanisms implied in onto-genetic development of the brain, Terrence WilliamDeacon argued that cere-bral reorganization always accompanies an increase in brain size.[15] The rela-tive sizes of the functional divisions of the brain are determined by results of the competition for space directed by the peripheral systems. Given that the peripheral sensory and motor systems did not undergo significant changes, they recruit a small proportion of the cortical space compared to what we would be expect in a primate brain as large as ours, so that other cortical areas and sys-tems can benefit from the extra space. The cortical nuclei and areas receive little or no information from peripheral nervous structures that have inherited this extra space because they are relatively isolated from peripheral restrictions.[16]

Deacon suggests that in the case of human beings, the prefrontal cortex has inherited the most new territory of all the cortical areas, perhaps because of the reduction in nearby motor areas.[17] Based on extrapolations from differ-ent sources, he concluded that the size of the human prefrontal cortex is ap-proximately double the expected size for a hominoid brain as large as ours. But this expansion is not homogenous for the entire prefrontal cortex, but has primordially affected its dorsal regions. Deacon affirms that the key factor in the appearance of human beings' symbolic capability is reorganization of their neuronal connections in the dorsal zones of the prefrontal cortex.[18]

Contrary to Deacon's reasoning, Holloway, based on his observations, concluded that the dimensions of the human prefrontal cortex are just about what we should expect for its size. With the aim to resolve this issue empiri-cally, Katerina Semendeferi and Antonio R. Damasio measured the overall brain size and that of the different regions of the brain in modern human be-ings, chimpanzees, gorillas, orangutans, and gibbons using magnetic reso-nance imaging.[19] They reconstructed the images to generate a three-dimensional reproduction, which allowed them to study the total brain volume and those of the frontal, temporal, occipital lobes and the combination of tem-poral and parietal lobes. The results revealed great homogeneity of the relative volumes in these sectors among those primates. The only significant differ-ences they found indicated that human beings have a smaller cerebellum than expected for their brain size, and that the frontal lobe of gibbons is smaller than expected. Their results did not suggest that there had been an appreciable increase in prefrontal cortex size throughout human evolution. Apparently, human beings' outstanding social behavior and cognition are not especially associated with an increase in the size of the prefrontal cortex.

James K. Rilling and Thomas R. Insel's work offers a final clue, sug-gesting the need to go beyond rough measures of brain size.[20] They carried out a magnetic resonance study using forty four specimens of eleven primate species. In addition to making a volumetric calculation, they investigated the relation between brain volume and gyrification, the degree that the cerebral cortex folds in upon itself to form sulci and gyri. Their results indicated that larger brain volume is positively correlated with the degree of gyrification. But two regions of the brain in human beings surpass the degree of gyrification predicted by this tendency: the prefrontal and posterior parietal-temporal regions. The authors suggested that this increased gyrification in these regions, appeared along the human evolutionary line, could constitute part of the neuronal underpinnings of some of the distinctive cognitive capabilities exhibited by human beings. Neuropsychology and neuroimaging provide possible ways to verify whether cognitive processes involved in social cognition are actually associated with these brain areas.

3. Cerebral Localization: The Case of Morality

A. Somatic Markers and Decision Making

The studies carried out by A. Damasio and colleagues on patients with damage to the medial and ventral portions of their frontal lobes has sparked a growing interest in the neuroaffective bases of social judgment.[21] With some variants, this patient case type is similar to that of Phineas Gage, a nineteenth century railway foreman, who entered the history of neuropsychology after an accidental explosion caused an iron bar of between two and three centimeters of diameter to pierce his cranium, entering through the base of the left cheekbone and exiting through the upper central part of the frontal bone. Due to this injury, Gage lost some encephalic mass from the medial prefrontal cortex. He survived the accident, although afterwards he was never able to lead a normal life. Despite apparently maintaining his capability to reason, he was unable to make correct decisions in the social sphere. For instance, he could not keep a job or was unable to refuse accepting excessive risks.

Damasio and his team argued that patients with injuries similar to Gage's suffer from emotional deficits. They are unable to effectively generate and use the so-called somatic markers. These are neuronal representations of body states imbuing the behavioral options with affective influence, guiding decision making. These patients' deficits allow them to keep normal cognitive functions, scoring within a normal range in intelligence quotient and other psychometric tests. In addition, these patients maintain their abstract social knowledge in spite of disastrous decision making in this area. Their affective or emotional deficits stop them from *feeling* how they should act. This indicates that social decision making is predominantly emotional and less reasoned than was previously thought.

The behavior of patients who have suffered injuries during their adult life causes more problems for them than for others. But a study by the Damasio team on two patients with prefrontal damage acquired during their early childhood found that these children engaged in immoral behavior: lies, thefts, aggression, threats, all without apparent remorse.[22] As previously, both patients fell within a normal range in cognitive tests, failing in tasks designed to test their skill in risky decision making. In addition, in contrast to patients injured as adults, they had difficulties establishing the moral/conventional distinction. In Lawrence Kohlberg's terminology, their mode of moral reasoning is "preconventional," aimed only at avoiding punishment. The damaged regions in these patients are crucial both for real time decision making, and for acquiring social knowledge and acquiring a disposition for normal social behavior.

These two patients exhibit behavior similar to psychopaths although their performance is associated with specific cerebral injuries. Also, psychopaths tend to use their aggressive behavior instrumentally as opposed to reactively.[23]

B. Studies of Functional Magnetic Resonance

Several research groups have recently used functional magnetic resonance (fMRI) to study moral decision making. Through this technique, they identify the brain regions that receive a greater amount of oxygen-rich blood. The technique indirectly indicates the zones of greatest neural activation in response to a given task. These tasks do not represent a set of unified efforts because the tasks proposed to subjects and the objectives of each group are widely diverse. Yet by combining them, we can extract a common neural substratum of moral decision making consisting of the ventromedial, prefrontal, and orbitofrontal cortices (vmPFC/OFC, representing reward/punishment and "hot" brain theory), posterior cingulate cortex (PCC, integrating emotion and memory) and the superior temporal sulcus (pSTS, theory of the mind and representing socially significant movements).[24]

First, Jorge Moll and collaborators showed their subjects simple sentences, some containing moral content ("They hanged an innocent person.") and others without it ("Walking is good for your health.").[25] Moll and collaborators compared judgments in response to simple moral allegations compared to judgments on sentences with a disagreeable emotional content ("He licked the dirty toilet." "Pregnant women tend to vomit.").[26] Finally, they compared the results of exposing their subjects to photographs with moral and emotional content.[27]

Moll's group wanted to find morality's correlation almost neo-phrenologically, contrasting moral emotions with basic emotions. In addition, in the studies using moral statements they indistinctly presented infinitive statements capable of suggesting a moral principle, such as "Older people are useless" along with others in third person referring to actions: "The boy stole his mother's savings." These two types of statements can have widely differing implications for brain theory, for example. This indistinct use of meaningfully different statement forms as a single type suggests that we must consider the results of their experiments with caution.

Another group, led by Hauke Heekeren, carried out two interesting studies. In the first, they minimized ambiguities and, using scenarios not involving personal injury or violence, they found that simple moral decisions, in contrast to decisions of a purely semantic nature, activated a network consisting of the superior temporal sulcus (pSTS), the ventromedial prefrontal cortex (vmPFC), the left lateral prefrontal cortex and both temporal poles.[28] Hawke and collaborators devoted their next paper to the study, in the same framework, of the influence of bodily injury in the cerebral processing of moral decisions. Presence of injury caused a lower response time and reduced activity of the temporal poles.[29] This indicates that physical injury reduces the depth of processing needed to reach a decision. The results are valuable because by proceeding systematically they set up the bases by which additional characteristics can be added to those collected in Table 1.

Comparison of the results of moral and non-moral tasks is not the only potentially productive channel of research. A group from Princeton directed by Joshua Greene decided to use neuroimaging techniques, not to locate the neuronal correlatives defining morality, but to check the explanatory hypothesis of a philosophic puzzle posed by the dilemmas known collectively as *trolley problems*. To introduce this kind of dilemma, let us consider the situation of Anne, who is standing beside the track, watching a maintenance group at work. Suddenly Anne hears a trolley approaching extremely fast, apparently without brakes, heading for those five workers. Next to her is a lever. If she pulls it, she will detour the tram into an adjacent rail where there is only one man. Should Anne pull the lever? The decision Anne faces is whether to pull the lever and save five lives in exchange for sacrificing one. In a second version, Mary faces the same dilemma as Anne except that the only way to stop the trolley, to save the five workers, is to push the sixth onto the track so that the trolley's automatic stop mechanism kicks in. By pushing him, Mary has condemned the sixth worker to a certain death, but will have saved the other five.

Table 1. Different possible conditions for moral tasks.

Condition	Variations
Agent (of the action judged)	First person (e.g. our decision on dilemmas such as how we should behave)
	Second person (moral laws and other imperatives and orders inasmuch as they imply moral obligation)
	Third person (we judge a third person's actions)
Bodily injury	Present
	Absent
Task type	Judge an action (statement)
	Decide a moral dilemma
Patient	A specific person or collective
	A non-specific person or collective

Philippa Foot introduced the trolley dilemma in the context of a discussion on abortion and the "doctrine of double effect,"[30] the principle that holds that sometimes implementing actions that have undesired effects as a consequence is permissible, if those actions are sub-products of a greater good. Yet Judith Jarvis Thomson developed diverse forms of these dilemmas and found that for most subjects, while Anne pulling the lever appeared acceptable, Mary's action of pushing an individual to save five other people's lives should be condemned.[31] On this schema, Greene and collaborators established a generalization of both types of dilemma by referring to them as "personal" and "impersonal."[32] Personal dilemmas have three characteristics: an *agent*, in the sense that the action must be carried out completely and not merely "edited"; a *damage* of a basic type, not elaborate, and a *specific victim*, not generic. "Impersonal" dilemmas may have one or two, but not all three of these elements.

The results indicated that responding to personal dilemmas versus impersonal dilemmas produced greater activation of areas typically associated with socio-emotional processing (including the medial frontal gyrus, the posterior cingulate gyrus, and the superior temporal sulcus). The opposite contrast generated greater activity in areas related merely to working memory (such as dorsolateral prefrontal and parietal areas). Concerning the answers to the dilemmas, they found that the response time of affirmative answers to personal violations—or judging in cases like Mary's that to fling the sixth worker onto the tracks is acceptable—increased significantly. The most plausible hypothesis is that subjects who chose that option had to overcome their negative emotional response when faced with moral violations of a personal nature such as those defined here.

In a second experiment, carried out in 2004, the research team tried to go even further. They distinguished between "easy" and "difficult" personal dilemmas, determined by response time.[33] An example of "easy" personal moral dilemma would be that of a single female adolescent who manages to hide her pregnancy and, once she gives birth, gets rid of her baby in the hope that the event passes unnoticed without compromising her or her family's life. Almost all subjects labeled this situation as inappropriate. In contrast, a "difficult" personal moral dilemma would be: in the context of war, a group of people meets in a room, hiding from enemy troops who want to eliminate them. In this situation, a baby starts to cry. The mother faces the possibility of suffocating her baby, knowing it will probably die in any case, thereby saving herself and the other refugees. Alternatively, if the mother does not suffocate the baby, she condemns the entire group to death, including the baby. Judgments of appropriateness of this dilemma evinced a more balanced distribution and response times were significantly higher than evinced in easy situations.

Comparison of the activated correlates of difficult and easy dilemmas revealed an increase of brain activity in two zones: the anterior cingulate cortex, related to the cognitive conflict (managing divergent stimuli), and the dorsolateral prefrontal cortex, characteristic of abstract reasoning processes. One step beyond this kind of contrast is dividing the difficult personal dilemmas into two groups according to the answer given in terms of the appropriateness of the moral violation. When the judgment was favorable to moral violation in the name of a greater good ("utilitarian" answer), activity again increased in centers related to abstract reasoning and cognitive control.[34]

From these studies, we can extract two main conclusions. First, moral judgment involves a whole network of coordinated cerebral areas, integrating ones typically related with emotion and others typically considered as bearing the capacity for "cold" cognition. Second, the neuronal activity in cerebral zones classically considered as purely "cognitive" predicts an "utilitarian" answer type, opposed to a deontological response, based theoretically on "rational" principles, derived through the powers of a "practical reason," but whose neural correlates are areas traditionally labeled as emotional.[35]

4. The "Genetic Cause"

In this final section, we turn our attention to the genetic mechanisms involved in social behavior. The most common research strategy used to address this issue has been to study genetic anomalies related to the disorganization of behavior and social intelligence.

Several studies have suggested that there is a relation between aggressive behavior in animals, as well as antisocial behavior in human beings, and an alteration in the metabolism of serotonin, dopamine, and noradrenalin. These observations suggest that genetic mutations affecting the metabolism of these neurotransmitters can lead to aggressive behavior such as impulsive aggression, pyromania, rape attempts, or exhibitionism.[36] The crucial factor in these metabolic alterations is decrease in the enzyme activity of monoamine oxidase (MAOA), which produces inactivation of those neurotransmitters.

The work of Avshalom Caspi and colleagues represents a noteworthy study of the relation between genetic and environmental factors involved in human social cognition and behavior.[37] They began their investigation based on the observation that although mistreatment during childhood increases the probability of criminal behavior during adult life, not every person mistreated during childhood becomes a delinquent or a criminal. They suggested that genetic susceptibility factors could explain this variability. They carried out an analysis to verify whether they could predict antisocial behavior from the interaction between the MAOA gene and the environment (mistreatment). Their results indicate that for people with high MAOA activity, childhood mistreatment is not strongly related with later antisocial behavior. People with a low MAOA activity show a significantly stronger relationship between childhood mistreatment and antisocial behavior.

The role of MAOA during the development of antisocial behavior is still open to question. Studies incorporating different samples and variations in the procedure and analysis of data have led to disparate conclusions. For example, Michael M. Vanyukov and colleagues did not find any relationship between the activity of MAOA and aggressiveness.[38] Ru-Band Lu and colleagues using a Chinese sample, and Håkan Garpenstrand and colleagues with a Swedish sample, also failed to find any such relationship.[39]

These discrepancies support Adrian Raine's arguments regarding interaction of social and biological factors in generating antisocial behavior.[40] After reviewing a wide range of studies the objective of which was to verify how these two factor types interacted, he admitted that a growing body of evidence supported some social and biological processes interacting to predispose toward antisocial behavior. The most significant finding did not refer to genetic factors, but found that interaction between complications in birth and negative family environments provide the predisposition for antisocial behavior during adult life. Raine also warned that we should not consider the establishment of relationships between variables as the final result, but as the beginning of understanding social and antisocial behavior.[41] Once the supposed relationships between diverse biological factors has been verified—which possibly include genetic and environmental factors—the meaning of the causal chains between these variables must be investigated.

5. Conclusion

In this study, we have reviewed recent scientific findings relating to the biological correlates of human social behavior. These findings lead to certain general conclusions. First, social cognition appears to be associated with an increase of relative brain size along the evolutionary lineage leading to our species. But determining the particular brain structures responsible for the appearance of this capability in human evolution is not easy. We should also accept that the chimpanzee brain is closer than ours to that of our common ancestors. This assumption, together with the ongoing identification of different functional areas in the human brain, might permits us to uncover hints that will allow an initial description of this evolutionary process.

Second, social cognition does not appear to be associated with a single specialized brain center, or even a distinctive kind of process. Instead, diverse cognitive and affective mechanisms appear to underlie this capability. Results from recent studies on the neural correlates of moral cognition demonstrate this diversity. Third, although information contained in genes apparently guides brain development, this alone does not determine the actual behavior output. As I demonstrated with the MAOA case, the outcome of the genetic contribution depends largely on its interaction with certain environmental conditions.

Although we know much more about the biological bases of social behavior and cognition than we did just ten years ago, each new research result opens new and interesting research avenues.

Notes

1. Edward O. Wilson, Edward O. Sociobiology: *The New Synthesis* (Cambridge, Mass.: Harvard University Press, 1975).

2. Vero Copner Wynne-Edwards, *Animal Dispersion in Relation to Social Behaviour* (Edinburgh, England: Oliver and Boyd, 1962).

3. George C. Williams, *Adaptation and Natural Selection: A Critique of Some Current Evolutionary Thought* (Princeton, N.J.: Princeton University Press, 1966); Wilson, *Sociobiology*; and Richard Dawkins, *The Selfish Gene* (Oxford, England: Oxford University Press, 1976).

4. Kevin N. Laland and Gillian R. Brown, *Sense and Nonsense* (Oxford: Oxford University Press, 2002).

5. William D. Hamilton, "The Evolution of Altruistic Behavior," *American Naturalist*, 97 (1963), pp. 354–356.

6. Robert L. Trivers, "The Evolution of Reciprocal Altruism," *The Quarterly Review of Biology*, 46 (1971), pp. 35–57.

7. E. Fehr, and S. Gächter, S. "Altruistic Punishment in Humans," *Nature*, 415 (2002), pp. 137–140.

8. Ralph L. Holloway, "Evolution of the Human Brain," *Handbook of Human Symbolic Evolution*, eds. Andrew Lock and Charles R. Peters (New York: Oxford University Press, 1996).

9. Ralph L. Holloway, "Toward a Synthetic Theory of Human Brain Evolution," *Origins of the Human Brain*, eds. Jean-Pierre Changeux and Jean Chavaillon (New York: Oxford University Press, 1995).

10. Leslie C. Aiello and P. Wheeler, "The Expensive Tissue Hypothesis: The Brain and the Digestive System and Primate Evolution," *Current Anthropology*, 36 (1995), pp. 199–221.

11. N. K. Humphrey, "The Social Function of Intellect," *Growing Points in Ethology: Based on a Conference Sponsored by St. John's College and King's College, Cambridge*, eds. P. P. G. Bateson and Robert A. Hinde (Cambridge, England: Cambridge University Press, 1976), pp. 303–317.

12. Daniel Clement Dennett, *The Intentional Stance* (Cambridge, Mass.: Bradford Books, 1987).

13. Sara F. Brosnan, and Frans B. M. deWaal, "Monkeys Reject Unequal Pay," *Nature*, 425(2003), pp. 297–299.

14. R. L. Holloway, "Human Paleontological Evidence Relevant to Language Behavior," *Human Neurobiology*, 2, 105-114.

15. Terrence William Deacon, *The Symbolic Species: The Co-Evolution of Language and the Brain* (New York: Norton, 1997).

16. Ibid.

17. Ibid.

18. Ibid.

19. Ibid.;

20. Ralph Holloway, *Evolution of the Human Brain*; and Katerina Semendeferi and Hanna Damasio, "The Brain and its Main Anatomical Subdivisions in Living Hominoids Using Magnetic Resonance Imaging," *Journal of Human Evolution*, 38 (2000), pp. 317–332.

21. James K. Rilling and Thomas R. Insel, "The Primate Neocortex in Comparative Perspective Using Magnetic Resonance Imaging," *Journal of Human Evolution*, 37 (1999), Poo, 191–223.

22. Antonio R. Damasio, *Descartes' Error* (New York: Putnam, 1994).

23. S. W. Anderson, A. Bechara, H. Damasio, D. Tranel, and A. R. Damasio, "Impairment of Social and Moral behavior Related to Early Damage in Human Prefrontal Cortex," *Nature Neuroscience*, 2 (1999), pp. 1032–1037.

24. R. J. Blair, "A Cognitive Developmental Approach to Morality," *Cognition*, 57 (1995), pp. 1–29.

25. J. D. Greene and J. Haidt, "How (and Where) Does Moral Judgment Work?" *Trends in Cognitive Sciences*, 6 (2002), pp. 517–523.

26. J. Moll, P. J. Eslinger, R. Oliveira-Souza, "Frontopolar and Anterior Temporal Cortex Activation in a Moral Judgment Task," *Arquivos de Neuro-Psiquiatria*, 59 (2001), pp. 657–664.

27. J. Moll, R. Oliveira-Souza, I. E. Bramati, and J. Grafman, "Functional Networks in Emotional Moral and Nonmoral Social Judgments," *Neuroimage*, 16 (2002), pp. 696–703.

28. J. Moll, R. Oliveira-Souza, P. J. Eslinger, I. E. Bramati, J. Mourao-Miranda, P. A. Andreiuolo, and L. Pessoa, "The Neural Correlates of Moral Sensitivity," *Journal of Neuroscience*, 22 (2002), pp. 2730–2736.

29. H. R. Heekeren, I. Wartenburger, H. Schmidt, H. P. Schwintowski, and A. Villringer, "An fMRI Study of Simple Ethical Decision Making," *NeuroReport*, 14 (2003), pp. 1215–1219.

30. H. R. Heekeren, I. Wartenburger, H. Schmidt, K. Prehn, H. Schwintowski, and A. Villringer, "Influence of Bodily Harm on Neural Correlates of Semantic and Moral Decision Making," *NeuroImage*, 24 (2005), pp. 887–897.

31. Philippa Foot, *Virtues and Vices* (London: Basil Blackwell, 1978).

32. Judith Jarvis Thomson, *Rights, Restitution and Risk: Essays in Moral Theory* (Cambridge, Mass.: Harvard University Press, 1986).

33. J. D. Greene, R. B. Sommerville, L. E. Nystrom, J. M. Darley, and J. D. Cohen, "An fMRI Investigation of Emotional Engagement in Moral Judgment," *Science*, 293 (2001), pp. 2105–2108.

34. J. D. Greene, L. E. Nystrom, A. D. Engell, J. M. Darley, and J. D. Cohen, "The Neural Bases of Cognitive Conflict and Control in Moral Judgment," *Neuron*, 44 (2004), pp. 389–400.

35. Ibid.

36. J. D. Greene, "From Neural 'Is' to Moral 'Ought': What Are the Moral Implications of Neuroscientific Moral Psychology?" *Nature Reviews Neuroscience*, 4 (2003), pp. 847–850.

37. H. G. Brunner, M. Nelen, X. O. Breakefield, H. H. Ropers, and B. A. van Oost, "Abnormal Behavior Associated with a Point Mutation in the Structural Gene for Monoamine Oxidase A," *Science*, 262 (1993), pp. 578–580; and A. Caspi, J. McClay, T. E. Moffitt, J. Mill, J. Martin, I. W. Craig, A. Taylor, and R. Poulton, "Role of Genotype in the Cycle of Violence in Maltreated Children," *Science*, 297 (2002), pp. 851–854.

38. Caspi, et al., "Role of Genotype in the Cycle of Violence in Maltreated Children."

39. M. M. Vanyukov, H. B. Moss, L. M. Yu, and R. Deka, "A Dinucleotide Repeat Polymorphism at the Gene for Monoamine Oxidase A and Measures of Aggressiveness," *Psychiatry Research*, 59 (1995), pp. 35–41; R.-B. Lu, W. W. Lin, J. F. Lee, H. C. Ko, and J. C. Shih, "Neither Antisocial Personality Disorder nor Antisocial Alcoholism is Associated with the MAOA Gene in Han Chinese Males," *Alcoholism-Clinical and Experimental Research*, 27 (2003), pp. 889–893; and H, Garpenstrand, E. Longato-Stadler, B. Klinteberg, E. Grigorenko, M. Damberg, L. Oreland, and J. Hallman, "Low Platelet Monoamine Oxidase Activity in Swedish Imprisoned Criminal Offenders," *European Neuropsychopharmacology*, 12 (2002), pp. 135–140.

40. A. Raine, "Biosocial Studies of Antisocial and Violent Behavior in Children and Adults: A Review," *Journal of Abnormal Child Psychology*, 30 (2002), pp. 311–326.

Eighteen

EVOLUTIONARY ORIGINS OF THE SOCIAL BRAIN

Merlin Donald

Human beings are cultural entities. We share mind. We construct cognitive collectivities called symbolic cultures. Raised in isolation from such collectivities, we have quite limited, nonsymbolic minds. Culturally isolated human beings are not much different from their large-brained anthropoid relatives. However, embedded in a cultural network from birth, human beings become something unique in the biological world: symbolizing intellects bonded to a community of minds.

Cultural networks are a vital link in the human cognitive process. They greatly affect the way we carry out our cognitive business. Cognitive scientists often portray culture as a secondary factor in cognition, a mere "content provider" for most of our conscious experience as adults. But this superficial account ignores the fundamental importance of culture in forming the mind. The deepest effects of enculturation are responsible for the basic structure of the unconscious and all conscious representational domains. Many of the surface phenomena of cognition, such as the specifics of gesture and language, tacit knowledge, archetypes, oral histories, and social ritual, come from culture. But so do the underlying cognitive foundations that make these possible, including the detailed algorithms that define habits of thought, the retrieval paths that direct memory, and even the functional systems that micro-manage attention. We acquire the most important of these from cultural immersion. Modern cultures also provide technologies that amplify cognition. External symbolic devices, such as books or computers, can relieve the brain's biological memory systems of some of their traditional burden and speed up mental processing, allowing the mind to build powerful representations of reality. All this changes how we think. The existence of fast, efficient external memory systems enables us to construct elaborate knowledge-networks and institutional structures that interlock many minds into social meta-organisms or mega-machines. These function as "distributed" cognitive networks, which are legitimate objects of study for cognitive science.

Unfortunately, cognitive science has generally ignored or denied the importance of culture, subscribing to what I have called "the myth of the isolated mind," the belief that minds are self-sufficient monads bounded by their physical container (usually the brain). Monads are isolated entities that supposedly look out at the world, and "solve" it, while remaining independent from it. Jean Piaget's approach to child development epitomized this approach; he viewed infants as budding scientists who observe and act on the world, remember the results of their experiments, and use this evidence to construct personal universes of considerable complexity.[1] As these (hypothetical) children pass through successive stages of development, they construct more and more complex concepts of time, space, and causality, achieving all of this alone. Although many of Piaget's experiments were brilliant, these solipsistic axioms proved to be wrong. The Russian developmentalist Lev Semenovich Vygotsky came closer to the truth, showing that many of the operations that Piaget thought essential for self-construction were not innate, but acquired from culture.[2] The mind gains much of its structure from culture. This is true especially of language and thought, which tend to develop in quite specific social contexts.

1. The Primacy of the Mimetic Adaptation

What type of cognitive change would have enabled a group of archaic hominids to start developing a communication system that led eventually to the invention of highly variable and arbitrary gestures and words, distinctive grammars, and symbolic cultures? When we consider the cognitive capacities of modern apes, which probably resemble those of our common Miocene ancestors, the most fundamental cognitive component missing from their repertoire would appear to be a generalized capability to refine action deliberately. Gestures and intentional vocalizations are ultimately actions of the musculature. In order to generate a variety of arbitrary gestures and sounds, primate motor behavior must somehow have evolved into a system that was more plastic, less stereotyped, and most importantly, subject to deliberate rehearsal and refinement. Languages must be learned and invented. Given the limitations of primate motor behavior, this called for an evolutionary breakthrough in hominid motor control.

In most species, the range of possible behaviors is largely fixed in the genes and closely attuned to its ecological niche. This results in what is sometimes called a "specialist survival strategy."[3] Specialization in evolution creates a remarkable diversity of behavior across species, but it produces virtual stereotypy on the behavior of any single species. This is even true of the higher mammals, where most species do not have enough variability in motor behavior for individuals to deviate significantly from an inherited standard motor repertoire and motor options are confined within a narrow morphological envelope.

Human beings have broken out of this morphological straitjacket. This is especially evident in the variety of human spoken languages. But it is also obvious in the range of styles, customs, sports, crafts, and games that human beings invent. Where would such flexibility have begun to evolve? This question leads us logically back to the fundamentals of human motor skills and procedural learning. To learn, vary, or refine any action, including speech, an individual must carry out a sequence of basic cognitive operations. Traditionally, these include rehearsing the action, observing its consequences, remembering these, and then altering the form of the original act, varying one or more of the parameters dictated by the memory of the consequences of the previous action, or by an idealized image of the outcome. We might call an extended cognitive sequence of this sort, whose inherent complexity should not be underestimated, a "rehearsal loop." This rehearsal loop is combined with an active process of metacognitive review, whereby actors direct their attention away from the outside world, and toward their own actions. In performing metacognitive review of a precise skill, such as speech, we must aim the focus of attention at the form of the act itself, not merely at its consequences.

Apes appear to be quite poor at rehearsal and metacognitive review. We can get them to repeat actions, as a function of reinforcement contingencies, and they can engage in socially facilitated imitation, But they cannot independently initiate and rehearse actions accurately for the sole purpose of refining their movement sequences. On the other hand, at some point in their early history, human beings developed a skill sequence known as throwing. Different species of primates can throw projectiles, but they do this crudely, and never practice deliberately to refine their accuracy and power. As a result, they do not create systematic variations or improvements on the way they throw. In contrast, even young children routinely engage in practicing and refining such skills, often for endless hours, and for no pragmatic purpose. It would be no exaggeration to say that this capability is uniquely human, and serves as the background for the creativity of human cultures and languages.

Early hominids presumably began their evolution with the same basic motor repertoire as most primates. They broke out of the limitations imposed by that repertoire, and eventually evolved the rich variability that served as the basis for inventing, among other things, the morpho-phonology of language. Language is the most complex learned skill in the human repertoire, and it is reasonable to infer that a capability for the purposive rehearsal and refinement of skill had to come into existence long before language, to support less complex skills, such as tool making and throwing. A cluster of more basic capacities, including gesture, imitation, and voluntary rehearsal itself, appears to have a common underlying neuro-cognitive architecture, and quite possibly evolved as a series of components of a single complex adaptation. Elsewhere, I have called these components "mimetic skill."[4] Mimetic skill, or mimesis, has its own evolutionary rationale, and its own representational principles.[5]

Mimesis involved a revolution in motor skill, but it also rested on a major change at a higher level of processing in the nervous system, that of metacognition, or self-review. In addition, it involved a corresponding modification of primate memory retrieval capability. The key to purposive rehearsal and morphological variability is voluntary recall: Hominids had to gain access to the contents of their kinematic memories. Apes appear quite poor at this. Presumably, they cannot rehearse actions, partly because they cannot recall them at will, and must depend on external cuing (from a trainer) to acquire a complex skill-sequence. If an animal depends on environmental cues to remember when and how to produce a particular action, skill development is extremely difficult and slow, because the animal cannot self-trigger the memory systems supporting the skill, and effectively hangs in suspended animation until the environment provides the necessary cues for the retrieval of a designated pattern of action. It usually takes thousands of trials to establish a reliable signing response in a chimpanzee.[6] In general, primates and other mammals have great difficulty in self-triggering their motor memories. Even enculturated apes, such as those described in the studies of E. Sue Savage-Rumbaugh and collaborators, rely heavily on their human caretakers for memory cues to trigger signing.[7] Human beings, in contrast, are able to "think about" or "imagine" things that are totally unrelated to the immediate environment, and seek out particular kinematic memory items without the need for the environment to come up with the relevant retrieval cues.

This suggests that mimesis resides in an imaginative capability unique to human beings. To be able to focus selectively on their actions, actors must assemble motor sequences in their imaginations. We recognize that this highly evolved capability is common among human beings. Coaches of professional athletes and teachers of musicians and actors rely heavily on this capability. For rehearsal to result in improved performance, imagining is insufficient. The subject must be able to edit the imagery generated in kinematic imagination before implementing it.

Human mimetic skills cut across all major sensory and motor modalities. In human beings, it is a domain-general capability. Neurophysiologists sometimes refer to a domain-general system as supra-modal. Supra-modal means "above modality," able to take inputs from many sources, and to implement an output in many sets of voluntary muscles. We can find a classic example of this capability in the action of writing. A writer may write the letter a with finger, wrist, elbow, lips, head, legs or trunk, or any combination of these. The motor template for the letter a can be mapped onto virtually any subset of the voluntary musculature. This is an example of supra-modal motor control in an action system producing an output that is culturally arbitrary in its form.

This type of control implies the existence of a modeling process in the brain that can generate variations in imagined actions, and try them out in performance, measuring them against a second-order motor model, or more accurately, an abstract "model of models." This evolutionary innovation would have had great adaptive value, in a variety of survival-related areas, because the entire range of voluntary action can be refined. This capability extends to such apparently non-utilitarian actions as standing on one's foot, making faces, or skipping stones.

The process that generates these kinds of action patterns relies on the same principle of perceptual resemblance that drives imitation, mime, and gesture. These are all components of mimetic skill. Mimesis is metaphoric, or holistic, in its cognitive style. We cannot easily reduce mimetic action to discrete or digital algorithms combined according to rules. Instead, it appears fuzzy in its logic, more like the visual recognition of faces. The "Gestalt," or overall pattern, is the primary driver.

Mimesis is the direct result of this fuzzy capability to generate variations of action under voluntary executive control and the logical first step toward language. Hominids could not have evolved a capability for language, even in its most elemental form, without meeting the cognitive preconditions for inventing a morpho-phonology. Mimetic capability would have allowed hominids to vary and elaborate upon the entire voluntary motor repertoire they inherited from the primate line. In addition, it provided a capability for considerable additional morphological invention. At this preliminary stage in the evolution of hominid motor capability, the expressive use of mimesis was probably restricted to action metaphor, mime, and rudimentary gesturing. Vocal skills would have been restricted at this stage to prosodic modulations of existing cries and calls.

On present evidence, this level of mimetic skill would have sufficed to explain the major cognitive achievements of archaic *Homo,* from about two million years ago until about 60,000 years ago. Mimesis would have served as a cognitive foundation for evolving a set of shared expressive customs and for triggering a legacy of nonverbal culture, which is still evident in human infants. In human infants, communication begins in mimetic exchanges with the mother. In adults, forms like dance, pantomime, and a public "theatre" of expression still play a major role in human life.

We should consider the evolutionary origins of the elaborate mimetically-driven systems of expression common to all human cultures to be distinct from the origins of language per se. Language was scaffolded on a mimetic foundation, but involved additional major adaptations, and, judging from present evidence, came much later in hominid evolution.

2. Bridging to Cultural Networks

The cognitive development of human beings depends upon their links with culture. The words, ideas, and habits of mind that dominate our conversations originate in cultural networks, as do the algorithms used in formal thinking and writing. Individual consciousness is a local funnel in this vast cultural landscape, receiving a narrow sample from an infinite number of possibilities. Viewed in this way, an individual mind is a wormhole in a vast culturally defined space.

To borrow a term from computing, every culture has a "network architecture" that directs the flow of knowledge among individuals, institutions, and external memory devices. But cultural networks are not minds because they have no integrative core equivalent to what we call the conscious self. They are better viewed as distributed networks, in the sense that they engage many minds and their cognitive activities are made possible only by interlinking those minds, often with the aid of technology, into large functioning networks. These are epitomized by the World Wide Web, which is only a recent variant in a long tradition of smaller, slower cultural networks, typified by the oral traditions of Stone Age society.

All cultural networks, even those of oral cultures, harness the cognitive resources of many individuals and impose a larger organization, often with a technological dimension, on the mental functioning of individuals. This greatly affects what an individual can achieve. Just as the powers of a computer are amplified when connected to a network, a human mind becomes more powerful by its connection to a cultural network. The extent of this amplification depends on the resources held by the culture. The cognitive properties of cultures can vary widely, due to differences in their network-level resources. In this sense, cultures are not all equal. Quite the contrary, some cultures confer a huge advantage on their members in cognitive matters.

The most important network-level resources of culture are undoubtedly writing and literacy, the invention of which revolutionized human cognition at the individual and network levels. Cultures equipped with a full range of literacy skills and technologies have an insuperable advantage over those that lack a writing system (the vast majority of known cultures have no indigenous writing). Literacy dictates a great deal about the cognitive powers of a culture. Some kinds of knowledge cannot develop without a writing system, and some kinds of formal thought-operations cannot happen without appropriate notations or technologies. Oral cultures are limited to the biological memories of their members and must rely on individual specialists, such as shamans and bards, to transfer their knowledge across generations. This imposes limitations on what such cultures can think and remember.

Once a culture has some form of writing, many new kinds of intellectual representations and transactions become possible, and institutional structures may become more complex. The earliest literate cultures, such as those of Egypt, Mesopotamia, and China, resembled one another in their style of cognitive governance, despite great differences in the substance of their traditions, because of the administrative options offered by writing technology. They evolved into highly centralized hierarchies with powers focused by a system of governing myths, which regulated every aspect of daily life. In such cultures, the cultural memory system slowly moved away from its traditional dependency on single individuals to assume a life of its own, sustained by institutions and symbolic technology.

Many kinds of memories, especially those related to agriculture, population, wars, and trade were stored in written records and other nonbiological memory media, such as monumental architecture. Eventually, the material records held by such societies greatly exceeded biological memory capability, and by about 1500 BCE, the first substantial libraries came into existence. This development gradually revolutionized the process of thought itself, which interlinked with formal institutions and a public process of scholarship and review. Metacognition, a self-supervisory skill that is the foundation of human individuality, became a community enterprise.

Institutions and social organizations are not conscious entities and we cannot say they have minds. But they are cognitive entities and they do perform cognitive work. They have beliefs, perceptions, and plans. They evaluate situations, and react creatively to challenges. Although they cannot function without the individuals that make them up, institutional structures rarely depend on single individuals over the long run. They dominate the minds of their members, and individuals assimilate institutional values to such an extent that they rarely violate them.

Institutions are real-world distributed networks, as opposed to the more limited ones created in computer simulations. They preserve particular problem-solving strategies (such as legal and scientific procedures), decision-making systems (such as corporate and parliamentary institutions), and representations of reality (such as works of art and scientific theories). These are stored and transmitted across generations with the aid of writing.

Some technologies amplify the intellectual powers of a society. These include systems of weights and measures, monetary systems, and cognitive machines, such as observatories, slide rules, sextants, clocks, and computers. Such technologies are crucial in defining the real intellectual power of a culture. They not only allow cultures to preserve more complex ideas and traditions, but change how they achieve this. Systems of external symbols can mediate some forms of thought. New notations (for instance, the zero, or the equal sign) can make possible some kinds of thought that were formerly impossible. Breakthroughs in the technologies of the visual arts or music, or revolutions in the public cognitive process, can produce the same revolutionary effects, as in the Greek habit of recording successive critical commentaries on texts, which created an institutionalized process of reflection on thought itself.

Viewed in this way, we might regard the culture of, say, France as an invisible knowledge-gathering apparatus that reaches over time and space into the minds of millions of people. The emerging global English-speaking culture is an even grander example of this, a sort of cognitive octopus with invisible tentacles into billions of minds. In some degree, we are all tethered to such a system, whether large or small. This has always been the human condition, but we have only recently become aware of the fact. It is difficult for us to accept the degree of our dependency, perhaps because intellectuals are so deeply beholden to cultural networks. We are its primary servants. We toil away in the bowels of culture, devoting entire lifetimes to some tiny region of the collective memory, or fine-tuning the algorithms of thought in some vanishingly small area. Our grand illusion of individuality is defined by its fixed place in a particular cultural network. Although it may appear that we lose our autonomy in this, we gain intellectual stature when wedded to a community of mind. All complex intellectual work results from a marriage of high-level neural circuitry with the algorithms of culture. We could not be the entities we are without this union. Even ideas that claim to subvert our cultural linkage, such as the annihilation of self, or the withdrawal of self from the world, are part of a specific cultural tradition, and have meaning only in that context.

Notes

1. Jean Piaget, *The Grasp of Consciousness: Action and Concept in the Young Child* (Cambridge, Mass.: Harvard University Press 1976).

2. Lev Semyonovich Vygotsky, *Mind in Society: The Development of Higher Psychological Processes* (Cambridge, Mass.: Harvard University Press, 1978); Tomasello, M. *The cultural origins of human cognition* (Cambridge, Mass: Harvard University Press, 1999).

3. Clive Gamble, *Timewalkers: The Prehistory of Global Colonization* (Cambridge, Mass.: Harvard University Press, 1994).

4. Donald, Merlin, *Origins of the Modern Mind: Three Stages in the Evolution of Culture and Cognition* (Cambridge, Mass.: Harvard University Press, 1991).

5. Merlin, *Origins of the Modern Mind*; "Précis of Origins of the Modern Mind with Multiple Reviews and Author's response," *Behavioral and Brain Sciences*, 16 (1993), pp. 737–791; "Mimesis and the Executive Suite: Missing Links in Language and Evolution," *Approaches to the Evolution of Language: Social and Cognitive Bases*, eds. J. R. Hurford, M. Studdert-Kennedy, and C. Knight (New York: Cambridge University Press, 1998), pp. 44–67; "Preconditions for the Evolution of Proto-languages," *The Descent of Mind: Psychological Perspectives on Hominid Evolution*, eds. Michael C. Corballis and S. E. G. Lea (New York: Oxford University Press, 1999), pp. 138–154; and *A Mind So Rare: The Evolution of Human Consciousness* (New York: W. W. Norton, 2001).

6. Patricia Marks Greenfield and E. Sue Savage-Rumbaugh, "Grammatical Combination in Pan Paniscus: Processes of Learning and Invention in the Evolution and Development of Language," *Language and Intelligence in Monkeys and Apes*, eds. S. Taylor-Parker and K. R. Gibson (New York: Cambridge University Press, 1990).

7. E. S. Savage-Rumbaugh, J. Murphy, R. A. Sevcik, K. E. Brakke, S. L. Williams, and D. M. Rumbaugh, "Language Comprehension in Ape and Child," *Monographs of the Society for Research in Child Development*, 58 (1993), pp. 1–221.

Nineteen

LANGUAGE ORIGINATED IN SOCIAL BRAINS

Luc Steels

1. Introduction

The question of the origins of language is today one of the central and hotly debated areas in human-related sciences and is directly relevant to the question how and why are brains became so profoundly social. All disciplines have something to say, from anthropology and psychology to linguistics, artificial intelligence, and complex systems science. Tremendous progress has been made recently, but no widely accepted consensus exists yet.[1] In my work, I have been engaged in different experiments with artificial systems (robots). They are endowed with several general cognitive mechanisms, for example categorization, associative memory, structure recognition, etc., and are then programmed to engage in language games, routinized local interactions which have a side effect that some sort of communication system with language-like features emerges. I have described these experiments in quite some detail in other papers and here I want to focus on the hypotheses that we tested and validated in these experiments.[2]

To develop an adequate theory for the origins of language, we must answer four critical questions:

(1) To participate in a language community you obviously need a highly sophisticated brain that can pull together a wide range of mental resources in the service of language. This configuration of mechanisms and knowledge structures is usually termed the language faculty. The first question is: What is the architecture and functioning of this language faculty, so that it can not only produce and interpret language but also participate in its creation? What does a "language-ready" brain have to be able to do?

(2) Language is a collective phenomenon, like paths and nests collectively built by an ant society or movements and trends in a stock market. It is a complex adaptive system shaped by many individuals, in turn influenced by the emergent language. This leads to the second question: What are the processes that govern the emergence and evolution of language at this collective level? For example, how does a lexicon become and remain shared, even if every language user may invent new words or

forget and misuse others? How can there be an increase in complexity, for example from a purely lexical language stringing together words without syntax, to a grammatical language that exploits syntax to express how the meanings of words are to be combined?

(3) Even supposing that we have a theory that can explain how "language-ready" brains create and coordinate languages of greater and greater complexity, a third question remains: Where does this language-ready brain come from? By what processes has it evolved? Can we find explanations that fit within the standard neo-Darwinian framework of genetic evolution by natural selection? Alternatively, are epigenetic processes at work, which rely on the recruitment and dynamic configuration of neural subsystems?

(4) The three questions above all relate to the issue how language may originate. They do not yet ask why this might have happened in our species and only in our species. This suggests a fourth question: What are the unique social and functional prerequisites that have supported the growth and evolution of language? Why did human beings start to speak?

All these research questions interact. Without an unambiguous idea of the language faculty, the study of its neurobiological embodiment and evolution is like groping in the dark. Without understanding how the laws of complex systems affects collective properties of language, we cannot be sure what the contribution of an individual language user can or needs to be, or what has to be available *a priori*. Without understanding what conditions might have prevailed at the dawn of language, we are at the risk of making the wrong assumptions of what mental mechanisms and strategies we can put into the models.

In the remainder of this paper, I discuss hypotheses for each of these four critical questions.

2. The Architecture of the Language Faculty

Everybody agrees that the language faculty includes three major subsystems:

(1) A *perceptual-motor system* that senses the world; segments incoming sensory data into different objects and events; extracts different features like size, speed, or loudness; and performs actions in the world, including the articulations required for speech;

(2) A *conceptual-intentional system* that sets and monitors communicative goals and conceptualizes reality for language or interprets conceptualizations by mapping them back to perceived reality, and

(3) A *language system* proper that maps conceptualizations into utterances in language production and reconstructs conceptualizations from utterances in language parsing.[3]

Each of these subsystems is in itself extraordinarily complex, consisting of many different subsystems, which all interact intimately with each other. To build a theory of the language faculty means to elucidate what all these subsystems are doing, what kind of information they require and produce, and how they do it.

Even supposing that we manage to make all the processes in the language faculty operational, including the learning processes that fill in the language-specific inventories for each of the subsystems, we would still have no explanation for the *origins* of language. We need something more. We need to find out what mental processes cause *new* elements to enter into a language. I argue, and this is my first major hypothesis, *that we should see the introduction of new conceptual or linguistic material as similar to invention.*

I consider the elements of language as tools, and these tools have been invented—and are still being invented and adapted—by intelligent human beings, using similar skills as those required for the invention of other tools like hammers or medicine. Most linguistic inventions are not entirely new; they are analogous to tool inventions in other domains. The first hammer was quite crude, a stone to push a pole in the ground. The human mind has this great ability to see how to improve a tool through experience. Some people must have noticed that you can get a better hammer when you introduce a handle, strengthen the head, cover the handle with some rubber coating against sweating, or change the size or shape of the head to fit better with a particular type of nail.

Sometimes an invention is lost or nobody understands it anymore, but then something else is invented to achieve the same functionality, perhaps in other ways. I argue that the same is true for concepts, words, and grammatical constructions. Speakers have invented them to deal with some particular need in communication and then continuously honed and fine-tuned them to achieve a higher rate of communicative success or to make the effort required for using them more manageable.

You might be surprised, but not all languages have grammatical markers for future tense. For example, in Chinese you have to hint at future tense by additional phrases or adverbs, like "yesterday" or "as I planned to." No specific future tense marker is used with the verb. So how can a language ever develop a grammatical way to express future?

A good candidate for hinting at future tense is a verb for desire. If you say, "I want to write a letter," you have not written the letter yet, you will do so in the future. Other candidates are verbs of movement ("I am going to London to see the queen"), verbs of possession (like Latin *habeo* (I have), which was the basis for the French *-ai* morpheme in *Je parlerai* (I will speak)), or verbs of obligation (like old German *skal* (owe), which was the basis for "shall"). Until about the sixteenth century, the English verb "will" was a main verb to express desire, as it still is in Dutch or German. If you say in Dutch, *Zij willen hun broer zien* (literally, They will their brother see), you mean that they want to see their brother and whether this will happen is uncertain. "Will" is still a main verb. In English, "will" has been grammaticalized into a future auxiliary verb. If you say, "She will write a letter," that person is going to do it. If you say "It will rain," nobody wants anything, "will" has lost its meaning of desire and shifted syntactic category from main verb to auxiliary. So that you do not say, "I don't will write him a letter," but "I will write him a letter."

Invention is only one side of the coin. Inventing a new tool for communication, such as a new word or a new grammatical marker, is fine enough. But if others cannot figure out its meaning and learn to use it themselves, the word will not propagate and it will die out. So learning (by understanding the intention) is crucial. It is even entirely possible that language learners unwillingly invent new features by believing that some aspect of an utterance, for example a particular word order or a particular intonation pattern, carries meaning, whereas it did not yet for the speaker. If the hearer then reuses the construction, another listener may pick it up and propagate it further in the population.

Invention requires that you can see the need for a tool and either create an entirely new one or adapt an existing tool for a new purpose. Intentional learning requires enough "theory of mind" to be able to guess what communicative goal somebody else wants to achieve and how she may have conceptualized the world, so that you can reconstruct the meaning and function of a tool's components, or what meanings and effects the words and grammatical constructions are supposed to have. A common reaction to the hypothesis that language originates through invention and intentional learning is that it requires too much intelligence and a conscious mind and so it assumes a much greater mental capability than we are normally willing to ascribe to early human beings or young children or maybe to most people period. I take this objection seriously.

Yet the kind of invention and intentional learning I have in mind is achieved by processes which do not involve consciousness nor impossible leaps of imagination. I am not at all thinking of intelligent conscious invention the way you would design a house or a new computer chip. Instead, the processes I have in mind take place at a subconscious level, even though you may occasionally consciously choose what your subconscious processes suggest.

Another common objection coming from some linguists is that language is not like a tool. They argue that the structure of language is not related to its function.[7] This is a surprising objection and counter-intuitive to non-linguists, because common sense tells us that language is a tool for communication and, derived from that, for representation and thought. I think this objection comes from not taking function and processing considerations into account. It is like looking at a car from a purely structural and descriptive point of view. Why it has wheels or a gear stick becomes impossible to understand. The function of the wheels becomes only obvious when you take into account that the car is designed to move. A gear stick makes sense only when you understand that a car has different "gears" to which the motor transmits power and that an engine's performance needs to be optimized by choosing the size of the gear depending on the speed of the car or the inclination of the road. The more you want to understand a car's components and the reason why they are installed, the more you have to delve into the operation and mechanics of the car. Why would this be different for understanding language and the language faculty that enables it?

3. Language as a Complex Adaptive System

My second hypothesis concerns collective dynamics. A few decades ago, the natural sciences discovered that quite often systems consisting of many elements interacting locally with a few others at the microscopic level could undergo a phase transition suddenly and spontaneously, in which a macroscopic structure emerges. For example, in the 1950s, Boris P. Belousov and Anatol M. Zhabotinsky discovered a chemical reaction, which spontaneously shows surprising spatial and temporal patterns. Order emerges out of chaos. The mixture of molecules they studied changes regularly among three colors, among three global states, like a clock. Poured into a dish, it produces the kind of beautiful spiral patterns, which are now on the cover of many books on chaos theory. Matter, which until then, people assumed to be dead, in the sense of moving to an equilibrium state and staying there, turned out to be full of activity, switching between unordered states, spontaneous order, and chaos, depending on contextual parameters. Molecules, which have only local interactions and no "awareness" of the global state, become coordinated.

The trick lies in a hidden positive feedback loop. Once things start moving in a designated way, the rest comes down like an avalanche. After investigators understood these phenomena and modeled them mathematically, scientists recognized similar self-organizing phenomena and discovered them in other chemical reactions and in physical systems like lasers or magnetic spin systems.

Self-organization is not the only morphogenetic process that creates structure in Nature. Another is selectionism, probably more familiar to many readers, as Charles Darwin appealed to selectionism to explain the origins of species. Selectionism, like self-organization, is completely general and applicable at many levels and to different types of systems, including economic or cultural systems. Another mechanism that has turned out to be quite useful is structural coupling, originally introduced by Humberto Maturana and Francisco Varela. It occurs when two autonomous systems become intimately attuned to each other without a central coordinator or prior determination, but only because input for one is output for the other and vice-versa. We see structural coupling in the tight integration between different cells in the body or in the coordination between independently evolving organisms, which still strongly depend on each other.

Yet another mechanism is level formation. It explains how higher-order structure may arise because individual units start to co-occur together and develop additional "glue" so that the whole becomes more than the sum of the parts. Given the ubiquity of all these generic morphogenetic mechanisms in Nature, scientists and mathematicians began to wonder whether any universal laws underlay them. This turns out to be the case and a body of knowledge has gradually developed into a true science of complex systems, which is still booming with excitement today, especially with the discovery of intriguing properties of evolving networks.

Is of all this relevant to our subject? I strongly believe so. This is my second hypothesis: *The same universal laws that explain the origins of order in natural systems are at work in socio-cultural systems, and especially in the origins and evolution of language.*[8] The elements at the microscopic level are the communicating agents, engaged in local verbal interactions with others and changing their internal states as a side effect of each interaction. Out of these local interactions, large-scale structures and behaviors emerge at the macroscopic level, the level of language itself.

The theory of complex systems suggests mechanisms for which we might look and add as ingredients to the artificial agent experiments. The universal laws make it possible to predict whether macroscopic structure will emerge. To take a mechanism discovered in some subfield of science, abstract from it the domain-specific details and then re-instantiate the same principles and apply them to the full glorious complicated detail of language is not so simple to do, but this is precisely the kind of exercise that I am advocating.

Here is, for example, how we can apply self-organization to the case of speech sounds. Suppose each individual agent produces sounds. If they ignored the others, no shared speech system would ever emerge. Suppose that agents align their speech sounds to those of others by slightly adapting their motor control programs and shifting their perceptual prototypes. This creates a hidden positive feedback loop and self-organization: The more some sounds are used, the more agents encounter them and because they align themselves to these sounds, a shared repertoire inevitably emerges and persists even if the population changes. So a global order, a shared sound system, appears, without one agent dictating to all others what sounds to use, and without any global overview by any of them, nor any prior genetic predisposition towards some sounds.[9]

Here is concisely how selectionism applies. Selectionism explains how "solutions" to a task can arise without explicit conscious intelligent design. It needs four ingredients: storage of the blueprints of solutions, instantiation of a solution from a blueprint, replication and recombination of blueprints with variation, and preferential choice to keep blueprints that lead to better solutions based on testing them for the task. Several ways exist in which we can apply this framework to language. One way, originally suggested by Richard

Dawkins and elaborated by the linguist William Croft, is to view language elements as memes that get replicated.[10]

We can view the basic elements of language (concepts, words, constructions) as "solutions" to the problems that speakers and hearers encounter if they try to communicative successfully. This is similar to viewing the structures and behaviors of an organism as solutions to the problems of survival in a particular ecosystem. Blueprints for solutions (like lexical entries) are stored as part of the language faculty of each agent and instantiated every time a sentence needs to be formulated or interpreted. This is similar to the genome, which is a kind of blueprint that guides the development and behavior of an organism.

In both cases, we should not take the term blueprint too literally, definitely not like the architectural blueprint of a house, because contextual processes and self-organization also play a big role. As a side effect of learning, the blueprint for a particular communicative solution is stored in the language faculty of the individual, and invention may recombine existing solutions to build up more complex hierarchical structures.

Invention and learning play the same role as replication and recombination of genomes. Invention, intentional learning, and instantiation of blueprints in actual language use with unavoidable inaccuracies, errors, and slips of the tongue, all conspire to introduce variation in language use. Seeing that selection also plays a role is not difficult. Language constructs that lead robustly and steadily to successful communication and that minimizes the cognitive effort of the individuals survive and the rest wither away.

So the selectionist framework fits perfectly for studying language as a dynamically evolving complex adaptive system. Its application is not just metaphorical because the framework predicts some of the properties the language faculty of communicating agents needs to have. The mathematical tools theoretical biologists have developed for analyzing the dynamics of selectionist processes become applicable.

Given that many conflicting constraints operating on language exist (for example, less effort for the hearer may imply more effort for the speaker), and that historical contingencies obviously exist, we cannot expect that language users will ever arrive at an optimal communication system. On the contrary, overwhelming evidence from the historical development of all human languages supports the conclusion that language users move around in the space of possible solutions. Sometimes languages optimize one aspect (for example dropping a complex case system), which then forces another solution with its inconvenience (for example using a large number of verbal patterns with idiomatic prepositions—as in English). Language, as a complex adaptive system, exploits the available physiological and cognitive resources of its community of users to handle their communicative challenges, but without ever reaching a stable state.

Here is a third example how universal notions of complex systems are relevant to understanding language emergence: the application of the notion of structural coupling to the coordination of different subsystems of the language faculty and especially to the coordination of the conceptual-intentional system and the language system. Suppose that the conceptual system has the capability to create new color distinctions. For example, you get two types of bananas, a green one and a yellow one, and discover that the yellow banana tastes better than the green one. So your conceptual system cuts up the continuous color space to have a boundary between these two color regions so that you can pick out the tasty bananas in the future. The same process occurs when you encounter delicious red apples and rotten brown ones, orange and black carrots, or purple and green (unripe) plums. But if individuals keep inventing new color distinctions to serve their individual needs, based on their personal history of interactions with the world, we would have no guarantee that the color distinctions become shared. Miscommunication is inevitable.

This has lead some people to suppose that color distinctions must already be genetically fixed in advance, which is unlikely given the profound cultural and individual differences in color categorization I discussed earlier. So we have a paradox for which structural coupling can come to the rescue.[11] The conceptual system suggests categories offered to the lexical system to be put into words, so an influence from conceptualization to language during production exists. But the lexical system also influences the conceptual system. Speakers may get feedback whether their hearers properly understood the categories they used, and if not, the speaker's conceptual system might adjust them.

The hearer has to figure out how the speaker uses words. So the hearers' lexical system tells their conceptual-intention system what categories should apply to the present case. If they do not, the conceptual system must adjust categories or create new ones. Our models have shown that this mutual influence is enough to efficiently coordinate both subsystems inside the language faculty. Perhaps more remarkably, the same mechanism is enough to coordinate the conceptual inventories across agents, even though each agent independently develops his own. Again, we see a macroscopic structure, a shared repertoire of perceptually grounded categories, emerges through local autonomous interactions between agents. No central control or prior disposition is required.

4. Recruitment Theory

My third hypothesis concerns the origins of the language faculty. Showing the information processing that a language faculty must be able to do to see the emergence of symbolic communication systems through universal morphogenetic processes, such as self-organization or selectionism, is insufficient. I also need to explain how this language faculty could have evolved. We know little about this extraordinarily difficult question despite intense speculation and debate. Only a few coherent theories exist, but one framework, defended by many linguists and evolutionary psychologists, does emerge. It starts from the hypothesis that the "human language faculty is a complex adaptation which evolved by natural selection for communication"; the interconnected areas of the brain involved in language form a highly specialized neural subsystem, a kind of language organ, which is genetically determined and came into existence through neo-Darwinian genetic evolution.[12] So I apply selectionism here at the level of the biological embodiment of the language faculty and not at the level of the language itself as I advocated in the previous section.

According to this vision, language is an instinct, not learned as such. The language organ grows like the liver or the fingers of a hand. The environment sets some growth parameters, for example, the way the liver of a heavy drinker becomes "fatty" to deal with excess alcohol. But none of the kinds of intelligence, invention, and intentional learning is ascribed to the language faculty the way I suggested earlier. Nor do we see any key role seen for the rapid cultural evolution of new language traits through grammaticalization as we view language change as surface variations on a static *Bauplan* (building plan; common properties of a systematic group) that captures the essence of language.

Steven Pinker, with like-minded psychologists and linguists, advances two types of arguments in favor of this language-as-adaptation hypothesis. The first type is based on examining the structure of language. Human languages exhibit some non-trivial universal trends, which could be the logical consequence of an innate language acquisition device that imposes quite specific structures on human languages. Otherwise, seeing how extremely young children based on apparently poor data so easily and routinely acquire the intricate complexity of human language is difficult. In addition, these same universal trends show up when new languages form, as in the case of Creoles. So far, so good—but two problems arise with this argument.

The first problem is that the universal trends are statistical trends, not universal laws. That means we observe some features in many languages, but we find many other languages (often the majority), which do not have them. A speech repertoire with the vowels *a, e, i, o,* and *u* is found in 28 percent of the world's languages, but the other 72 percent have other systems. Some have only three vowels; others have nine. R-colored vowels (like in American pronunciations of "sir") occur only in 1 percent of the world's languages. The language of the Khoi-San in the Kalahari Desert uses clicks and produces some vowels while inhaling. Mandarin Chinese or Somali use tones. French exploits the nasal cavity (as in the vowel *un* (one)). Ian Maddieson and Peter Ladefoged, who have been the principle experts in this area and built the UPSID database on which we usually base discussions on speech trends, point out that although there are 177 vowels and 645 consonants, this classification groups phonemes which are not always exactly identical. They argue that any sound the vocal tract can produce and the auditory system systematically recognize (after training) is used in one language or another. So if you have to design a language faculty with an innate set of speech sounds, how would you do that? Which ones would you include or exclude?

Similar issues arise with any other aspect of language including conceptualization. If you want to create a bias for color categories, what would that bias be? Although some statistical trends appear to exist, as first shown by Brent Berlin and Paul Kay in the 1960s, tremendous differences not only among languages but also among individuals speaking the same language are also evident. For example, British psychologists Debi Roberson and Jules Davidoff studied the Berinmo of Papua, New Guinea, who conceptualize the yellow-blue-green region of English into two regions named *nol* and *wor* along lines that do not coincide with those of English at all. Roberson and Davidoff replicated their study with the Himba, a semi-nomadic culture in equatorial Africa, and established yet another profoundly different color map. So if you want to bias color concepts, whose categorization are you going to chose? Why would the color categories of English have any bigger claim on being innate than those of the Himba or the Berinmo?

The situation is not much better for grammar. Adaptationists assume that minimally the syntactic and semantic categories of languages, such as the parts of speech (noun, speech) or possible cases (nominative, dative, accusative) are innately determined and provide a strong bias on language acquisition. They argue that these have to be part of the language instinct that has evolved through natural selection. But what about the observation that many languages do not make a distinction between adjectives and nouns, do not have a notion of subject or direct object, categorize events and event types into quite different semantic roles, maintain quite different subtle usages for the dative, and so on. Decades of research in generative linguistics to capture the universal grammar that underlies all human languages have not at all yielded a consensus view, despite that most studies focus only on English or a few other European languages. Some linguists have made the unavoidable conclusion that syntactic and semantic categories are language- and maybe even speaker-dependent. Like pieces of chess, grammatical categories only make sense within a designated system. If we pull a chess piece from a chess game and insert it into a set of checkers, what does it mean? If I wanted to design a language system, which has the "innate" syntactic and semantic categories programmed in but is not ridiculously biased towards English, which ones should I program into it?

A second problem arises. Even assuming that universal trends exist, does this necessarily mean that they are the result of innate predispositions? My earlier discussion on complex adaptive systems should alert the reader that this is not necessarily the case. That universal trends in language are a consequence of universal morphogenetic processes (like self-organization, selectionism, structural coupling) is entirely possible. These processes would operate within the constraints that human beings have: the physical constraints of the real world, human embodiment, the resources and limitations of the human brain (for example, memory, and processing speed), and the nature of the communication task. Without going to the bottom of this line of explanation, we cannot know for sure what has to be innately specified and what is emergent. Many highly complex patterns in nature are not the result of innate predispositions but a side effect of epigenetic, behavioral, and environmental factors. Is the same style of explanation relevant to language? It would be foolish and narrow-minded to exclude it.

For example, are the trends we find in the vowel systems of the world's languages a consequence of innate predispositions? Or, are they the consequence of morphogenetic processes constrained by the human vocal tract, the auditory system, the physics of the sound medium with its unavoidable noise, the limits to the precision of motor control, the nature of human categorization processes, and memory? A lot of basic biological structure develops under genetic influence, such as the structure of the larynx, the vocal chords, the glottis, and the circuitry to perform fine-grained high-speed control or auditory categorization. The point I am arguing is that the vowels do not have to be innate. The generic machinery exists, but not the contents on which it operates. Once a group starts to self-organize a speech system with this kind of machinery and subject to the same constraints as human beings, they arrive automatically at the sort of speech systems we find in human languages.

I argue that the same explanatory framework is true for all other trends observed in languages: color categories, syntactic and semantic categories, and typical grammatical patterns. I realize that we have to show precisely how that is possible and many of our experiments do that. Claiming that something is innate (for example, an inventory of speech sounds) does not resolve the difficulty. You cannot merely shift responsibility to the evolutionary biologist. You must show scenarios that demonstrate how the distinction between dative and accusative, active and passive, voiced and voiceless, or past perfect and future continuous may become innate. I have never seen a convincing evolutionary argument or a simulation for any of these.

Arguing that a quasi-optimal system is in place (for example that the vowels are optimally distributed over the space of possible sounds the vocal tract can make or that the ear can perceive) is not sufficient either. We have to show how linguistic agents can autonomously discover these solutions without central control, a global view, or prior bias. Or, if you are an adaptationist, you have to show how genetic evolution and natural selection have found them and how the genes can exert sufficiently control over the fine-grained structure of the brain so that the brain circuits become biased towards them.

The second type of arguments in favor of the language-as-adaptation hypothesis comes from molecular and population genetics. They rest on the identification of genes that have undergone selection in the human lineage, and have an unmistakably identified effect on language. The most promising (and only) example in this respect is the FOXP2 gene which is linked to a unique constellation of language impairments identified in the multi-generational KE-family.[13] At the time of its discovery, it was hailed as "the" or "the first" language gene by the popular press. Since then, a growing number of questions have been raised which show that things are not that simple, as is so often the case in biology.

First, pinning down exactly the language organ is supposed to be in the brain is difficult. Brain imaging studies overwhelmingly show that speaking or listening involves the activation of many brain areas, not just those traditionally associated with language: Broca's and Wernicke's area. Even for just speaking, the cerebellum and thalamus gets involved along with other motor areas. Conversely, the traditional "language areas" are also active in many other non-linguistic tasks; they are definitely not only specialized for language. For example, Broca's area is heavily involved in selecting and monitoring all sorts of motor control patterns, not only those related to speech production. Interestingly, different brain areas can take over the functionalities of these areas if brain damage occurs, as long as the brain still has enough vitality and plasticity to recuperate. The most amazing example in this respect is that the neural activities associated with Broca's and Wernicke's area can shift from the left hemisphere of the brain where they are typically located in right-handed people to the right hemisphere. So the picture is blurred. No obvious language organ exists akin to, say, a patently delineated liver.

Second, we have to be careful about a direct mapping between genes and brain areas.[14] Those involved in this research know this, but that message usually gets lost in popularization. The FOXP2 gene is not uniquely relevant for language but plays a crucial role in the development of many areas of the brain and leads to many impairments if affected, especially in the motor domain. The gene plays also a role in the development of the lungs, the gut, and the heart. To say that FOXP2 is a language gene is misleading, you might as well call it a gene for lungs. FOXP2 is a transcription factor, which has the potential to affect a potentially large number of genes. In the brain, its function is probably more generic, perhaps regulation of post migratory neuronal differentiation.

Does all this mean that the language-as-adaptation hypothesis is invalid? Not necessarily. It just means that we cannot elevate this hypothesis to dogma yet. Science can only benefit from exploring and comparing many hypotheses. An alternative hypothesis exists: *the recruitment theory of language origins*. It argues that the origins of the human language faculty might be explainable as a dynamic configuration of brain mechanisms, which grows and adapts, like an organism. Instead of being genetically pre-wired, the brain may be recruiting available cognitive/neural resources for optimally achieving the task of communication. Achieving this task implies maximizing expressive power and communicative success while minimizing cognitive effort in terms of processing and memory. The mechanisms that get recruited are not specific for language. They are exaptations in Stephen Jay Gould's terminology and instantiated and configured dynamically by each individual. Consequently, genetic evolution by natural selection is not the causal force that explains the origins of language. Genetic evolution still plays a role, partly to evolve the basic building computational blocks such as categorization or detection of hierarchical structure, and partly to evolve brains that have the kind of intense plasticity that recruitment requires. I personally do not believe that genetic evolution has fixed the vowels of languages or whether the subject of a sentence is likely to come before or after the verb, or any of the other constraints on language that are usually ascribed to an innate language faculty.

One example of recruitment concerns egocentric perspective transformation (computing what the world looks like from another viewpoint). This activity is normally carried out in the parietal-temporal-occipital junction of the brain and used for a wide variety of non-linguistic tasks, such as prediction of the behavior of others or navigation. All human languages have ways to change and mark perspective (as in "your left" versus "my left"), which is only possible if speaker and hearer can conceptualize the scene from the listener's perspective. That, in turn, implies that they have recruited egocentric perspective transformation as part of their language system. By recruitment, I mean that information can flow from one subsystem to another and so that the signals make sense on both ends.

Another example of a universal feature of human languages is that the speaker can express emotional states by modulating the speech signal. For example, in case of anger, the speaker may increase rhythm and volume, use a higher pitch, or a more agitated intonation pattern. This requires that the neural subsystems involved in emotion (such as the amygdala) are linked into the language system so that information on emotional states can influence speech production and so that information from speech recognition can flow towards the brain areas involved with emotion. I would argue that the specific links are not predetermined, but are the result of a recruitment process that relies on the plasticity of the human brain to establish links in all directions and then choose the ones needed to participate in language.

Another example relates to the core of grammar. Language is unique compared to animal signaling systems because it uses recursive structure: words group in phrases, which group in bigger phrases and a bigger phrase can reoccur as component in a phrase of the same type. For example, "the big box" is a noun phrase, which can be part of the noun phrase "the ball next to the big box," which can in turn be part of a still bigger noun phrase: "the speed of the ball next to the big box."

Hierarchical structure implies that language production must involve a hierarchical planning process and that parsing requires the ability to recover hierarchical structure. But is this capability unique for language? Definitely not. Whenever we plan a series of actions, we have to be able to conceive and monitor hierarchical structure. Whenever we are recognizing events in the world, and especially complex actions performed by other human beings, we need hierarchical event recognition. So we find it difficult to maintain that hierarchical processing is unique. It may not even be unique to the human species. The language faculty recruits the ability to do this kind of hierarchical processing and then instantiates it for the domain of syntax.

I argue that the brain functionalities necessary to create a symbolic communication system could be entirely epigenetic, driven by the need to build a better, more expressive, and more efficient communication system as opposed to being genetically pre-determined and evolved through natural selection. Because such profound differences between languages exist, we cannot exclude that different languages call upon different functionalities. If we compare the needed language faculty, we may end up with quite different neural systems. We may even see differences between individuals speaking the same language, as alternative ways to achieve the same functionality may exist. The historical choices a language community may have made force newcomers to recruit designated neural resources and subsystems, and so in some sense, a human community encourages the brains of newcomers to configure themselves in designated ways. If a language exploits the pitch differences between vowels, such as the tone system in Chinese, then everyone speaking that language must develop feature detectors able to sense and reproduce this, something not at all simple to do if you are not accustomed to it. If a language does not exploit word order for syntax, as early forms of Latin or present-day Australian aboriginal languages, then the language system has to set up the parsing process quite differently, keeping in memory disconnected individual units, which might only link into hierarchical structure when all words have been heard.

The recruitment theory resonates with other proposals for the origins of the language faculty. For example, the biologist Eörs Szathmary has proposed the metaphor of a growing "language amoeba," a pattern of neural activity essential for processing linguistic information and grows in the "habitat" of a developing human brain with its characteristic connectivity pattern.[15] Many researchers, including those who believe that some parts of the language faculty are innate, agree that a multitude of non-linguistic brain functions gets recruited for language—if we take the language faculty in a broad sense, including conceptualization of what to say.

5. The Human Revolution

The reason something like human language developed might appear obvious. Almost any task requiring cooperation can profit from having a powerful communication system: to plan joint action, coordinate effort and activity is ongoing, or discuss afterwards what went wrong and how we could improve things. Then why species closely related to us do not have language as well? Part of it has to do with lacking the mental capability for language. But if the same selectionist pressures acted on chimpanzees, whose brains appear tantalizingly similar to those of human beings, with whom they share 98.77 percent identical genomes, did not both species undergo similar evolution?

Consider two additional puzzles: Communication gives information away which is potentially exploitable by the listener. Fine for the listener. But what does the speaker gain? Speakers may give information away that is useful for them or perhaps disclose their intentions so that others know what they are going to do, so the listeners can use that information for personal gain. In a Darwinian world driven by selfish genes, only those organisms survive that maximize their individual fitness. So cooperation and communication presents a problem. We cannot take cooperation for granted.

People chatter away on the bus with neighbors they have never seen before and may never see again, apparently unaware of such a potentially dangerous open attitude towards information sharing. Then how can hearers avoid manipulation by speakers? In a symbolic communication system, cheating is easy. For example, it does not cost you anything to say with great conviction that you are powerful or angry and in that way entice others to give you food or sexual favors. I am constantly amazed by how some people apparently get sucked into sending large amounts of money or disclose their personal information solely based on some e-mail message promising large gains. In a Darwinian world, such an attitude would be a disaster. A cheater could clobber up all resources to the detriment of the rest, leaving the others to be eaten alive.

So how do animals cope with this danger of a fully cooperative attitude? They cope in two ways. First, they only unselfishly cooperate and communicate freely under designated conditions, such as kinship selection—I help you because you share enough of my genes that I consider unselfish cooperation and communication to be beneficial in the propagation of my genes.

More directly relevant here is that if animals communicate, they invariably use signal-based communication instead of symbol-based communication. Signals are bodily changes or auditory and bodily gestures that have an influence on the behavior of others. The peacock tail or the alarm calls of vervet monkeys are two typical examples. Signals are analog in the sense that the intensity of the signal correlates with the intensity of what is expressed; the bigger the peacock, the stronger the bird, the louder the alarm call, the greater the threat.

Signals are not under conscious control, neither for the sender nor for the receiver; their evolution is nearly always genetically driven. The peacock cannot just grow a longer tail. The dog cannot refrain from barking when it sees another dog threateningly near. Emotional signaling in human beings (getting white from anger, red from shyness, crying from sadness) falls within this class. Unless you are an excellent actor, you cannot just turn white when you want to without feeling authentic anger; unless you have a heart of stone, you cannot remain untouched when a person cries in your arms. Signals are honest. If a peacock could grow a longer tail by will, it could signal, "Look how powerful I am," without actually being sufficiently powerful. If you could just turn white when you want to, you could cheat other people into believing that you are angry when you are not.

In contrast, symbolic communication, like human language, does not link in a reflex-like way to internal states, but is produced and interpreted on demand, through a rich system of conceptualizations. This makes possible lying, doubt, or ignoring what someone else says, whereas these actions are impossible to do with signals. We establish the meaning of symbols through a cultural consensus. Whether we call fish "fish," *poison* (French), or *oryu* (Chinese) is entirely arbitrary.

Symbols are not costly; the cost of producing a signal does not keep it honest. Whether you say "I did not cheat at the exam" or you say, "I cheated at the exam" requires equal amounts of efforts even if statement is true and the other is false. It can be adapted easily to new communicative needs; it can handle great semantic complexity; we can learn it quickly. These features make symbolic communication powerful. But the power comes with enormous risks that animals generally cannot take.

All this helps us to understand why animals do not have symbol-based communication, but not yet why human beings do have it. Here I propose my fourth hypothesis: *Human beings developed symbol-based communication because they underwent a kind of revolution that allowed them to surpass the Darwinian world of selfish genes. They became social. They became fundamentally cooperative and capable to establish and follow a rule of law, even if that law goes against their interest.* A game of chess is an example of the rule of law. Players agree to follow the rules; everything is allowed, as long as you follow the rules. You may not hit somebody else on the head with a chess piece or use telepathic forces.

Language is like the rule of law. You agree to abide by rules of the language game that you tacitly accept. You accept the conventions and contribute to them yourself. In jointly creating a language, you have to be entirely honest (in your use of the language) and cooperative, otherwise symbol-based communication system collapses.

The sociality assumption is crucial for understanding why we profusely speak not only with our kin, but with anyone. We hold a tacit assumption that others will not exploit us, that we can give away information, and that eventually everybody will benefit from the free flow of information. Those that display a greater capability to acquire new information gain prestige in the group when they make the information available to others. This does not mean that no one will exploit other people. Unfortunately, this happens all too often and language plays a key role in manipulation and cheating. But if human language would be an honest, costly signaling system, it would not be possible to use it for this purpose. Granted, human beings do not always follow the rule of law. We are constantly tempted, especially those of us who have amassed more power or have fewer moral objections compared with others, to try to set up or change the rules to our advantage or to circumvent the rules. But if we are caught, the communal reaction is severe.

This raises the question how sociality might have developed in our species. How have our brains become so profoundly social? Where does this unusual cooperative attitude and capability to set up the rule of law come from? How did it develop and why? I personally have no particular theory, although I believe the theories of some anthropologists such as Leslie C. Aiello, Chris Knight, and Camilla Power go a long way.[16] They base their answers on biological arguments. As brain size expanded, energy cost for bringing up helpless children grew. Mothers had to break through the male dominance structures that are still the norm in chimpanzee groups in order to entice males to help feed their children. This necessarily required a cooperative attitude among females to raise the children and form coalitions against males but also among males to hunt the large game that became necessary. Once language or other forms of symbolic representation became established even in a very simple form, it was an enormously powerful instrument to help organize human society, formulate and enforce the rule of law, and help everybody to see the world in similar ways.

6. A Revolution in Linguistics

I have introduced hypotheses for each of the four issues introduced in the beginning of this paper. All of them are obviously controversial and some readers may have become sufficiently upset that they have torn pages out of this book in total disagreement! The experiments that we have been doing with artificial agents attempt to operationalize each hypothesis and prove that if we endow artificial agents with the mechanisms they imply, we see the emergence of communication systems with features similar to human languages. So what is the nature of language and its origins that is beginning to emerge? Language did not jump from nothing by a freak genetic mutation that suddenly caused a human child to have a language organ, enabling it to speak a grammatical language which its parents presumably could not understand (as apparently Derek Bickerton suggested).[17] Neither did human beings stumble on language by accident and then transmitted culturally by imitation, the way human beings presumably stumbled on the idea of roasting coffee beans to make a stimulating drink or on chewing ginger to alleviate stomach pain.

Language is an invention created by intelligent human beings and propagated based on intentional learning. To engage in language, the brain self-configures an enormously complex language faculty, recruiting the many functionalities required from perceptual-motor processing and conceptualization to parsing and production. Human embodiment, the challenges of the communication task, and the ecologies and environments in which human beings find themselves all conspire to drive the emergent communication system in particular directions and explain why we see some universal trends.

We cannot underestimate the depth of change I am advocating here compared with mainstream linguistics. Noam Chomsky famously set the goals of the field in the late fifties and sixties as follows:

> Linguistic theory is concerned primarily with an ideal speaker-listener, in a completely homogeneous speech-community, who know its language perfectly and is unaffected by such grammatically irrelevant conditions as memory limitations, distractions, shifts of attention and interest, and errors (random or characteristic) in applying his knowledge of this language in actual performance.[18]

These goals were entirely appropriate at a time when the cognitive revolution was beginning to make everybody aware that we could best study mental processes as information processes. A good first step was to isolate a single individual and study the knowledge this individual might appear to have at any given moment under ideal circumstances. But if we keep pursuing only these goals, as many mainstream linguists continue to do, we discard the possibility of finding explanations for the origins of language.

We can no longer apply or observe the universal morphogenetic processes like selectionism or self-organization that underlie the origins of so many other complex structures in nature. First, these collective processes always rely on a population, for example a population of organisms in natural selection or a population of molecules in molecular self-organization. So we also need to take a population view in our models of language. Doing so is entirely natural because language is a phenomenon found in a community of people, not a single individual. Second, morphogenetic process always requires variation among the elements and their behavior. So we should not consider the kind of population we need in our models to be homogeneous. Again, doing this is entirely natural because studies have proven that in a human language community, neither the competence nor the performance of all individuals is homogeneous. Third, we cannot restrict our attention to a synchronic view, only looking at a snapshot of a language at a designated point in time. If we did so, we would not see that language is forever changing.

Linguistic theory should, therefore, incorporate change at its foundation, not only change over long periods of time as studied in historical linguistics, but rapid change even within the confines of a single dialogue. Every verbal interaction changes the language and through these cumulative changes, language grows and evolves.

Apart from leading to a more naturalistic approach to language, this complex adaptive systems approach brings language more in line with contemporary science. Instead of a science of being, trying to capture the essential properties of a static idealized entity, it becomes a science of becoming. To use the terminology of the French philosopher Gilles Deleuze, language is a multiplicity. It is forever in the making.

Acknowledgment

The research underlying this paper was conducted at the Sony Computer Science Laboratory in Paris and the Artificial Intelligence laboratory of the University of Brussels (VUB). I thank Oscar Villaroya for his continuous encouragement, the organization of the tremendous Social Brain symposium, and his deep thinking on the issues I discussed in this paper.

Notes

1. Alison Wray, ed., *The Transition to Language* (Oxford: Oxford University Press, 2002); E. J. Briscoe, ed., *Linguistic Evolution through Language Acquisition: Formal and Computational Models* (Cambridge, UK: Cambridge University Press, 2002); Angelo Cangelosi and Domenico Parisi, eds., *Simulating the Evolution of Language* (Berlin: Springer-Verlag, Berlin, 2001); James W. Minett and William S.-Y. Wang, *Language Acquisition, Change and Emergence: Essays in Evolutionary Linguistics* (Hong Kong: City University of Hong Kong Press, 2005); and Caroline Lyon, Chrystopher L Nehaniv, and Angelo Cangelosi, eds., *Emergence of Communication and Language* (Berlin: Springer Verlag, 2006).

2. Luc Steels, "A Self-Organizing Spatial Vocabulary," *Artificial Life*, 2:3 (1995),

pp. 319–332; Luc Steels, F. Kaplan, Angus McIntyre, and Joris Van Looveren, "Crucial Factors in the Origins of Word-Meaning," *The Transition to Language*, ed. Alison Wray (Oxford: Oxford University Press, 2002); and Luc Steels, "Evolving Grounded Communication for Robots," *Trends in Cognitive Science*, 7:7 (July 2003), pp. 308–312.

3. Steven Pinker and Ray Jackendoff, "The Faculty of Language: What's Special about it? *Cognition*, 95 (2005), pp. 201–236.

4. Rosalind Thornton and Kenneth Wexler, *Principle B, VP Ellipsis, and Interpretation in Child Grammar* (Cambridge, Mass.: The MIT Press, 1999).

5. Elizabeth Closs Traugott and Bernd Heine, *Approaches to Grammaticalization*, vol. 1 and 2 (Amsterdam: John Benjamins Publishing Company, 1991).

6. Michael Tomasello, *The Cultural Origins of Human Cognition* (Cambridge, Mass.: Harvard University Press, 1999).

7. Frederick J. Newmeyer, *Language Form and Language Function* (Cambridge, Mass.: The MIT Press, 1998).

8. Luc Steels, "Language as a Complex Adaptive System, Lecture Notes in Computer Science," *Parallel Problem Solving from Nature–PPSN VI*, ed. Marc Schoenauer, et al. (Berlin: Springer-Verlag, Berlin, 2000).

9. Bart De Boer, "Self-Organization in Vowel Systems," *Journal of Phonetics*, 28:4 (2000), pp. 441–465.

10. William Croft, *Radical Construction Grammar: Syntactic Theory in Typological Perspective* (Oxford: Oxford University Press, 2001).

11. Luc Steels and Tony Belpaeme (2005) "Coordinating Perceptually Grounded Categories through Language: A Case Study for Color," *Behavioral and Brain Sciences*, 24:6 (2005), pp. 469–489.

12. Steven Pinker, "Language as an Adaptation to the Cognitive Niche," *Language Evolution: The States of the Art*, eds. Morten H. Christiansen, and Simon Kirby (Oxford: Oxford University Press, 2004), p. 16.

13. W. Enard, M. Przeworski, S. E. Fisher, C. S. Lai, V. Wiebe, T. Kitano, A. P. Monaco, and S. Paabo, "Molecular Evolution of FOXP2, a Gene Involved in Speech and Language," *Nature*, 418 (2002), pp. 869–872.

14. Karin Stromswold, "The Heritability of Language: A Review and Metaanalysis of Twin, Adoption, and Linkage Studies," *Language*, 77:4 (2001), pp. 647–723.

15. Eörs Szathmary, "Origin of the Human Language Faculty: The Language Amoeba Hypothesis," *New Essays on the Origins of Language*, eds. Jurgan Trabant and Sean Ward, *Trends in Linguistics, Studies, and Monographs*, 133 (2001), pp. 41–55.

16. Luigia Carlucci Aiello, "Terrestriality, Bipedalism and the Origin of Language," *Evolution of Social Behaviour Patterns in Primates and Man*, eds. Walter Garrison Runciman, John Maynard-Smith, and Robin Ian MacDonald Dunbar (Oxford: Oxford University Press, 1996), pp. 269–289; Chris Knight, *Blood Relations: Menstruation and the Origins of Culture* (New Haven, Conn.: Yale University Press, 1991); and Camilla Power and Leslie C. Aiello, "Female Proto-Symbolic Strategies," *Women in Human Evolution*, ed. Lori D. Hager (New York: Routledge, 1997), pp. 153–171.

17. Derek Bickerton, "The Language Bioprogram Hypothesis," *Behavioral and Brain Sciences*, 7 (1984), pp. 173–222.

18. Noam Chomsky, *Aspects of the Theory of Syntax* (Cambridge, Mass.: MIT Press, 1965), p. 3.

Twenty

THE APE IN THE ANTHILL

Derek Bickerton

Many evils mar the world we inhabit: war, injustice, exploitation, tyranny, terrorism, and more. Most, if not all, of us of us would like to end those evils; we long for a world of peace, justice, and freedom. Why, with all the wonders of science and technology at our command, are we still unable to achieve this ideal?

The most fundamental cause of our failure lies in a far deeper failure: failure to realize the true predicament of our species. Science can help us to understand the precise nature of that predicament; whether we can then resolve its contradictions is up to us.

We are fortunate in that the progress of science, especially the progress of those branches of science that pertain to the evolution of our species, has now reached a stage where we can understand our place in nature. Previous centuries could not. We can distinguish three stages in our slow and difficult progress towards self-understanding.

In the first epoch, which extended from the emergence of our species to the Renaissance, we had no notion of either prehistory or historical change. As far as we knew, the world had always been as it was then. When Adam and Eve first donned clothing, the clothing they donned was no different from modern clothing ("modern" here meaning "in use at whatever period we were looking back from"). We can see this from any mediaeval painting of biblical or classical events. The shepherds of Bethlehem or the senators of Rome will be dressed alike in contemporary versions of mediaeval dress.

The second epoch stretched from the Renaissance to Charles Darwin's time. People still had not developed a notion of prehistory, which meant we still had no notion that human beings had any ancestors that were not human. Through the recovery of classical learning, we gained some understanding that the superficial aspects of human behavior could and did undergo change. Our perception of time had changed, not radically, but enough to allow some depth; now historical paintings strove for accuracy in representing the costumes of their subjects' times. But the human beings who wore them remained the same throughout history.

The third epoch extends from Darwin's time to the present. During that period, we became aware of two crucial things: that time had a depth amounting to countless millions of years, and that instead of being created from dust and a rib; we had descended as just one branch of the family of primates, having the great apes as our cousins.

How did those epochs differ in their interpretation of the human predicament—the clash between the desire for a purer, freer world and the reality
of a world riddled with conflict and injustice?

During the first epoch, people believed things were just that way and we
had nothing that we could do about it, although if you followed this or that
religious prescription, things might improve or become more bearable. During
the second epoch, people believed that the growth and spread of human reason
and the decline of irrational superstitions, along with institutional changes,
would make things significantly better. ("Let us strangle the last king with the
guts of the last priest."[1])

During the third epoch, people held one of two equally unsubstantiated
beliefs. The first merely continued and developed the faith of the Enlightenment, the spread of reason. "Humanists" view the world's problems arising
from conflict between two aspects of human nature: our "primitive"—
emotional, instinctive, aggressive, irrational—inheritance from ape ancestors,
and our "civilized"—rational, controlled, peace-loving—characteristics, those
we made from our unique culture. As time passed, or primitive selves would
fade, our civilized selves would emerge victorious.

The second belief, more modern and held most closely by self-described
"sociobiologists" or "evolutionary psychologists," denied the humanists' dichotomy. This group believed that human beings are merely the product of
millions of years of evolution: a species of ape with the same drives basic
behaviors as our primate cousins. Our vaunted culture, far from battling with,
and further still from conquering these behaviors, formed merely an elaborate
disguise for them. The worlds of business and politics served as substitutes for
the primeval savanna. Men in three-piece suits re-enacted all the strategies,
subterfuge, and rituals of masculine chimps. If a better world were a legitimate goal, we could not hope to achieve it until we fully understood and came
to terms with our fundamentally ape nature.

As so often happens with apparently conflicting beliefs, both of these
camps shared the same false assumption. Both assumed that the course of
human development was a single straight line. Each shared with the two previous epochs a belief in continuity: no longer continuity without change, but
still continuity. Regardless of whether our primitive nature was a curse to be
extirpated or an inescapable reality, the same fundamental primate nature per-
sisted throughout both views, with no constraints on it other than those imposed by our ever-growing "civilization." An ape had grown up and become
more intelligent, more self-conscious, and less tolerant of some of its own
apish ways. That was all.

The circumstances under which our human ancestors lived have been
radically altered in ways no other primate, or for that matter no other species
of any kind, had ever previously experienced. Our struggles to adjust to this
radically different, unprecedented situation constitute the direct cause of all
the problems that now vex our species, and that may well end by destroying it.

Here is what happened. Among all animals, only human beings developed language. Language gave us not merely an efficient means of communication, but also an enhanced cognition. We eventually reached a point at which, unlike other species, we could make radical changes in our behavior without first undergoing genetic changes. The most fateful of these changes occurred when, at the end of the last Ice Age, human beings began to collect the seeds of cereal plants and deliberately cultivate them.

Agriculture already had a history of many millions of years. Several species of ants had practiced agriculture; they fed on fungus cultivated in the nest. These ants underwent several changes in the history of their species. They had increased enormously in numbers, with nests numbering their inhabitants in the millions. They had developed a high degree of specialization, with as many as five castes determined solely by the roles they performed in the agricultural process. Like ants in general, their modes of social organization differed in almost every detail from those of every primate species.

People tend to think that ants having some sort of nature that causes them to do what they do. People tend to hold similar beliefs about every species. That is not true. Ants that practice agriculture descend from ants that were homeless and roamed around foraging, just as our own ancestors did. At some stage, those ancestors started, just as ours did, to assemble piecemeal the behaviors that, in sum, amount to the anthill and the agricultural way of life. It took them many times longer to do this. For each step, genetics had to catch up. Thanks to our language and culture, we developed agriculture far faster, far too fast for genetics to catch up. But the principle is the same.

You become what you do.

The adoption of agriculture by human beings radically changed the circumstances under which they lived. In the first place, human numbers increased just as ant numbers had done: instead of depending on a changing and uncontrollable environment for food, human beings created heir own environment, one that they controlled, ensuring (apart from occasional droughts and famines) a potentially unlimited supply of food. The increase in their numbers in turn forced profound changes in the ways in which they behaved and reacted to one another.

Consider the differences that resulted in these categories of endeavor:

Social structure: Before agriculture, human—like other primates—societies' organizational patterns were based on small groups, with a fluid and flexible social structure and few status differences within those groups. After agriculture, societies organized in much larger groups, with a rigid, hierarchical structure of many levels and with marked status differences between levels.

Division of labor: Before agriculture, gender determined division of labor. Society expected any man or woman to perform any or all of the roles appropriate for their sex. After agriculture, a complex system of

specialized functions developed, with soldiers, farmers, millers, trans-
porters, bureaucrats and more—just as with ants. In some societies took
this process even further, into the formation of a hereditary caste system.

Personal possessions: Before agriculture, persons' personal possessions
were limited to those they could carry. Afterwards, personal possessions
multiplied to include real property, personal ornament, money, and
things people could accumulate without limit. This trend increased the
gap between those who had possessions and those who did not.

Land: Before agriculture, land was open, without boundaries. Tribes
routinely hunted over the same areas. While they might regard some
fruit trees as belonging to different groups, the land on which the trees
grew was common to all who roamed over the land. After people
adopted agriculture, people owned land and jealously defended it from
those who would take it by force.

Personal interaction: Before agriculture, human beings lived as other
primates did, in communities where everyone was more or less closely related—communities small enough for everyone to know everyone else intimately. Afterwards, human beings lived in ever-growing communities
where many of the people they saw daily were strangers whom they might
never see again.

In small face-to-face communities, people had to tolerate a diverse array
of types, regardless of whether they had anything in common with them (apart
from kinship). In post-agricultural communities, people found associating
with anyone outside their class difficult. Even within their class, people could
choose to associate only with those with whom they shared similar back-
grounds and interests. This freedom further subdivided society into mutually
suspicious groups and raised the general level of intolerance.

The people concerned did not consciously desire or select these vast and
multiple changes. Instead, all followed as inescapable consequences of the
different—antlike—system of food extraction human beings had developed.
Instead, members of our species have been, for the last ten thousand years,
struggling to adapt, without time for genetic adaptation, to a way of life far
closer to that of social insects than to that of the primate species from which
human beings had originally evolved. Instead, members of our species have
been, for the last ten thousand years, struggling to adapt, without time for genetic adaptation, to a way of life far closer to that of social insects than to that
of the primate species from which human beings had originally evolved. Problems of war, injustice, intolerance, vast disparities in resources, and all the
other ills that plague humanity are the natural and unavoidable consequences
of this sudden change that has no parallel in the four billion years of Earth's
existence. The demands of the ape nature we have inherited and the ant nature

forced on us by agriculture are irreconcilable. Our ape nature urges us to be selfish, free-living individuals, who pursue our good and the good of our immediate family by the light of our own thinking; our ant nature urges us to be pacific and regimented, without personalities or significant individual desires, and to sacrifice ourselves for the greater good of the myriad. That describes the problem succinctly.

Can science do more than explain the problem? Can it resolve, or ameliorate it? Realistically speaking, only two ways of resolving the problem exist. Unfortunately, the vast majority of people would accept neither of them.

We could abandon technical civilization and revert to our ape way of life. We could revert to the hunting-gathering lifestyle our species practiced for most of its life on Earth. This would involve some radical changes, like reducing the human population to the natural carrying capacity of Mother Earth—removing, peacefully or otherwise, over 99 percent of people living today. Call this "Rollback 10,000 years."

Alternatively, we could genetically adapt ourselves to an ant's way of life. We could become eusocial, living as a species in a highly complex form of social organization akin to that of ants, with only one breeding female and a small number of idle inseminators per city, so we would all share biological relatedness. We could develop a hierarchical system of occupational castes. We would still have wars, like ants do, but war would not cause us to worry. We could try to do things less radically, selectively breeding out the courageous, the creative, the innovative, the non-conforming, and the individualist tendencies among us (sometimes I look around and think, maybe this is already happening). That way, we would lose everything that makes us distinctively human. Call it "Ape into Ant."

If we will not accept either Rollback 10,000 or Ape into Ant, then things will never change. The same old injustices will persist, temporarily vanquished in one place only to reappear, as vigorous as ever, in another. The ape is in the anthill with no way out. That is what we have to understand and accept.

Note

1. Attributed to Denis Diderot by Jean-François de La Harpe in *Cours de Littérature Ancienne et Moderne* (Paris: F. Didot Frères, 1840).

Twenty-One

HUMAN COGNITION AND THE
RECOGNITION OF HUMANITY

Robert Ginsberg

Arcadi Navarro has served us well in showing how the Darwinian struggle for existence in natural evolution might have room for cooperation.[1] Charles Darwin, in his *Origin of Species*, celebrates the beauty and wonder of the operation of universal laws in biology.[2] His aesthetic point of view turns the struggle for survival into a process of perfection, although individuals are killed and species rendered extinct. In the last paragraph of his revolutionary book on evolutionary theory, Darwin does acknowledge "the war of nature" as underlying the development of higher beings.

Since Darwin applies the laws of evolution to instincts in addition to physical traits, we may hope that the human species has selected the instinct for social cooperation for its perfection. Mutual aid might be in our genes, alongside competitive killing. Caring for one another might be perfectly natural. But the adoption of an official policy for breeding human beings, and eliminating undesirable specimens, is not in the interests of humanity.

Social Darwinism makes the case that the struggle for survival extends, and should extend, from nature into society. Let the weak be eliminated, let the strong prosper. This point of view leads to unpleasant results when practiced by cutthroat capitalism and traditional dictatorship.

We can argue that human evolution is no longer active, or that if it continues, it is out of our hands. Thomas Henry Huxley, responding to the Darwinian revolution, makes the case that humanity has replaced natural selection by ethics.[3] The surest sign of our rejection of the survival of the fittest is the hospital. We insist on not eliminating the weakest, a principle for which I am most grateful. The moral realm is a human creation that stands opposed to nature.

But many people have been killed on supposedly moral grounds. People often use moral assertions and religious doctrines as ideological instruments to divide humanity. Aggression and excessive egoism cloak themselves in the language of righteousness when people engage in oppression and extermination. We are back to the problem of the biology of the brain.

Let us see if we can find the grounds for peaceful cooperation by going beyond the brain to the mind, or better, to the heart. Join me in the search, as we test the limitations and possible contributions of Cognitive Science.

The cognitive trigger for shifting behavior from conflict to cooperation is the sudden change of heart, which is simultaneously a self-recognition and a recognition of the Other as also a self. Despite our opposition, we are, at heart, selves, side by side. Initially, each of us may have been an object, an obstacle, that blocked the other's path, but we become revealed as fellow subjects.

My recognition of the self that you are enlarges the self that I am and that I can become. Whatever you are that differs from whatever I am, you are a human being. And so am I! My discovery of your humanity alerts me to my humanity.

Such recognition is re-cognizing. It re-minds, re-forms, reforms our knowledge-system. Not an addition to what we know or a calling back into mind of what we knew, it is a radical change in who we are as knowers.

Cognitive Science distinguished itself in the twentieth century as the rigorous study of the process of knowing. Cognitive Science in the twenty-first century will explore the process of the knower, how the knower becomes more fully human. Engaged in that humanistic activity, Cognitive Science will become the discipline of Cognitive Value Inquiry. The Value Inquiry Movement welcomes Cognitive Science to its mansion!

I know that you are human. More than that, I know you as a human being, even though I do not know you personally. You are unknown to me, except in one essential way: your humanity. But your humanity is also my humanity. What I know about you may be minimal. But I know you essentially. Though we may oppose each other in a thousand heart-felt ways, at heart, we share in humanity.

"Knowledge about" differs from this kind of knowing. Usually, we think that the more we get to know about something, or someone, the better we know that object: knowledge as acquisition.

The quantity of possible observations of an object is, in principle, endless, but in sum, never equals knowing the distinctive identity of the unique subject. Henri Bergson makes this argument in his beautifully expressed "Introduction to Metaphysics."[4] A shift is required in my stance of knower from the position of subject over against an object to the reality of subject-with-subject. Martin Buber differentiates this encounter of I-Thou from the relationship of I-it.[5]

Intersubjectivity is a knowing that changes me from being an acquisitive, inquisitive subject wandering in the endless field of objects, to residing purely in the subjective ground that we share as human beings. We overcome objectivity, which separates us, when we come over to being at home with one another, thanks to heart-to-heart encounter.

I am better for discovering your humanity. The knower, in this case, realizes itself more fully by the experiencing of knowing, the revelation of reality. I am transformed by your humanity—our humanity.

This awakening restructures the rest of my knowledge. We had suspended objectivity in the shock of mutual recognition, but it returns to serve in a thousand ways our revealed intersubjectivity. Thanks to objective knowledge, you and I can accomplish so many things in the world to celebrate and serve our humanity that our hearts fill with joy. We redirect all our knowledge to fulfillment of humanity.

What is this humanity that I discovered in you and which I share? You are a being of inestimable value. Though you may be fittingly paid money for your work, you are priceless for what you are. Immanuel Kant made this point about the foundation of morality. We are all ends in ourselves, he discovered, never means alone.[6] You, like I, are the value-giver who assigns worth to things, yet you, like I, are not a thing, but a person, a self, a human being, a will, a subject.

In recognizing that you have unlimited worth, I am immediately moved to respect you. To respect your humanity is to experience the awe when faced with the sacred. The categorical imperative that flows from the sacral is: Do not harm humanity. Humanity is no mere abstraction, a philosopher's concept. Instead, humanity is present here and now in the unique and concrete person you are, to use the words of Miguel de Unamuno, a living being of "flesh and bone, who is born, suffers, and dies."[7]

Respect for humanity means that I must not harm you, who are the living presence of humanity. Above all, respect for your humanity requires that I not kill you. That obligation appears easy to fulfill, especially if I am inclined toward nonviolence, if I do not own firearms, and if I appeal to the police in any dispute that threatens violence.

What may not be as easy is my obligation to prevent the institutions of which I am a member from killing people. Any state, which executes people, even for serious crimes, is engaged in a serious crime. Just as the state forbids premeditated killing, so we should forbid premeditated killing by the state. The business of the state is protecting life, not taking it. From respect for human life, I may have to take action to change political institutions. Conscience, one of the highest forms of knowing, obliges engagement: consider Henry David Thoreau, Mohandas K. Gandhi, and Martin Luther King, Jr.

I may also have to change social institutions, the practices, and attitudes of groups within society. Educating others to the rights of all is the best way to assure respect for humanity.

The dictate of not harming obviously applies to renunciation of torture. Torture, even of torturers, is a violation of humanity and can never be justified. The violation of the victim's human dignity is simultaneously a denial of the dignity of the torturer and of all other human beings who are thereby turned into potential further victims. My obligation is to rid the world of torture and slavery, rape, genital mutilation, ethnic cleansing, gender discrimination in marriage or employment, and every other form of oppression. Any action in the world that victimizes a human being is a crime against all of us. Since I am a member of the world, I must set the world aright. This is full-time work!

The killers are at work, while I sit in a café or speak in a lecture hall. The world constantly makes victims. Knowing of their plight, we must respond with immediate assistance. This follows from recognition of the humanity of the Other. The fundamental cognition of humanity provides the grounds for a doctrine of human rights. The rights of humanity are universal, undeniable, imperative.

Such rights are not paper castles. They engender actions. Knowing activates. Cognition instigates change. Cognitive Science must turn its attention to this inescapable connection between knowing and activity in the world. Knowledge for the sake of knowledge is worthy. But knowledge for the sake of humanity is worthier.

The Other whose humanity I discovered is not just you, but every Other—a tremendous revelation. Suddenly, my humanity is magnified six billionfold. I thought that I was facing only you, directly in front of me, but the intersubjectivity in which I am at home covers the whole world. If I stagger back for a moment, almost overwhelmed by my responsibilities to everyone, I recover with recognition of the wonder of global humanity.

Before, I may have recognized myself as member of a group, a nationality, or a religion, which left billions of people outside of it. Now, I know that I am a permanent member of the most comprehensive, the most valuable community in the world, from which no one can be excluded: the family of humanity. Any nation, any religion that denies the humanity of anyone must be restrained in the name of everyone. A global self-corrective agenda unfurls itself as we face the world. We have work to do in saving the world!

This is the work of joy. Cognitive Science must acknowledge joyful knowing, knowing inseparable from immediate growth of the knower: participatory, exhilarating, exultant, epiphanic, sacral, sublime. To know that we are all human is wonderful. The joy of such knowing turns into love, the knowing of the heart. "The heart has its reasons, of which the reason knows naught."[8]

Epistemology drives its way to the metaphysical: knowing comes to being. Being comes to knowledge.

How can we trigger the recognition from which universal love, fulfilled selfhood, global intersubjectivity, respect for human rights, and activated improvement of the world all spring? Many paths are available. I will point to three of them.

(1) Introspective meditation, such as that conducted by René Descartes, may bring the individual to the turning point for knowledge in discovery of an unshakeable reality.[9] Thinkers may rethink the Cartesian Cogito Science, "I think, therefore I am." Jean-Paul Sartre and Simone de Beauvoir would have it read, "I think, therefore we exist."[10] Albert Camus, "I think, therefore we rebel."[11]

Because Descartes started with the self-contained ego, he could only move analogically to the existence of others. Others were an afterthought. I contend that by philosophical discipline we can find within us the co-presence of Others, because each of us is, at heart, situated in intersubjectivity.

Thought is socially grounded. We do not deduce Otherhood; we discover it within ourselves. We exist, therefore I think. Cognitive Science should assist people everywhere on Earth to conduct such an interior inquiry.

(2) The arts may open our hearts to the dignity of the Other by making us feel the presence of that Other in ourselves. Art is the adventure of internal discovery. It enlarges our selfhood by revelation of the souls of others.

Cognitive Aesthetics may study how great works of art accomplish this, so that teachers may assist people to broaden their humanity through encounter with the arts.

The magnificent frescoes gathered from Catalonian churches at the *Museu Nacional d'Art de Catalunya* fuse the viewer's soul with the souls of the anonymous makers of these holy images. The soulful vision of these masterpieces has remained with me since first I laid eyes upon them, when, in 1961, I visited Barcelona as a poor student. Pablo Picasso's protest against wanton destruction in his enormous painting, *Guernica*, awakened my heart, whenever, as a boy, I visited it during its exile in New York. In its permanent home in Madrid, it continues to awaken hearts.

World Civilization, which we are creating in the twenty-first century, calls for celebration of great achievements of cultures from around the Earth. A Universal Forum of Cultures, an Olympics of Creativity, must be a model for continuation on every continent and in every year. We should insist on "cultures" in the plural, as representing the enriching diversity that peoples contribute to humanity.

(3) But revelation of our shared humanity may occur immediately, without philosophical discipline or absorption in the arts. Unexpected breakthroughs happen in life as unforgettable moments that change the heart. The inexplicable occurs. Do not ask me to explain it.

Zen reminds us to not be so mindful that we close the heart to what is already present. The disclosure of reality is not conceptual, nor even discursive, but the event by which both the subject and the object are present as subjects. Zen experience opens us to profound appreciation of the world and everyone in it. Cognitive Science should respect such Cognitive Revelation.

I have been sketching a prospectus for the development of Cognitive Inquiry that may be adopted by such organizations as the *Centre de Recerca en Ciència Cognitiva* at the *Universitat Autònoma de Barcelona*.

From the discovery of humanity within each of us follows our moral and social duties, our political and international obligations, our task as teachers of humanity, and our love of life. But, you ask, can we attach so much to an act of knowing? Can such a knowing actually occur?

The answer, my friend, is in your heart.

Notes

1. Arcadi Navarro, "Conflict and Cooperation in Human Affairs," paper presented to the Universal Forum of Cultures, The Social Brain: Biology of Conflict and Cooperation, Barcelona, Spain, June 2004, (see this volume chap. 7).

2. Charles Darwin, *The Origin of Species by Means of Natural Selection*, vol. 49, *Great Books of the Western World*, ed. Robert Maynard Hutchins (Chicago, Ill.: Encyclopædia Britannica, Inc., 1952).

3. Thomas Henry Huxley, *Evolution and Ethics, and Other Essays*, vol. 9 in *Collected Essays* (London: Macmillan, 1894).

4. Henri Bergson, "*Introduction à la Métaphysique*," *La Pensée et le Mouvant*, in *Œuvres*, ed. André Robinet (Paris, Presses Universitaires de France, 1970); Translated by T. E. Hulme as *Introduction to Metaphysics*, 2nd ed. (Indianapolis, Ind.: Bobbs-Merrill, 1955).

5. Martin Buber, *Ich und Du* (Leipzig: Insel-Verlag, 1923). Translated by Ronald Gregor Smith as *I and Thou*, 2nd ed. (New York: Charles Scribner's Sons, 1958).

6. Immanuel Kant, *Grundlegung zur Metaphysik der Sitten*, ed. Theodor Valentiner (Stuttgart: Philipp Reclam, 1962). Translated by Lewis White Beck as *Foundations of the Metaphysics of Morals* (Indianapolis, Ind.: Bobbs-Merrill, 1959).

7. Miguel de Unamuno, *Del Sentimiento Trágico de la Vida en los Hombres y en los Pueblos*, 11th ed. (Madrid: Espasa-Calpe, S.A., 1967). Translated by Anthony Kerrigan as *The Tragic Sense of Life in Men and Nations* (Princeton, N.J.: Princeton University Press, 1972).

8. Blaise Pascal, *Pensées*, *Œuvres Complètes*, ed. Jacques Chevalier (n.p.: Bibliothèque de la Pléiade, 1954). Translated by John Warrington as *Pensées* (London: Dent, 1960).

9. René Descartes, *Discours de la Méthode*, ed. Étienne Gilson (Paris: Librairie philosophique J. Vrin, 1967). Translated by Laurence J. Lafleur as *Discourse on Method* (Indianapolis, Ind.: Bobbs-Merrill, 1956).

10. Jean-Paul Sartre, *L'Existentialisme est un Humanisme* (Paris: Les Éditions Nagel, 1966). Translated by Bernard Frechtman as *Existentialism* (New York: Philosophical Library, 1947); and Simone de Beauvoir, *Pour une Morale de l'Ambiguïté* (Paris: Gallimard, 1974), translated by Frechtman as *The Ethics of Ambiguity* (Secaucus, N.J.: Citadel Press, 1972).

11. Albert Camus, *L'Homme Révolté* (Paris: Gallimard, 1951). Translated by Anthony Bower as *The Rebel: An Essay on Man in Revolt* (New York: Vintage, 1992).

ABOUT THE AUTHORS

SCOTT ATRAN, Research Director, National Center for Scientific Research, Paris, Adjunct Professor of Psychology, Anthropology, and Natural Resources, University of Michigan, and Visiting Professor, John Jay College of Criminal Justice, New York City.

LAWRENCE W. BARSALOU, Samuel Candler Dobbs Professor of Psychology, Emory University, Atlanta, Georgia.

ERIC BREDO, Professor, Department of Leadership, Foundations, and Current and Policy, University of Virginia.

DEREK BIKERTON, Professor Emeritus, Department of Linguistics, University of Hawaii.

CAMILO JOSÉ CELA CONDE, Professor of Human Evolution and Director, Laboratory of Human Systematics, University of Balearic Islands.

DANIEL C. DENNET, Distinguished Arts and Sciences Professor, Professor of Philosophy, and Director of the Center for Cognitive Studies at Tufts University.

MERLIN DONALD, Professor and Chair in Cognitive Science at Case West Reserve University, Cleveland, Ohio.

ROBERT GINSBERG, Professor Emeritus of Philosophy and Comparative Literature, Pennsylvania State University, and Director, International Center for the Arts, Humanities, and Value Inquiry.

ANTONI GOMILA, Lecturer in Thought and Language, University of the Balearic Islands.

STEVAN HARNAD, Professor, School of Electronics and Computer Sciences, University of Southampton, United Kingdom.

SANDRO NANNINI, Professor of Theoretical Philosophy, University of Siena.

ARCADI NAVARRO, Ramón y Cajal Program Researcher, Pompeu Fabra University, Spain.

KATHERINE NELSON, Distinguished Professor of Psychology Emerita, City University of New York Graduate Center.

SHAUN NICHOLS, Professor of Philosophy, University of Arizona.

F. JOHN ODDLING-SMEE, Lecturer in Human Sciences, Mansfield College, Oxford.

FÉLIX OVEJERO, Professor, University of Barcelona.

DAVID PREMACK, Visiting Professor, CREA Ecole Polytechnique, Paris, France.

EMILY A. PARKER, Doctoral Candidate, Department of Philosophy, Emory University, Atlanta, Georgia.

NÚRIA SEBASTIÁN GALLÉS, Professor, Autonomous University of Barcelona.

LUC STEELS, Professor Computer Science University of Brussels, and Director SONY Computer Science Laboratory, Paris.

WILLIAM A. ROTTSCHAEFER, Professor Emeritus, Philosophy, Lewis and Clark College, Portland, Oregon.

ADOLF TOBEÑA, Professor of Psychiatry and Medical Psychology, Autonomous University of Barcelona, and Cochairman, Research Unit on Cognitive Neuroscience, Autonomous University of Barcelona–IMAS, Spain.

INDEX

abilit(ies)(y), 31, 34, 136
  adaptive a., 171, 225
  a. based in brain, 22, 50
  cognitive a., 12, 27, 78, 177, 203, 204
  a. to make commitments, 108
  empathic a., 65, 93, 94, 135
  imitation and representation a., 11
  a. to lie, 95
  linguistic a., 23, 28, 120, 235
  mathematical a., 51
Abraham (biblical), 102
abstraction, 39, 76–78, 80, 179, 251
academic circles, 63
accidents, 124
act(ion)(or)(s), 34, 35, 53, 70, 73, 83, 85,
     93, 102, 132, 155, 182–186, 208,
     216–218, 224
  adaptive a., 191
  altruistic a., 202
  complex a., 235
  consequences of a., 179
  cooperative a., 174
  correct a., 139
  dilemmas, courses of a. in, 153, 155, 209
  direct a., 88
  emotional consequences of a., 127, 205
  a. engendered by rights, 252
  a. governed by alternate criteria, 144
  joint a., 236
  knowing, a. of, 253
  lying, a. of, 237
  martyrdom or missionary a., 110, 112
  mental a., 183
  a.-metaphor, 219
  mimetic a., 218
  moral a., 8, 85, 88, 125, 133, 136, 137,
     163, 209, 210
  motor a., 136
  musculature, a. of, 216
  notionally equivalent but physically
     dissimilar a., 164
  offensive and defensive a., 32
  a. vs. omission, 155

  a.-patterns, 218
  personality theories of a., 137
  political a., 251
  a. producing best outcome, 152, 154
  profits from a., 175
  punative a., 175
  rational a., 110
  rewarded a., 162
  rules as subproduct of a., 142
  sacrificial a., 132
  social a., 205
  social/organizational contexts of a., 137
  sophisticated vs. disreputable a., 162
  suicidal a., 94, 105, 112
  terrorist a., 95, 105, 108, 111, 147
  utilitarian a., 218
  vicitimizing a., 251
  voluntary a., 113, 184, 186, 218, 219
activit(ies)(y), 4, 11, 38, 40, 53, 54, 87,
     137, 191, 227, 236, 250, 252
  a.-based perspective, 53
  cognitive a., 219
  earthworms, a. of, 191
  enzyme a., 211
  externally (experientially)-driven a., 27
  mental a., 152
  scientific a., 1
  social a., 52
  synaptic a., 20, 22
Adam (biblical), 243
adaptation(ist)(s), 11, 144, 156, 190–192,
     203, 219, 230, 232, 233
  language-as-a. hypothesis, 231, 233, 234
  mimetic a., 216, 217
adequacy, 132, 136
adjective(s), 70, 232
adolescents, 93
adults, 38, 219
  children compared with a., 25, 28, 41,
     42, 44, 73, 92, 162, 208
adverbs, 70, 225
aeration, 191

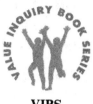

VIBS

The **Value Inquiry Book Series** is co-sponsored by:

Adler School of Professional Psychology
American Indian Philosophy Association
American Maritain Association
American Society for Value Inquiry
Association for Process Philosophy of Education
Canadian Society for Philosophical Practice
Center for Bioethics, University of Turku
Center for Professional and Applied Ethics, University of North Carolina at Charlotte
Central European Pragmatist Forum
Centre for Applied Ethics, Hong Kong Baptist University
Centre for Cultural Research, Aarhus University
Centre for Professional Ethics, University of Central Lancashire
Centre for the Study of Philosophy and Religion, University College of Cape Breton
Centro de Estudos em Filosofia Americana, Brazil
College of Education and Allied Professions, Bowling Green State University
College of Liberal Arts, Rochester Institute of Technology
Concerned Philosophers for Peace
Conference of Philosophical Societies
Department of Moral and Social Philosophy, University of Helsinki
Gannon University
Gilson Society
Haitian Studies Association
Ikeda University
Institute of Philosophy of the High Council of Scientific Research, Spain
International Academy of Philosophy of the Principality of Liechtenstein
International Association of Bioethics
International Center for the Arts, Humanities, and Value Inquiry
International Society for Universal Dialogue
Natural Law Society
Philosophical Society of Finland
Philosophy Born of Struggle Association
Philosophy Seminar, University of Mainz
Pragmatism Archive at The Oklahoma State University
R.S. Hartman Institute for Formal and Applied Axiology
Research Institute, Lakeridge Health Corporation
Russian Philosophical Society
Society for Existential Analysis
Society for Iberian and Latin-American Thought
Society for the Philosophic Study of Genocide and the Holocaust
Unit for Research in Cognitive Neuroscience, Autonomous University of Barcelona
Yves R. Simon Institute

Titles Published

1. Noel Balzer, *The Human Being as a Logical Thinker*

2. Archie J. Bahm, *Axiology: The Science of Values*

3. H. P. P. (Hennie) Lötter, *Justice for an Unjust Society*

4. H. G. Callaway, *Context for Meaning and Analysis: A Critical Study in the Philosophy of Language*

5. Benjamin S. Llamzon, *A Humane Case for Moral Intuition*

6. James R. Watson, *Between Auschwitz and Tradition: Postmodern Reflections on the Task of Thinking.* A volume in **Holocaust and Genocide Studies**

7. Robert S. Hartman, *Freedom to Live: The Robert Hartman Story*, Edited by Arthur R. Ellis. A volume in **Hartman Institute Axiology Studies**

8. Archie J. Bahm, *Ethics: The Science of Oughtness*

9. George David Miller, *An Idiosyncratic Ethics; Or, the Lauramachean Ethics*

10. Joseph P. DeMarco, *A Coherence Theory in Ethics*

11. Frank G. Forrest, *Valuemetrics**: *The Science of Personal and Professional Ethics.* A volume in **Hartman Institute Axiology Studies**

12. William Gerber, *The Meaning of Life: Insights of the World's Great Thinkers*

13. Richard T. Hull, Editor, *A Quarter Century of Value Inquiry: Presidential Addresses of the American Society for Value Inquiry.* A volume in **Histories and Addresses of Philosophical Societies**

14. William Gerber, *Nuggets of Wisdom from Great Jewish Thinkers: From Biblical Times to the Present*

15. Sidney Axinn, *The Logic of Hope: Extensions of Kant's View of Religion*

60. Palmer Talbutt, Jr., Rough Dialectics: *Sorokin's Philosophy of Value*, with contributions by Lawrence T. Nichols and Pitirim A. Sorokin

61. C. L. Sheng, *A Utilitarian General Theory of Value*

62. George David Miller, *Negotiating Toward Truth: The Extinction of Teachers and Students*. Epilogue by Mark Roelof Eleveld. A volume in **Philosophy of Education**

63. William Gerber, *Love, Poetry, and Immortality: Luminous Insights of the World's Great Thinkers*

64. Dane R. Gordon, Editor, *Philosophy in Post-Communist Europe*. A volume in **Post-Communist European Thought**

65. Dane R. Gordon and Józef Niznik, Editors, *Criticism and Defense of Rationality in Contemporary Philosophy*. A volume in **Post-Communist European Thought**

66. John R. Shook, *Pragmatism: An Annotated Bibliography, 1898-1940*. With contributions by E. Paul Colella, Lesley Friedman, Frank X. Ryan, and Ignas K. Skrupskelis

67. Lansana Keita, *The Human Project and the Temptations of Science*

68. Michael M. Kazanjian, *Phenomenology and Education: Cosmology, Co-Being, and Core Curriculum*. A volume in **Philosophy of Education**

69. James W. Vice, *The Reopening of the American Mind: On Skepticism and Constitutionalism*

70. Sarah Bishop Merrill, *Defining Personhood: Toward the Ethics of Quality in Clinical Care*

71. Dane R. Gordon, *Philosophy and Vision*

72. Alan Milchman and Alan Rosenberg, Editors, *Postmodernism and the Holocaust*. A volume in **Holocaust and Genocide Studies**

73. Peter A. Redpath, *Masquerade of the Dream Walkers: Prophetic Theology from the Cartesians to Hegel*. A volume in **Studies in the History of Western Philosophy**

74. Malcolm D. Evans, *Whitehead and Philosophy of Education: The Seamless Coat of Learning*. A volume in **Philosophy of Education**

75. Warren E. Steinkraus, *Taking Religious Claims Seriously: A Philosophy of Religion*, Edited by Michael H. Mitias. A volume in **Universal Justice**

76. Thomas Magnell, Editor, *Values and Education*

77. Kenneth A. Bryson, *Persons and Immortality*. A volume in **Natural Law Studies**

78. Steven V. Hicks, *International Law and the Possibility of a Just World Order: An Essay on Hegel's Universalism*. A volume in **Universal Justice**

79. E. F. Kaelin, *Texts on Texts and Textuality: A Phenomenology of Literary Art*, Edited by Ellen J. Burns

80. Amihud Gilead, *Saving Possibilities: A Study in Philosophical Psychology*. A volume in Philosophy and Psychology

81. André Mineau, *The Making of the Holocaust: Ideology and Ethics in the Systems Perspective*. A volume in **Holocaust and Genocide Studies**

82. Howard P. Kainz, *Politically Incorrect Dialogues: Topics Not Discussed in Polite Circles*

83. Veikko Launis, Juhani Pietarinen, and Juha Räikkä, Editors, *Genes and Morality: New Essays*. A volume in **Nordic Value Studies**

84. Steven Schroeder, *The Metaphysics of Cooperation: A Study of F. D. Maurice*

85. Caroline Joan ("Kay") S. Picart, *Thomas Mann and Friedrich Nietzsche: Eroticism, Death, Music, and Laughter*. A volume in **Central-European Value Studies**

86. G. John M. Abbarno, Editor, *The Ethics of Homelessness: Philosophical Perspectives*

87. James Giles, Editor, *French Existentialism: Consciousness, Ethics, and Relations with Others*. A volume in **Nordic Value Studies**

129.   Paul Custodio Bube and Jeffery Geller, Editors, *Conversations with Pragmatism: A Multi-Disciplinary Study.* A volume in **Studies in Pragmatism and Values**

130.   Richard Rumana, *Richard Rorty: An Annotated Bibliography of Secondary Literature.* A volume in **Studies in Pragmatism and Values**

131.   Stephen Schneck, Editor, *Max Scheler's Acting Persons: New Perspectives* A volume in **Personalist Studies**

132.   Michael Kazanjian, *Learning Values Lifelong: From Inert Ideas to Wholes.* A volume in **Philosophy of Education**

133.   Rudolph Alexander Kofi Cain, Alain Leroy Locke: *Race, Culture, and the Education of African American Adults.* A volume in **African American Philosophy**

134.   Werner Krieglstein, *Compassion: A New Philosophy of the Other*

135.   Robert N. Fisher, Daniel T. Primozic, Peter A. Day, and Joel A. Thompson, Editors, *Suffering, Death, and Identity.* A volume in **Personalist Studies**

136.   Steven Schroeder, *Touching Philosophy, Sounding Religion, Placing Education.* A volume in **Philosophy of Education**

137.   Guy DeBrock, *Process Pragmatism: Essays on a Quiet Philosophical Revolution.* A volume in **Studies in Pragmatism and Values**

138.   Lennart Nordenfelt and Per-Erik Liss, Editors, *Dimensions of Health and Health Promotion*

139.   Amihud Gilead, *Singularity and Other Possibilities: Panenmentalist Novelties*

140.   Samantha Mei-che Pang, *Nursing Ethics in Modern China: Conflicting Values and Competing Role Requirements.* A volume in **Studies in Applied Ethics**

141.   Christine M. Koggel, Allannah Furlong, and Charles Levin, Editors, *Confidential Relationships: Psychoanalytic, Ethical, and Legal Contexts.* A volume in **Philosophy and Psychology**

142. Peter A. Redpath, Editor, *A Thomistic Tapestry: Essays in Memory of Étienne Gilson*. A volume in **Gilson Studies**

143. Deane-Peter Baker and Patrick Maxwell, Editors, *Explorations in Contemporary Continental Philosophy of Religion*. A volume in **Philosophy and Religion**

144. Matti Häyry and Tuija Takala, Editors, *Scratching the Surface of Bioethics*. A volume in **Values in Bioethics**

145. Leonidas Donskis, *Forms of Hatred: The Troubled Imagination in Modern Philosophy and Literature*

146. Andreea Deciu Ritivoi, Editor, *Interpretation and Its Objects: Studies in the Philosophy of Michael Krausz*

147. Herman Stark, *A Fierce Little Tragedy: Thought, Passion, and Self-Formation in the Philosophy Classroom*. A volume in **Philosophy of Education**

148. William Gay and Tatiana Alekseeva, Editors, *Democracy and the Quest for Justice: Russian and American Perspectives*. A volume in **Contemporary Russian Philosophy**

149. Xunwu Chen, *Being and Authenticity*

150. Hugh P. McDonald, *Radical Axiology: A First Philosophy of Values*

151. Dane R. Gordon and David C. Durst, Editors, *Civil Society in Southeast Europe*. A volume in **Post-Communist European Thought**

152. John Ryder and Emil Višňovský, Editors, *Pragmatism and Values: The Central European Pragmatist Forum, Volume One*. A volume in **Studies in Pragmatism and Values**

153. Messay Kebede, *Africa's Quest for a Philosophy of Decolonization*

154. Steven M. Rosen, *Dimensions of* Apeiron: *A Topological Phenomenology of Space, Time, and Individuation*. A volume in **Philosophy and Psychology**

155. Albert A. Anderson, Steven V. Hicks, and Lech Witkowski, Editors, *Mythos and Logos: How to Regain the Love of Wisdom*. A volume in **Universal Justice**

Printed in the United States
By Bookmasters